"The chapter authors review structured programs for forensic populations, ranging from adults and juveniles who have committed sexual aggression, to substance abusers, to psychotic individuals who have committed violent crimes. I recommend this book for anyone interested in practical, hands-on lessons from experienced practitioners who are on the front lines of treatment for these challenging cases".

Philip H. Witt, Ph.D., A.B.P.P. (forensic),
Somerset Psychological Group, USA

Innovative Treatment Approaches in Forensic and Correctional Settings

This book describes targeted therapeutic interventions, programmatic approaches, and system-wide transformations of forensic mental health services.

Interventions include creative applications of a variety of multidimensional and theoretically grounded approaches. These include variations of cognitive-behavioral therapy (CBT), dialectical behavior therapy (DBT), psychodynamic, psychosocial, Risk-Needs-Recovery (RNR) and Good Lives Models, and other approaches. Contributors from several countries address key topics such as aggression, sexual violence, substance use, trauma-informed care, competency restoration, and other specialized treatment areas. Clinical examples are included throughout, which include current data and research and suggestions for further research for use by clinicians working in a range of settings with a variety of treatment population subsets.

This book is essential for administrators and clinicians seeking effective and state-of-the-art approaches.

Michael Siglag, Ph.D., is a licensed psychologist with over 35 years of clinical and forensic experience working in psychiatric, forensic, and correctional settings in direct service, leadership, and consulting roles.

International Perspectives on Forensic Mental Health
A Routledge Book Series
Edited by Patricia Zapf
Palo Alto University

The goal of this series is to improve the quality of healthcare services in forensic and correctional settings by providing a forum for discussing issues and disseminating resources related to policy, administration, clinical practice, and research. The series addresses topics such as mental health law; the organization and administration of forensic and/or correctional services for persons with mental disorders; the development, implementation, and evaluation of treatment programs and interventions for individuals in civil and criminal justice settings; the assessment and management of violence risk, including the risk for sexual violence and family violence; and staff selection, training, and development in forensic and/or correctional systems.

Published Titles

Diversity and Marginalisation in Forensic Mental Health Care
Edited by Jack Tomlin and Birgit Vollm

Safeguarding the Quality of Forensic Assessment in Sentencing
A Review Across Western Nations
Edited by Michiel van der Wolf

Globalization, Displacement, and Psychiatry
Global Histories of Trauma
Edited by Sanaullah Khan and Elliott Schwebach

Approaches to Offender Rehabilitation in Asian Jurisdictions
Edited by Chi Meng Chu and Michael Daffern

Innovative Treatment Approaches in Forensic and Correctional Settings
Edited by Michael Siglag

Innovative Treatment Approaches in Forensic and Correctional Settings

Edited by Michael Siglag

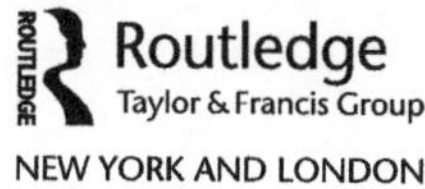

NEW YORK AND LONDON

Designed cover image: Daria Zaseda © Getty Images

First published 2024
by Routledge
605 Third Avenue, New York, NY 10158

and by Routledge
4 Park Square, Milton Park, Abingdon, Oxon, OX14 4RN

Routledge is an imprint of the Taylor & Francis Group, an informa business

Library of Congress Cataloging-in-Publication Data
Names: Siglag, Michael, editor.
Title: Innovative treatment approaches in forensic and correctional settings / edited by Michael Siglag.
Description: New York, NY: Routledge, 2024. |
Series: International perspectives on forensic mental health |
Includes bibliographical references and index.
Identifiers: LCCN 2023051602 (print) | LCCN 2023051603 (ebook) |
ISBN 9781032420387 (paperback) | ISBN 9781032420394 (hardback) |
ISBN 9781003360926 (ebook)
Subjects: LCSH: Prisoners—Mental health services. |
Prison psychology. | Forensic psychiatry.
Classification: LCC RC451.4.P68 I478 2024 (print) |
LCC RC451.4.P68 (ebook) | DDC 365/.6672—dc23/eng/20240215
LC record available at https://lccn.loc.gov/2023051602
LC ebook record available at https://lccn.loc.gov/2023051603

ISBN: 978-1-032-42039-4 (hbk)
ISBN: 978-1-032-42038-7 (pbk)
ISBN: 978-1-003-36092-6 (ebk)

DOI: 10.4324/9781003360926

Typeset in Sabon
by codeMantra

Contents

Acknowledgment

Thank you to each of the authors who contributed to this volume for sharing their personal and professional perspectives and for providing windows into their work.

To all of those who have participated in the treatment interventions described here, my thanks as well. Hopefully, many others will benefit in the future from aspects of your treatment being shared.

Finally, I want to thank my family for their support during the many hours I've spent working on this project.

Contributors

Geraldine Akerman. Honorary Professor Dr Geraldine Akerman is a Consultant Forensic Psychologist at HMP Grendon working for Oxford Health Mental Health NHS Trust. She has worked in the prison service for over 24 years with adult males and young men in custody. Geraldine is a visiting lecturer at Cardiff Metropolitan University where she was awarded Honorary Professorship and at the University of Birmingham. Geraldine has publications about therapeutic communities, working with those convicted of sexual offenses, and the importance of culture within establishments. Geraldine is the past chair of the Division of Forensic Psychology, a Co-founder of the YouTube channel 'Let's Talk Forensic Psychology' and Co-Director of the Forensic Psychology Network.

Shelby Arnold, Ph.D., is a Staff Psychologist at the Beck Institute Center for Cognitive Therapy. She received her PhD in Clinical Psychology with a concentration in Forensic Psychology from Drexel University. Dr. Arnold has worked in a variety of forensic clinical settings, ranging from forensic assessment clinics to inpatient forensic hospitals and correctional settings to community diversion. She currently collaborates with a diverse set of forensic partners across the spectrum of forensic involvement to implement CT-R in their settings. Her areas of research interest include evidence-based practices for justice-involved individuals, community diversion, and other alternatives to standard prosecution, particularly for individuals with mental health challenges. She has published numerous peer-reviewed articles and book chapters on these topics and is the co-author of *Problem-Solving Courts and the Criminal Justice System*, published by Oxford University Press.

Ricardo Barroso, Ph.D. is a Clinical Psychologist, Associate Professor at the University of Trás-os-Montes and Alto Douro (Portugal), and Researcher at the Psychology Center of the University of Porto (CPUP). For several years, he has dedicated special attention to interpersonal violence prevention programs and to the processes of psychological intervention in sexual offending behaviors in adolescents and adults. As part of his professional activity, he has been a consultant for national (e.g., Ministry of Justice of Portugal) and international (e.g., United Nations) governmental organizations. The current President of the Portuguese Society of Psychiatry and Psychology of Justice. Executive member of "Grupo VITA" (www.grupovita.pt), a technical group that is monitoring situations of sexual violence against children and vulnerable adults in the context of the Catholic Church in Portugal.

Mickey Bash, M.A., is a Clown Doctor, part of the "Dream Doctors" association in Israel. Mickey is a Drama Therapist, a graduate of acting school, a dancer, and a performer. He works as a Clown Doctor in 'Sha'ar Menashe', an Israeli state psychiatric facility. He also works in a general hospital, "Haemek", with children and adults in various wards.

Dr. John M.W. Bradford, MB ChB, DPM, FFPsych, MRCPsych, FRCP(C). Dr. Bradford was the Professor and Head of the Division of Forensic Psychiatry, Department of Psychiatry, Faculty of Medicine, University of Ottawa. He was cross-appointed as a Professor in the Department of Criminology. He is an Emeritus Professor at the University of Ottawa. He is currently a Full Professor at McMaster University. He is a senior scientist at the Royal Institute of Mental Health Research.

Dr. Bradford is a graduate of Medicine and received a Diploma in Psychological Medicine from the University of Cape Town, South Africa. He holds specialist degrees in Psychiatry from South Africa, the UK, the USA, and Canada. He has an added qualification in Forensic Psychiatry [US] and is a Founder of Forensic Psychiatry granted by the Royal College of Physicians and Surgeons of Canada.

Dr. Bradford has published over 150 peer-reviewed papers; more than 55 chapters in academic books, including textbooks; presented at over 350 peer-reviewed international and national conferences; and co-authored five books.

Dr. Bradford has received every available forensic psychiatry award in the United States and Canada, besides the Guttmacher Award [USA]. These awards are the Silver Apple Award, the Red Apple Award, the Golden Apple Award, the Seymour Pollock Award, the Isaac Ray Award from the United States, and the Bruno Cormier Award from Canada.

Heidi Camerlengo, Ed.D., is a licensed psychologist working in an outpatient forensic evaluation program at the Ann Klein Forensic Center in West Trenton, New Jersey. Prior to this appointment, Dr. Camerlengo worked as a clinical psychologist for over 17 years at Ancora Psychiatric Hospital in Hammonton, New Jersey, providing a variety of mental health services to a forensically involved population. She is the developer of the Community Reintegration Group. Heidilynne55@yahoo.com

Dr. Gary A. Chaimowitz, MB ChB, MBA, FRCP(C). Professor of Psychiatry and Forensic Psychiatry Academic Division Lead, McMaster University, and Head of Service of Forensic Psychiatry, St. Joseph's Healthcare, Hamilton. Dr. Chaimowitz has Royal College of Physicians and Surgeons of Canada Forensic Psychiatry Founder status, an MBA (University of Toronto), and is a Certified Physician Executive (Certifying Commission on Medical Management 1999) – Diplomate American College of Physician Executives. He obtained the Chartered Director (C.Dir.) designation from The Directors College (2022). He is a Distinguished Fellow of the Canadian and American Psychiatric Associations. He is the President of the Canadian Psychiatric Association. Continuing medical education activities include organizing the Canadian Psychiatric Association International Professional Development Conference, The International Forensic Psychiatry Lecture Series, and the Forensic Psychiatry Risk and Recovery Conference.

Dr. Chaimowitz has been awarded the Ontario Medical Association Life Membership Award (2022), the International Association of Forensic Mental Health Services Rüdiger Müller-Isberner Award (2021), the Canadian Psychiatric Association C. A. Roberts Award for Clinical Leadership (2016), the Association of General Hospital Psychiatric Services Jane Chamberlain Award (2016), the Ontario Medical Association Section Service Award (2016), the Canadian Academy of Psychiatry and the Law Bruno Cormier Award (2015), and the St. Joseph's Healthcare Hamilton Mission Legacy Award (2015).

Susie Chung, Ph.D., BCBA, is a licensed psychologist and Board Certified Behavior Analyst with expertise in forensic mental health evaluations as well as the treatment of severe problem behaviors in developmentally disabled individuals and psychiatric patients. In her over 20 years of experience, she has worked in three forensic psychiatric hospitals in different states, including the Ann Klein Forensic Center in New Jersey, where she currently conducts competency to stand trial and criminal responsibility evaluations in the outpatient evaluation program. Dr. Chung led the development of the competency restoration program at Ann Klein and has presented on this program with her colleagues at two national conferences. schungphd@comast.net

Melissa Coelho is a registered social worker practicing in Hamilton, Ontario. She received her Master of Social Work degree from the School of Social Work at the University of Windsor and is trained in several evidence-based approaches. She has provided psychotherapy for individuals and couples, utilizing cognitive-behavioral therapy models and drawing from the tenets of behavioral approaches. In addition, Ms. Coelho has an extensive background as a psychiatric social worker, case manager, and mental health crisis worker. She has also partnered with police services for consultation. She is a strong advocate for her clients, including mentally ill adults, individuals with dual diagnoses, and those with concurrent disorders.

Nancy Fenning, B.A., has an extensive background working with psychiatrically hospitalized individuals. She began employment at Ancora Psychiatric Hospital in Hammonton, New Jersey, since 2005, when she was hired as a social worker on a chronic inpatient unit. In 2007, Ms. Fenning began working in the secure care forensic unit, where she co-facilitated the Community Reintegration Group. She is currently retired from state service. Fenningnancy@yahoo.com.

Patrícia Figueiredo is a psychologist with a Ph.D. in Psychology. She is an Assistant Professor at the School of Psychology and Life Sciences (EPCV) at the Centro Universitário Lusófona - Lisboa (CUL-L) and an Integrated Member at the Hei-Lab. Collaborating researcher in the Neuropsychophysiology Laboratory of the Faculty of Psychology and Education Sciences of the University of Porto. She has a Master's degree in Clinical Psychology from the Universidade de Trás-os-Montes e Alto Douro. She has conducted research and psychological interventions in the area of aggression and violent behaviors and is a co-author and researcher of PREVINT (https://www.prevint.pt/en).

Dr. Kyrsten Grimes received her Ph.D. in Clinical Psychology from the University of Toronto, Scarborough. Dr. Grimes is registered with the College of Psychologists of Ontario, practicing in the areas of clinical, forensic, and neuropsychology. She is a psychologist at Waypoint Centre for Mental Health Care, the only highly secure forensic mental health program in the province. Dr. Grimes is continuously active in clinical research, focusing on the metacognitive and neurocognitive predictors of psychosis to develop more targeted psychological interventions for schizophrenia in forensic settings.

Russell S. Horton, MPA, is a compliance reporting specialist for the Washington State Department of Social and Health Services' Office of Forensic Mental Health Services. In this role, he contributes to the implementation of the Trueblood Contempt Settlement Agreement through data and management analysis, compliance reporting to the federal court and state legislature, and collaborating with internal and external partners to enhance implementation and compliance-related decision-making. Previous government experience includes serving with the Washington

State Senate and several years as staff to a Member of Congress. Prior to his work on the Trueblood implementation, Rusty spent more than a decade working in private non-profit higher education in the Offices of the Registrar, where he developed expertise in admissions, transfer, and systems policies and practices within higher education. Rusty has given numerous professional conference presentations across North America and has presented his scholarly research internationally. He has several publications to his credit, including peer-reviewed articles.

Rusty completed a Bachelor of Arts in Political Science and German from Western Washington University and a Master of Public Administration from Seattle University.

Ellen Inverso, Psy.D., is a co-developer of recovery-oriented cognitive therapy (CT-R) and a licensed psychologist practicing in Pennsylvania. An internationally recognized expert in CT-R, Dr. Inverso provides large-scale training and consultation to mental health providers for individuals given serious mental health condition diagnoses. She has developed transformative strategies for implementing CT-R in inpatient units, community residences, schools, forensic facilities, and assertive community treatment (ACT) teams. She was named the Pennsylvania Psychological Association's 2020 Early Career Psychologist of the Year for her innovative and influential work in Pennsylvania and in systems across the United States. She is the co-author of the book *Recovery-Oriented Cognitive Therapy for Serious Mental Health Conditions*, through Guilford Press.

Dione Johnson is a dually licensed clinical psychologist in Pennsylvania and New Jersey. Having earned her doctoral and master's degrees from Fuller Theological Seminary in California, Dr. Johnson specializes in forensic and community psychology. Dr. Johnson has experience with the New Jersey State Parole Board doing mental health parole evaluations, has directed mental health programs in jails and prisons, and provides expert testimony in forensic cases. Dr. Johnson is also an ordained minister. She often integrates psychology with faith principles in helping individuals make and sustain necessary positive changes in their lives. All communication with Dr. Johnson should be forwarded to truthheartwdoc@gmail.com.

MSc. Kateřina Klapilová, Ph.D. (ECPS) is the head of the Centre of Sexual Health and Intervention at the National Institute of Mental Health, Klecany, CR, and an assistant professor at the Faculty of Humanities, Charles University, Prague. She is a founder and guarantor of the first primary intervention program for people with paraphilic interests in the Czech Republic (the Parafilik program) and a guarantor of SexHelp: the National Helpline for Sexual Health. She has a long history of research on human sexuality. Her main research aims include the national representative surveys of problematic sexual behaviors and preferences, research in communities with unusual sexual preferences, the development of psychodiagnostic tools in sexology, and the testing of social and health care innovations in the field of sexual offending prevention. She is a leading member of several national societies related to sexual health and sexual violence prevention (e.g. CSSM, SS CLSJEP) and an active member of international societies in the same area (e.g. ISSM/ESSM, EFS, IASR, IATSO, and ESMN COST).

Lucie Krejčová is a senior researcher at the National Institute of Mental Health and the Faculty of Humanities, Charles University in Czechia. Her areas of research interests include testing of physiological sexual responses by application of psychophysiological measures, basic research on female sexuality, paraphilic sexual interests, and national surveys of sexual behavior and preferences. She also works on testing the effectiveness of evidence-based treatments and social interventions in the fields of sexual health and sexual offense prevention.

Dr. Angela Li, BHSc (Honours), M.D., is a third-year psychiatry resident in the Department of Psychiatry and Behavioural Neurosciences at McMaster University. She completed her undergraduate degree in the Bachelor of Health Sciences (Honours) program and medical school training at the Michael G. DeGroote School of Medicine at McMaster University. In addition to her interest in forensic psychiatry, she has also published in scholarly journals on the topic of political healthcare advocacy, and her other research interests include substance use disorders and harm reduction. She has served as the resident research representative in the McMaster Department of Psychiatry and Behavioural Neurosciences Research Advisory Committee and Resident Research and Scholarship Committee. She also served as a resident representative in the Competency-Based Medical Education Working Group. She currently serves as the Forensic Psychiatry Representative for her general psychiatry residency training program. She is also involved in many initiatives related to resident medical education in her residency program.

Aura MacArthur is the Director of the Washington State Department of Social and Health Services' Behavioral Health Administration's Project Management Office. Prior to this role, she served as the senior Project Manager responsible for facilitating the negotiation of the contempt settlement agreement, managing the class action member notification process, designing and building the necessary infrastructure to support the implementation of the elements across multiple agencies and entities, and eventually hiring a team of project managers to work with her in supporting each of the elements' implementation in Phases 1 and 2. Previous government experience includes 19 years with DSHS across three administrations, five years in various administrative roles with the Department of Corrections, and two and a half years as a 911 dispatcher with the Washington State Patrol.

Aura received both an Associate in Business and an Associate in Arts from Pierce Community College and obtained her Bachelor of Science from Western Governor's University.

Liam E. Marshall, Ph.D., RP, ATSAF, Waypoint Centre for Mental Health Care, the University of Toronto Department of Forensic Psychiatry, and Rockwood Psychotherapy & Consulting. Liam Marshall received his Doctoral and other degrees from Queen's University in Kingston, Canada. He has been providing treatment and conducting research on offenders and offenders with mental health issues for more than 25 years. Liam has more than 100 peer-reviewed publications and is the co-author/co-editor of four books. He is a board member and reviewer for many international journals and has made numerous international conference presentations on offender and mental health issues. He has provided consultation to governments and delivered training for therapists and staff working with offenders in 26 countries. Liam has been named a Fellow of the Association for the Treatment of Sexual Abusers (ATSA) for his contributions to the organization's goals. He is currently the Director of Rockwood Psychotherapy & Consulting, a researcher and clinician at Waypoint Centre for Mental Health Care, and an Assistant Professor in the Department of Forensic Psychiatry at the University of Toronto.

Louis Martelli, B.A., began his career providing a full range of mental health services to juvenile sex offenders in a New Jersey Juvenile Justice Commission residential setting. In 2003, he began employment as a social worker at Ancora Psychiatric Hospital in Hammonton, New Jersey, working with forensically involved patients in a secure care unit, where he co-facilitated the Community Reintegration Group for over eight years. In 2018, Mr. Martelli transferred to a geriatric unit at this same institution, where he currently serves as a treatment team leader. Lmartelli77@yahoo.com.

Sarah M. McKay, Psy.D., is a licensed psychologist in Oregon and a Certified Forensic Evaluator. She completed her doctoral degree at the California School of Professional Psychology in San Francisco, California, and completed her APPIC internship at the Alexandria Veteran's Affairs Healthcare System in Alexandria, Louisiana. She has worked at the Oregon State Hospital since 2016. Dr. McKay was one of several individuals who worked on the DBT unit at Oregon State Hospital before, during, and after the credentialing process and provided full-fidelity DBT to patients residing on the unit. While working on the unit,

Dr. McKay went through extensive training in DBT hosted by the Portland DBT Institute, credentialed through the Linehan Board of Certification. Currently, she works as one of the hospital's Risk Psychologists specializing in violence, stalking, and fire-setting risk assessments.

Daniel Mendonça is a Clinical Psychologist. He has a Master's degree in Criminal Sciences and Deviant Behavior from the Faculty of Medicine of the University of Lisbon. He has been a member of the probation services of the Portuguese Ministry of Justice since 2001. From 2009 to 2016, he worked in the Department of the General Directorate of Reintegration and Prison Services, responsible for supervising the activity of the juvenile detention centers, and was part of the team of the Project for the Assessment of Risk of Recidivism and Criminogenic Needs, responsible for adapting the YLS/CMI instrument and training technicians to apply it. From 2016 to the present, he has worked in a Social Reintegration Team in Lisbon, exclusively with young offenders, both in the assessment of risk and needs and in the monitoring of these young people, within the scope of educational tutelary measures applied by the courts.

Etay R. Nachmias, M.A., is a Clown Doctor, part of the "Dream Doctors" association in Israel. Etay is an Art Therapist, an Actor, and a Performer. He works as a Clown Doctor in 'Sha'ar Menashe', an Israeli state psychiatric facility. He also works in a general hospital, "Carmel", with children and adults in various wards.

Dr. Andrew T. Olagunju, M.B.B.S., M.Sc., Ph.D., FWACP, FMCPsych. Dr. Olagunju is an Assistant Professor at the Department of Psychiatry and Behavioural Neurosciences, McMaster University, and a Psychiatrist at the affiliated hospitals. He is a Research Fellow at the University of Adelaide, Australia and a Collaborator on the Global Burden of Diseases project, University of Washington, USA. Dr Olagunju is a member of the Advisory Board for the Institute of Neurosciences, Mental Health, and Addiction, Canadian Institute of Health Research. He is an associate editor for the Journal of Climate Change and Health and Frontiers in Psychiatry.

Previously, he was a senior lecturer at the College of Medicine, University of Lagos, and an Affiliate in Research with King's College London.

Dr. Olagunju currently devotes his time to evidence-based clinical practice, medical education, and cutting-edge research. His research works are contained in over 200 peer-reviewed publications (90,000+ citations, H-index=71) and have been awarded several recognitions. He is a European Union Commission Erasmus Mundus scholar and an Australian Government Research Training Scholar.

Dr. Olagunju is a founding board member of the Patela Care Foundation, a non-governmental organization with mainstream health programs for underserved populations to alleviate suffering and poverty and promote equitable access to health services.

His hobbies include traveling, hiking, and gardening.

Christina Oliveira-Picado, BScN, RN, CPMHN(C) is a registered nurse at St. Josephs Healthcare, Hamilton, ON. Christina has held a variety of positions as an inpatient nurse, community case manager, and substance abuse treatment specialist with the Forensic Program. She is a trained addiction treatment specialist and has participated in provincial projects on addiction problems. She has a special interest in working with individuals with concurrent disorders, with a focus on individualized care and recovery.

Ms. Ashley Palmer holds a Bachelor of Arts Honours in Therapeutic Recreation degree from the University of Waterloo. Since 2009, she has worked as a Recreation Therapist at St. Joseph's Healthcare Hamilton for the Forensic Psychiatry Program. In 2021, she expanded her portfolio, transitioned to support the patients in the Acute Stabilization Unit, and helped launch and coordinate support with the Specialized Therapeutic Recreation Team. Ashley also has a range of recreation-related experience in mood disorders, acute care, corrections, and the acquired brain injury population. Ashley holds the titles of Senior Recreation Therapist and Foster/Lead Handler for the Forensic Psychiatry Program's Resident Dog. Ashley was the recipient of the TRO 2021 Innovation in TR Award and the Innovation in Professional Practice Award through St. Joseph's Healthcare Hamilton in 2022. Outside of work, Ashley enjoys traveling and spending time with her family, friends, and her dog, Oreo, and the new Forensic Dog, Scout.

Jeffrey Palmer, Psy.D., is a licensed psychologist with 15 years of experience in inpatient forensic assessment and mental health treatment. He has worked alongside his colleagues in bringing a structured competency restoration program to Ann Klein Forensic Center, New Jersey's state forensic psychiatric hospital, where he is currently employed. Jeffpalmer1976@gmail.com

Marek Páv, MD, PhD, MBA, is a psychiatrist and sexologist in charge of clinical management at Bohnice Psychiatric Hospital in Prague, affiliated with the First Faculty of Medicine, Charles University and General University Hospital in Prague, Czech Republic. His main professional interests include forensic psychiatry and sexology (with fifteen years of experience as a forensic expert), violence risk assessment, acute psychiatry, and therapy for people with paraphilic preferences. His research aims to evaluate therapeutic programs' effectiveness, risk assessment tools, the Czech Republic's forensic population mapping, and research on violent behavior. He is involved in projects of the Ministry of Health and the Ministry of Justice dealing with the transformation of forensic psychiatry and sexology services. https://www.researchgate.net/profile/Marek-Pav

Hilik Peri, M.A., is a supervising clinical psychologist in Israel. Hilik works as a Senior Clinical Psychologist in a maximum security forensic ward in 'Sha'ar Menashe', an Israeli state psychiatric facility, where he also supervises the work of medical clowns. In his private practice, he also works with children and adolescents. hilikperi@hotmail.com

Eduarda Ramião is a psychologist with a Master's degree in Clinical Psychology from the University of Trás-os-Montes and Alto Douro, Portugal. She is a Ph.D. student in the Ph.D. Program in Psychology at the Faculty of Psychology and Education Sciences of the University of Porto, in the Laboratory of Neuropsychophysiology. She has conducted research and psychological interventions in the fields of psychopathy, behavior problems, aggression, and violence.

Merrill Rotter, M.D., is a forensic psychiatrist working at Albert Einstein College of Medicine, where he is an Associate Clinical Professor of Psychiatry and Director of the Division of Law and Psychiatry for the Department of Psychiatry. Trained in clinical psychiatry at Columbia and in forensic psychiatry at Yale, Dr. Rotter leads a program of teaching, research, and clinical service for Einstein as well as the New York State Office of Mental Health (NYSOMH). In his OMH role, Dr. Rotter is Senior Forensic Advisor to the Commissioner of Director of NYS OMH and Director of the Division of Forensic Services at Bronx Psychiatric Center. Dr. Rotter is the creator and Project Director of SPECTRM, a research, training, and treatment program aimed at helping to meet the needs of individuals with mental illness who have a history of incarceration. Dr. Rotter has researched, presented, and published in areas related to forensic training, violence risk assessment, treatment and management of mentally ill offenders, the insanity defense, criminal recidivism, and mental health diversion and re-entry.

Benjamin A. Rubin, Psy.D., is a licensed psychologist who specializes in forensic psychology, assessment, and treatment. Dr. Rubin received his Psy.D. in Combined School-Clinical Psychology from the Ferkauf Graduate School of Yeshiva University. He completed a pre-doctoral internship at the Child Guidance Center of Southern Connecticut and post-doctoral fellowships in psychoanalysis at the New York Psychoanalytic Society and Institute and the Derner Institute of Advanced Psychological Studies at Adelphi University. Dr. Rubin has presented at national and international professional conferences on forensic mental health assessment, the Rorschach, practical applications of psychoanalytic theory, psychological testing, and ethics. Dr. Rubin formerly served as Director of Forensic Services at Rockland Psychiatric Center, a New York State Office of Mental Health psychiatric facility. He is currently in independent forensic practice as the Director of Measured Minds LLC. He is a co-author of the Rorschach Performance Assessment System (R-PAS).

Paul S. Saks, Ph.D., is currently the Chief of Psychology at Rockland Psychiatric Center, is an Adjunct Assistant Professor of Psychology at John Jay College of Criminal Justice/The City University of New York, and does forensic consulting in his private practice. His career with the New York Office of Mental Health spans almost twenty years and includes positions at Mid-Hudson Forensic, Manhattan, and Bronx Psychiatric Centers. He has published on topics that include interpreting the language of psychotic patients, the assessment of psychotic disorders in State Psychiatric Hospitals and the impact of trauma on metaphor.

Kristina Shatokhina, M.Sc., Ontario Tech University, Department of Forensic Psychology

Kristina Shatokhina is a Doctoral student at Ontario Tech University, supervised by Dr. Leigh Harkins. Through her research, she aims to better understand the factors that motivate the commission of sexual violence as well as treatment engagement. Her doctoral dissertation investigates multiple-perpetrator sexual offending, elucidating the driving forces of group influence. Her Master of Science, also completed at Ontario Tech, focused on applying the Integrated Risk Assessment and Treatment System (IRATS) to the prediction of sexual and violent recidivism, as well as treatment attrition. Over the last several years, Kristina has worked and volunteered for organizations including the Correctional Service of Canada, the Centre for Addiction and Mental Health – Forensics Division, and the Salvation Army – Correctional and Justice Services.

Dr. Peter Sheridan, B.Sc., M.A., Ph.D., CPsych., received his B.Sc. with Specialization in Psychology from Trinity College, University of Toronto, and his M.A. and Ph.D. in Clinical Psychology from York University. He completed his internships at the Wellesley Hospital and at the Forensic Service, Centre for Addiction and Mental Health (formerly the Clarke Institute of Psychiatry). Dr. Sheridan is registered with the College of Psychologists of Ontario to provide clinical and forensic psychological services. He is a staff psychologist in the Forensic Psychiatry Program at St. Joseph's Healthcare Hamilton, where he provides a range of services, including psychological assessment, risk assessment, and treatment, for individuals found Unfit to Stand Trial or Not Criminally Responsible on Account of Mental Disorder. He has provided clinical services for both the provincial and federal ministries of corrections and has facilitated community interventions for sexual abuse survivors and perpetrators of partner abuse. He is trained in client-centered, psychodynamic, CBT, and DBT approaches to treatment.

Ashley Strathern, Psy.D., graduated with her doctorate in clinical psychology from Immaculata University. She is a licensed psychologist working in an outpatient forensic evaluation program at the Ann Klein Forensic Center in West Trenton, New Jersey, where she conducts competency to stand trial and mental state at the time of the offense evaluations. Prior to that, she worked in an inpatient unit providing treatment, conducting various forensic psychological assessments, and developing and implementing a competency restoration treatment program. Dr. Strathern, who also works in private practice where she specializes in the treatment of children and adolescents, has presented with her colleagues on the restoration program at two national conferences. Dr.Ashley.Strathern@gmail.com

Zach Yeoman, Psy.D., Somerset Psychological Group, PA. Zachary Yeoman received his master's and doctoral degrees from the Illinois School of Professional Psychology. He is a clinical and forensic psychologist licensed in both New Jersey and New York. He conducts psychological evaluations and provides expert testimony and training on various psycholegal issues, including risk assessment and treatment of those who commit sexual offenses. He co-authored several articles and one book chapter related to the evaluation and treatment of those who sexually offend.

About the Editor

Michael Siglag, Ph.D. I received my Ph.D. in clinical psychology from the University of Detroit and am a licensed psychologist in New Jersey and Pennsylvania. My professional roles have included clinician, forensic evaluator, expert witness, supervisor, and administrator in both civil and forensic settings. I have initiated and promoted numerous innovative treatments and programs, including supervising a state-award-winning Cognitive Remediation program. Leadership roles have included chairing a psychiatric hospital Psychology Department, directing an APA-accredited pre-doctoral internship program, and serving on New Jersey's State Board of Psychological Examiners. I have written and presented on topics such as group therapy, psychosocial rehabilitation, treatment approaches for individuals struggling with psychosis, trauma issues, and hospital systems. Prior to editing this book, I co-edited a book about clinical psychologists' work in inpatient mental health settings that was published by Routledge in 2019. Throughout my career, I have provided psychological services and worked to advance clinical and forensic psychological services in settings where resources often don't match needs.

Introduction

Innovative Treatment Approaches in Forensic and Correctional Settings

Michael Siglag, John M.W. Bradford, and Andrew T. Olagunju

Mental health professionals who work with individuals in forensic psychiatric and correctional facilities often need to develop treatment approaches that differ from those implemented in other settings. Interventions in forensic-correctional settings must strike a balance between addressing identified clinical treatment needs and managing challenging or dangerous behaviors and physical safety concerns. To provide appropriate treatment while managing risk, clinicians often adapt established interventions and develop innovative programs and therapy interventions. The interventions developed under such conditions can be well-grounded in theory, built upon established and evidence-based methodologies, and effective. However, despite the effort, knowledge, creativity, and resources put into their development and often demonstrable therapeutic benefits, many of these interventions never receive exposure outside of the treatment settings where they are applied. After a pressing clinical or administratively prioritized need is addressed, the limited resources applied to such programs may be redeployed. Interventions may be discontinued, stripped of resources, or altered until they become unrecognizable. Such interventions may disappear without ever being adequately documented and without formal research demonstrating or validating their effectiveness.

The primary goals of this book are to present an array of current innovative interventions and to provide windows into the systems that support such interventions. Interventions described here range from specific approaches developed to treat individuals with specialized clinical or management needs in specific treatment settings to broader systemic transformations that influence the treatment and management of forensic and correctional populations in a variety of settings.

Through the exposure provided in this volume, it is hoped that the value of the innovative interventions identified here will gain wider recognition. Such recognition can contribute to the broader implementation of such programs, increasing the range of settings and the number of individuals who may benefit from these treatment interventions. Chapters in this book

DOI: 10.4324/9781003360926-1

that include examples of systemic support and change will help provide models for those working in complicated systems to implement such new, innovative, and needed programs and interventions.

This broad introduction provides a current perspective concerning forensic-correctional populations and settings, as well as the multiple levels of forensic-correctional treatment that this book addresses. This overview will assist international readers working in diverse forensic-correctional settings to determine how the interventions described here will best meet their clinical and professional needs and identify the systemic resources necessary for successful implementation.

Mental health professionals working in forensic-correctional settings apply psychological and behavioral management theories to individuals presenting a wide range of cognitive, behavioral, and mental health issues. Such individuals' behavior and mental health issues have often led to their involvement in both the mental health treatment system and the legal-correctional system, including the application of laws relevant to competency and criminal responsibility or sanity. Approaches to addressing the issues presented by such individuals through a mental health lens are continually evolving and expanding. Forensic-correctional work involves interaction and collaboration between legal professionals and multiple mental health treatment specialties. Involved professions and paraprofessionals include clinical and forensic psychologists and psychiatrists, neuropsychologists and social workers, specialists in other therapy and rehabilitation fields, nursing staff with specialized clinical training, and other colleagues in the mental health field.

In recent years, the roles and importance of treatment of individuals with mental health issues who are involved with the criminal justice system in forensic and correctional settings have grown for several reasons. One factor has been the significant reduction of psychiatric inpatient beds in the United States and internationally. This reduction has resulted in an increased transition of many individuals formerly hospitalized in public mental health treatment facilities to other types of facilities, including jails and prisons, forensic mental health facilities, and community settings. Two related results of this shift are: (1) an increased concentration of individuals in inpatient psychiatric facilities who suffer from severe emotional disturbance, as well as possessing legal charges that pose obstacles to discharge and (2) the incarceration of large numbers of people with mental illness in various types of correctional facilities. These two factors have contributed to an expanding inpatient forensic-correctional population with needs for mental health treatment services.

In general, forensic-correctional treatment populations include individuals who are found unfit to stand trial, not considered criminally responsible for their legal charges due to mental disturbance, mentally ill offenders in correctional facilities, and individuals whose aggressive behavior is unmanageable in adult mental health service settings (Al Marzooqi et al., 2022; Askola et al., 2022; Crocker et al., 2017; Olagunju et al., 2018). Settings where specialized inpatient care and psycho-legal services for offenders with mental illness are provided include secure forensic, correctional and general psychiatric units or hospitals. Although the concentrations of beds devoted to such populations vary across countries, thousands of psychiatric beds are allocated internationally to forensic-correctional populations. In their study, Beis et al. reported that 4,540 beds in the United Kingdom, 3,797 beds in several European countries, 13,244 beds in some North and South American countries, 19,721 beds in some Asian countries, 2,538 beds in three African countries, and 901 beds in Oceania are allotted for forensic patients (Beis et al., 2022). More often, inpatient forensic-correctional psychiatric care is integrated with comprehensive outpatient and community-based mental health services to treat mental-behavioral health issues, manage and mitigate risk, and reduce recidivism (Al Marzooqi et al., 2022; Chaimowitz et al., 2020a; Olagunju et. al., 2022).

While there are commonalities in forensic-correctional mental health work between the United States and other countries, international legal systems differ, sometimes in significant ways. This book includes chapters describing the international practice of forensic-correctional mental health treatment in the United States, Canada, the Czech Republic (Czechia), Portugal, Israel, and elsewhere, highlighting some of the similarities as well as differences between forensic-correctional mental health treatment practices that have emerged in various countries.

The scope and delivery of forensic-correctional mental health services vary widely across jurisdictions worldwide. These variations in forensic-correctional mental health systems stem from several factors. Among the most significant of these factors are international differences in legal frameworks (e.g., common law, civil law, Islamic law, and former communist country legal system regulations) across jurisdictions. Such differences play an important role by impacting the definition and extent to which the concepts of fitness to stand trial, criminal responsibility, risk, and mental disorder are applied in adjudicating processes. Whether forensic-correctional services are recognized as a distinct subspecialty can also impact the ways in which these services are provided, as well as the training of healthcare professionals such as psychiatrists and psychologists needed to carry out these specialized services (Beis et al., 2022; Bioku et al., 2021; Olagunju et al., 2018). Furthermore, a country's gross domestic product, healthcare spending allocation, and cultures of risk containment often contribute to the variability in forensic-correctional mental health services and resources (Askola et al., 2022). Despite these variations, there is a consensus that forensic-correctional psychiatric services represent an important component of public mental health systems that conduct psycho-legal assessments and provide treatment for individuals with mental disorders within the criminal justice system in secure settings in order to ensure a degree of public safety (Al Marzooqi et al., 2022; Olagunju et al., 2018).

The forensic mental health work addressed in this volume includes examples from a range of settings, including forensic hospitals, jails, prisons, civil hospital settings, and the community. The focus ranges from interventions addressing the problems of a single individual to the transformation of state-wide forensic mental health services. It includes examples of well-established approaches as well as unique and cutting-edge approaches. It provides examples and models relating to the provision of services relevant to forensically and correctionally involved individuals on multiple levels. The approaches described in this book are grounded in a variety of theoretical models. Interventions are described that incorporate and integrate biopsychosocial, cognitive-behavioral, psychoanalytic, systemic, and other approaches.

The book is divided into three sections and includes 17 chapters. The three sections of the book reflect a variety of intervention levels. These sections are: (Part 1) focused treatment interventions; (Part 2) treatment that involves broader and more programmatic elements; and (Part 3) interventions or systemic innovations that involve broad changes and the introduction of new interventions and approaches across treatment delivery systems.

Part 1 (Targeted Therapeutic Interventions) includes descriptions of targeted treatments addressing specific treatment issues and the beneficial effects on people engaged in those treatments. Treatments, patient benefits, systemic supports and obstacles, and organizational impacts relevant to these treatments are described in the chapters in this section. Treatment issues include stalking behavior, sex offending, violence mitigation, substance abuse, the impact of past traumatic experiences, and other issues.

Part 2 (Programmatic Approaches) covers treatment programs that are larger in scope. The interventions described in this section address multiple dimensions of treatment, rather than a targeted problem. Individuals sharing similar treatment issues may be housed together. These programs often have units devoted to their implementation. Entire sections of hospitals, forensic settings, or correctional facilities are devoted to these treatment programs or interventions. In some instances, they take place in separate specialized facilities and have their own administrative structure and personnel. Chapters in this section include applications of cognitive therapy (CBTp), dialectical behavior therapy, trauma-informed treatment, community reintegration, and approaches addressing issues such as paraphilia, adolescent sexual behavior problems, violence mitigation with a 'seriously mentally ill' population, and legal competency restoration.

The third section, Part 3 (System Wide Intervention and Transformation), includes chapters describing a range of interventions with system-wide applications and systemic changes impacting treatment. This section includes examples in which state or federal judicial or legislative initiatives have broadly impacted the provision of forensic treatment. These chapters describe interventions and systemic changes being implemented across multiple settings that are part of a larger treatment system. Interventions described in this section include recovery-oriented cognitive therapy, innovative treatment options for 'seriously mentally ill' inmates housed in secure correctional settings, and approaches to community re-entry. This section includes a chapter describing the transition and reorganization of services in a large-scale mental health service system, affecting forensic services throughout an entire state.

In all sections of the book, the authors describe therapeutic approaches, programs, and systemic initiatives they have developed and/or applied in their own work. All of the approaches described in this book apply to forensic-correctionally involved individuals. Interventions are described that have been carried out in: (1) civil psychiatric hospitals housing forensically involved patients; (2) forensic psychiatric hospitals; (3) correctional facilities housing adults or juvenile populations; and (4) specialized facilities such as sex offender treatment facilities. The chapters also describe interventions relating to the interface with, and transitions between, forensic-correctional settings and community settings.

Chapters in this book that focus on treatment interventions include several elements that are particularly valuable for clinicians who will carry out such interventions. These elements are also valuable for clinical and administrative leaders in organizations that need to prioritize treatment resources. These elements include:

- Description and delineation of specific treatment goals/needs that the therapeutic intervention is intended to address (e.g., violence risk mitigation, competency restoration)
- Systemic challenges that might need to be addressed and systemic supports that will help facilitate the implementation of the program
- Description of both key components and actual implementation of the intervention or program
- An explanation of the intervention's theoretical or conceptual grounding
- Demonstration of program effectiveness and ideas about future research

Treatment in forensic and correctional settings is a growing and evolving field. This book is not intended as a comprehensive and static handbook of therapies and programs. This book grows out of the perspective that therapy approaches and programs will continue to evolve and develop and from the expectation that ongoing systemic transformations will continue to take place in response to changing needs. The development of innovative treatment approaches in forensic and correctional settings is a continual process. Treatment options and data indicating demonstrable benefits will continue to grow. It is expected that in the future, more innovations, advances, and systemic transformations will emerge. The current volume is intended to provide a sampling of current innovative therapeutic approaches and programs, as well as pioneering steps being taken to initiate and implement structural change in system-wide therapy delivery. Significant aspects of forensic psychological work being carried out in a variety of settings and developing treatment trends are described by authors with specific areas of forensic psychology experience and expertise.

Increasing clinicians' and administrators' awareness of the treatment approaches described in this book provides numerous opportunities. These include: (1) expanding practitioners' treatment options in forensic and correctional settings; (2) directly helping individuals housed and treated in these facilities who may participate in such treatments; (3) improving the treatment results for the facilities in settings where these treatments can be carried out; and (4) allowing for the development of more and stronger empirical evidence regarding these interventions. In addition, chapters providing examples of unit, hospital, and system-wide transformations that incorporate a range of innovations provide practical models and highlight some of the obstacles that may need to be overcome when seeking to improve services in various settings.

The array of treatment approaches described in this volume represent methods for addressing problems presented by a variety of forensic-correctional populations in a range of settings and in several countries. Chapter authors in this volume describe approaches incorporating transtheoretical concepts such as recovery and trauma-informed care, which have widely influenced many treatment approaches. Such approaches include cognitive-behavioral, psychodynamic, and other theoretical models such as Risk-Needs-Recovery (RNR), one of the prevailing approaches in numerous jurisdictions, including Canada, the United Kingdom, and Australia (Crocker et al., 2017). Other models include the Good Lives Model and the Recovery Model (Lutz et al., 2022), developed for the treatment of specific forensic-correctional populations. Recovery, risk management, and mitigation of recidivism are critical and common goals for forensic-correctional psychiatric populations, transcending theoretical models.

Treatment outcomes can be highly variable depending on multiple factors, including the unique characteristics of specific treatment populations, the complexities of individual patients, practitioner training, and setting resources and support. Several intervention models described in this book have been developed to manage these risk complexities, promote recovery, and facilitate desired outcomes. The development and refinement of treatment approaches persist, and continued research to determine and build upon effective interventions is needed to keep pace with ongoing developments.

There has been movement in recent years toward more patient-centered care and treatment and increasing patients' engagement through the provision of meaningful involvement in a range of activities in forensic-correctional mental health service delivery. There has also been increased emphasis on improving the social milieu and comfort of the inpatient wards to support the safety of patients and staff (Crocker et al., 2017). These movements and emphases are also represented in the current volume, demonstrating how these developments have paved the way for a range of therapy interventions that build upon both current research and well-established approaches.

The treatment approaches presented in this volume are examples of an evolution in forensic-correctional mental health treatment, including non-traditional innovative interventions such as incorporation of Eye Movement Desensitization and Reprocessing, an animal-assisted intervention, and a poetry therapy model, as well as more traditional therapy approaches incorporating behavioral, cognitive-behavioral, and other theoretical approaches (e.g., RNR, the Good Lives Model, the Recovery Model). The interventions presented here are among those most currently being provided to treat individuals in forensic-correctional settings who have previously engaged in behaviors that have resulted in harm to others and may continue to pose a continued risk to others' safety. The goals of interventions described here include aiding in the learning of prosocial behaviors, improving safe social interactions, helping individuals develop a sense of purpose, and enhancing community reintegration. The benefits of successfully engaging individuals in such treatments include improving the safety of all individuals participating in such treatments. The results of providing appropriate and effective treatment include enhancing treatment effectiveness in the settings where the treatments take place.

In the context of forensic-correctional work, outcomes vary widely. Even with effective treatment, many individuals will remain in restrictive settings for extended periods of time or may not be eligible or able to regain freedom to live in the community. For such individuals, successful implementation of interventions may help improve their mental health, reduce dangerous or concerning behaviors, and increase safety and quality of life, both for those housed in such settings and for those working in such settings. For other individuals who may safely progress to less restrictive settings and communities or who reside in the community, appropriate and effective treatment and support can provide long-term benefits for individuals and the community, relating to both mental health and safety. The goal of this book is to contribute to both of these outcomes.

References

Al Marzooqi, S., El Sheikh, A., Al Shehhi, N., Al Mesmari, A., Al Zaabi, M., Haweel, A., Wang, J., Prat, S.S., Chaimowitz, G.A., & Olagunju, A.T. (Winter 2022). Forensic-Correctional Psychiatric Services in Abu Dhabi: Lessons From a Descriptive Analysis of the Attributes of a Sample of Service Users. *Psychiatr Danub*, *34*(4): 635–643. https://doi.org/10.24869/psyd.2022.635.

Askola, R., Louheranta, O., & Seppänen, A. (2022). Factors Affecting Treatment Regress and Progress in Forensic Psychiatry: A Thematic Analysis. *Front Psychiatry*, *13*: 884410. https://doi.org/10.3389/fpsyt.2022.884410

Beis, P., Graf, M., & Hachtel, H. (2022). Impact of Legal Traditions on Forensic Mental Health Treatment Worldwide. *Front Psychiatry*, *13*: 876619. https://doi.org/10.3389/fpsyt.2022.876619

Bioku, A.A., Alatishe, Y.A., Adeniran, J.O., Olagunju, T.O., Singhal, N., Mela, M., Bradford, J.M., Chaimowitz, G.A., & Olagunju, A.T. (2021). Psychiatric Morbidity among Incarcerated Individuals in an Underserved Region of Nigeria: Revisiting the Unmet Mental Health Needs in Correction Services. *J Health Care Poor Underserved*, *32*(1): 321–337. https://doi.org/10.1353/hpu.2021.0026.

Chaimowitz, G. A., Mamak, M., Moulden, H. M., Furimsky, I., & Olagunju, A. T. (2020a). Implementation of risk assessment tools in psychiatric services. *J Healthc Risk Manag.*, *40*(1), 33–43. https://doi.org/10.1002/jhrm.21405

Chaimowitz, G.A., Mamak, M., & Olagunju, A.T. (December, 2020b). Aggressive Incidents Scale (AIS) – A Measure of Aggression That Manages Violence Risk. Rossiiskii psikhiatricheskii zhurnal. *Russ J Psychiatry*, *6*: 36–44. https://doi.org/10.24411/1560-957X-2020-10605

Crocker, A.G., Livingston, J.D., & Leclair, M.C. (2017). Forensic Mental Health Systems Internationally. In *Handbook of Forensic Mental Health Services* (pp. 3–76). Routledge/Taylor & Francis Group. https://doi.org/10.4324/9781315627823-2

Lutz, M., Zani, D., Fritz, M., Dudeck, M., & Franke, I. (2022). A Review and Comparative Analysis of the Risk-Needs-Responsivity, Good Lives, and Recovery Models in Forensic Psychiatric Treatment [Review]. *Front Psychiatry*, *13*. https://doi.org/10.3389/fpsyt.2022.988905

Olagunju, A.T., Oluwaniyi, S.O., Fadipe, B., Ogunnubi, O.P., Oni, O.D., Aina, O.F., & Chaimowitz, G.A. (May-June, 2018) Mental Health Services in Nigerian Prisons: Lessons from a Four-Year Review and the Literature. *Int J Law Psychiatry*, *58*: 79–86. https://doi.org/10.1016/j.ijlp.2018.03.004.

Part I

Targeted Therapeutic Interventions

1 A Semi-Structured Manualized Treatment Program (SSMTP) for Substance Abuse

Andrew T. Olagunju, Angela Li, Christina Oliveira-Picado, Peter Sheridan, and Gary A. Chaimowitz

Introduction

The prevalence of substance use disorders is very high globally. Alcohol use disorder is the most prevalent, with an estimated 1320.8 cases per 100,000 people, followed by opioid use disorder (353.0 cases per 100,000) and cannabis use disorder (289.7 cases per 100,000). The prevalence of cocaine use disorder is 82.6 cases per 100,000 and amphetamine use disorder is 70.4 cases per 100,000 (Degenhardt et al., 2018). Within the forensic population, 30–75% of patients have been found to meet the criteria for severe mental illness and a concomitant DSM-IV or DSM-5 substance use disorder (Crocker et al., 2015; McFadden et al., 2022). The prevalence of alcohol use disorder is 10 times higher in the criminal justice population than in the general population. Within the forensic population, there is a twofold increase in the lifetime prevalence of cannabis use disorder, a 40-fold increase in the lifetime prevalence of amphetamine use disorder, and a 60-fold increase for opioid use disorder (Kivimies et al., 2012; Slavin-Stewart et al., 2022). An increase in substance use appears to be associated with a greater risk of recidivism and poor outcomes with respect to symptom remission, functional recovery, and community reintegration (Al Marzooqi et al., 2022; Joe et al., 1990; Olagunju et al., 2018, 2022).

Substance abuse in persons with severe mental illness is an important factor contributing to incarceration (Mueser et al., 2000). This raises the issue of violence and criminality associated with concurrent disorders. The most important predictors of violence among individuals with major mental illness include a history of violence, acts of aggression prior to the onset of illness (Hodgins & Côté, 1993; Mueser et al., 2003), and substance abuse (Swartz et al., 1998). Active symptoms of psychotic disorders are associated with the risk for violence, and comorbid substance abuse is a major mediator of the risk for violence (Fazel et al., 2009). Substance use also appears to be a risk factor and motivator for absconding from forensic mental health units (Campagnolo et al., 2019; Olagunju et al., 2022).

DOI: 10.4324/9781003360926-3

Globally, the most frequently utilized treatment approach for substance use disorders in the forensic setting is psychoeducation, which has been demonstrated to be largely ineffective with no associated cognitive or behavioral change (McFadden et al., 2022). However, in the general inpatient psychiatric population, the efficacy of cognitive behavioral therapy (CBT) and motivational interviewing in the treatment of concurrent substance use disorders has been consistently demonstrated (Drake et al., 2004; McFadden et al., 2022). Further development and research in the growing field of evidence-based treatment approaches for substance use disorders in forensic settings is needed. Furthermore, substance use disorders and psychiatric disorders in forensic and correctional settings were traditionally addressed sequentially by separate mental health and drug and alcohol services (Ogloff et al., 2004; Bioku et al., 2021; Olagunju et al., 2022). However, the literature recommends that individuals who have concurrent disorders should have access to integrated treatment provided simultaneously for psychiatric and substance-related issues within one service setting by staff trained to address both issues (Canada, 2001; Drake et al., 2004; Ogloff et al., 2004).

There are pharmacological therapies that have been approved and shown to be effective for the treatment of alcohol and opiate abuse disorders, including disulfiram, acamprosate, and opiate agonists such as methadone and buprenorphine (Olagunju & Slavin-Stewart, 2023). However, currently, there are no pharmacologic agents approved for treating stimulant, cannabis, or benzodiazepine use disorders (McGovern & Carroll, 2003). Although some medications, such as bupropion, methylphenidate, mirtazapine, and other psychostimulants, have been used in small trials as replacement medications, most clinicians are reluctant to consider this option due to abuse potential and liability (Mooney & Haglund, 2014). There have been no controlled studies examining the efficacy of these agents with concurrent disorders in this population. There needs to be careful consideration regarding the potential risks of hepatotoxicity, a lowered seizure threshold, and possible medication interactions.

The above-mentioned gaps and the need to mitigate substance misuse in our forensic psychiatric population motivated the development of the semi-structured manualized treatment program (SSMTP). In this chapter, we describe the development and use of SSMTP using selected themes to provide an overview of the literature on substance misuse/use disorders in the forensic psychiatric population, the theoretical underpinning of SSMTP, its program structure, implementation, and recommendations.

Forensic Mental Health Services in Canada and Substance Misuse

Forensic mental health services in Canada are described in the literature, including in this volume (Chaimowitz et al., 2022; Olagunju et al., 2023). Briefly, the forensic psychiatric population includes individuals found unfit to stand trial (UST) or not criminally responsible (NCR). Following a court pronouncement, individuals with a UST or NCR finding fall under the purview of their provincial Criminal Code Review Board. The review boards are independent, quasi-judicial administrative tribunals, holding hearings to review individuals under their jurisdiction to render dispositions for their management. Possible dispositions include detention, conditional discharge, and an absolute discharge order wherein the accused is no longer subject to the oversight of the review board (Chaimowitz et al., 2022). The conditions and privileges outlined within a disposition can include measures to manage the risk of substance misuse. Hence, the management of substance use and the associated risk is very important in forensic psychiatric services. Hospital privileges are graduated with various degrees of supervision (e.g., escorted, accompanied, and indirectly supervised) and determined by the individual's mental status, treatment response, behavior, and breach of conditions in their disposition. In Canada, the goals of forensic mental health services include treatment of active mental health conditions, rehabilitation or recovery, management of risk, and safe reintegration of people into the community.

Theoretical Underpinnings of the Semi-structured Manualized Treatment Program

Addressing the needs of the forensic psychiatric population using an integrated approach can be an effective way to manage risk. A variety of treatment modalities, including individual and group therapies, CBT, motivational enhancement/interviewing (MI), and contingency management, have been shown to be effective interventions for individuals with concurrent disorders (Drake, 2006). A 2022 systematic review on the effectiveness of psychosocial interventions on prisoners with mental health and substance use disorders demonstrated that MI, interpersonal psychotherapy, CBT, positive psychology interventions, music therapy, and acceptance and commitment therapy significantly improved outcome measures, including symptom severity of substance abuse, depression, anxiety, and deliberate self-harm. Positive effects were also observed on secondary outcome measures such as motivation, aggression, attendance at follow-up, compliance with treatment, and recidivism (Thekkumkara et al., 2022).

Research regarding mandated treatment interventions generally indicates that, despite required attendance, positive outcomes are achieved in a variety of areas. Although more research is required in the area of substance abuse treatment, it has been shown that those who do not enter treatment of their own free will seem to do as well as those who enter voluntarily (Mueser et al., 2003). It is therefore important for clinicians not to dismiss individuals who are mandated to receive treatment. |||Therapy provided by staff with strong interpersonal skills and the development of a therapeutic alliance will enhance engagement and have been associated with an increase in positive treatment outcomes (Canada, 2001). Evidence suggests that the client–counsellor relationship, through multiple treatment episodes, has more influence on engagement and improved outcomes than the methods, tools, and instruments employed (Hubble et al., 1999; Minkoff, 2000). The available research provides evidence supporting the effectiveness of various therapy models, which may be accounted for by common factors between these therapy models (Johnson & Tran, 2020; Moos, 2007). This suggests that common factors within different therapy models are more influential on treatment effectiveness than specific therapy models. Another future avenue of research within this field may be to clarify unique factors that contribute to the effectiveness of specific therapy models.

Program Structure for Forensic Patients

The forensic psychiatry program (FPP) at St. Joseph's Healthcare Hamilton was started in 1972. It consists of two general secure units, two higher security units, one assessment unit, one outpatient unit, and an acute stabilization unit to manage incarcerated individuals with active psychosis. If an individual is identified as having a substance use disorder or history of substance misuse, the treatment team refers such patients to the SSMTP, which can be provided either individually or in a group context. Pre-treatment screening is conducted to assess client needs, make decisions about the appropriateness of various sessions, and introduce the program.

Group interventions are divided into three categories: *Level 1*, *Level 2*, and structured relapse prevention (SRP) (*Level 3*). The intervention begins with a pre-treatment program called "Level 1". The goal of this phase is to evaluate clients' substance use and attitude towards change, increase their understanding of the effects and risks of substance misuse, and improve their motivation or commitment to altering their substance use patterns. There are six sessions, occurring twice per week, with homework between sessions. Clients are expected to participate in group discussions and complete questionnaires about their substance use (described in the program evaluation section) to assist in the evaluation of the intervention.

Level 2 is an intensive treatment program addressing substance abuse and dependency. The goal of this phase is to identify triggers to use, develop and employ strategies to cope and manage behavior without substance use, develop a plan to anticipate lapses, and identify needs and resources for support. It consists of 14/15 sessions occurring twice weekly for 7–8 weeks. Group participants are expected to complete homework between sessions. Some of the worksheets used during the sessions are adapted from the manual, *Group Treatment for Substance Abuse: A Stages-of-Change Therapy Manual -Second Edition* published by Velasquez et al. (2015). The time spent on each of these topics is flexible to the group's needs (Table 1.1).

Table 1.1 Level 2: Overview of sessions

Session	*Content objectives*	*Process objectives*
1	Introduction and orientation of group members Group norms/confidentiality Pre-group questionnaires Pros and cons of substance use Review previously identified goals or set goals related to substance use Review of common culturally held ideas and biases related to substances	Develop therapeutic alliance No challenge/confrontation Emphasize personal choice Develop personally relevant goals Reinforce the decision to make changes
2	Review broad categories of substances of abuse Review common language related to: –abuse, addiction, dependence, tolerance, use, and misuse –continuum of addiction to different substances –thoughts, urges, and cravings	Develop therapeutic alliance Employ supportive, non-judgmental approach Facilitate openness and self-awareness Reinforcement Personal identification
3	Discussion of strategies in a variety of domains: cognitive, behavioral, substitution, interpersonal, and environmental Identify stressors and triggers leading to the last use or relapse Identify risk factors for social pressure related to drug abuse Identify triggers: focus on people, places, and things, including feelings/emotions Identify alternatives to using substances meaningful activities to replace them, how achievable are the replacements	Reinforcement of self-awareness and self-monitoring Encouragement Employ realistic and gentle challenging Take the opposing position (Devil's Advocate)

(*Continued*)

Table 1.1 (Continued)

Session	*Content objectives*	*Process objectives*
4	Identify emotions leading to substance use Manage positive and negative emotions without use Identify how thoughts influence behavior Manage thoughts Manage cravings and urges Identify hierarchy of risk situations Apply effective coping strategies for each risk area	Encourage self-esteem Reinforce self-reflection, self-efficacy, self-awareness, and self-monitoring
5	Review communication styles (passive, aggressive, and assertive) Identify effective communication skills and strategies Practice effective communication between group members Discuss and analyze the feelings associated with effective communication	Self-awareness of personal style Soliciting and giving feedback Develop trust within the group Reinforcement
6	Effective refusals Increase confidence in refusal Manage criticism Manage setbacks when trying to make changes	Soliciting and receiving feedback Develop self-awareness Practice through role play Self-awareness of emotions and criticism Affirm progress Reinforcement

(*Continued*)

Table 1.1 (Continued)

Session	*Content objectives*	*Process objectives*
7	Development and identification of effective coping strategies Develop personalized strategies for solving problems Link previous experience and current efforts towards change Practice skills in a low-risk environment Self-assessment of outcomes Self-reflection on success Learn how to celebrate success without substances	Soliciting and giving feedback Openness and self-monitoring Reinforce flexibility Non-defensive, non-confrontational approach, challenge ideas
8	Review of Marlatt's stages of change Identification of the cycle of relapse Identification of relapse warning signs Review of seemingly irrelevant decisions Review high-risk situations and plan to manage them	Self-esteem and self-efficacy Reinforcement
9	Develop relapse prevention plan Identify past successful or unsuccessful strategies and what needs to change	Reinforce self-efficacy Encourage and reinforce critical evaluation of the current lifestyle
10/11	Enjoying life Reflecting on feeling well without substances Lifestyle balance/needs assessment Identify barriers	Review and reinforce long-term goals Reinforce self-efficacy Identify that relapse starts prior to use Encourage and reinforce critical evaluation of the current lifestyle Challenge ideas of "no risk" for relapse
12/13	Identification of support systems and self-help groups to join Develop an action plan Review the action plan and next steps Review and reinforce long-term goals	Highlight the importance of prior sessions Putting it all together Reinforce self-monitoring and awareness, self-efficacy, and self-liberation
14/15	Feedback for group leaders Post-group questionnaires Celebration	Self-empowerment Confidence enhancement Self-determination and efficacy

Level 3 is SRP. In brief, SRP is a counselling approach that utilizes cognitive-behavioral treatment to aid clients in learning coping skills to effectively manage day-to-day substance use triggers and risk situations. Our sessions have been adapted from the *Structured Relapse Prevention: An Outpatient Counselling Approach* manual by Herie and Watkin-Merek (2006).

This level is designed for individuals with moderate-to-severe substance dependence and is delivered in one 60–90-minute group session weekly over approximately eight weeks. Following completion of Levels 1 and 2, clients are encouraged to participate in Level 3 to review the effectiveness of their relapse plan and re-evaluate triggers and strategies to manage their substance use. They can repeat Level 3 as often as required.

In Level 3, participants are encouraged to discuss personal struggles related to relapses, apply strategies to manage high-risk situations, and enhance personally relevant reasons to abstain. During the first session, participants are asked to identify high-risk situations for relapse, such as boredom, intimate relationships, etc. The following sessions are focused on reviewing the relevant worksheets that have been adapted for concurrent disorders for each high-risk scenario in the Herie & Watkin-Merek manual (Herie & Watkin-Merek, 2006).

Implementation

History of Implementation

Historically, the treatment focus of patients in forensic psychiatry settings was mental health symptoms. The FPP psychologists met with individual patients to address their specific needs, which included substance abuse counselling. They developed the structure and the majority of the content for the outline of the group, although it changed over time to reflect the discussions and needs of group members. As the program expanded, the number of patients requiring support increased significantly, and it was difficult for the psychologists to focus on substance abuse groups in addition to other requirements of their role. Other addiction services were available in the community, but patients were often unable to access them due to a lack of freedom to attend community agencies. Staff from other disciplines, such as nursing or social work, participated as facilitators/co-leaders in group sessions. This assisted and supported professional development and skill building, leading to the creation of a semi-structured, manualized treatment program for substance use in the FPP.

Initial challenges in implementation included the lack of dedicated staff to lead the program as well as time constraints related to multiple requirements of the role. In terms of patient population, the group was not homogeneous, and this was challenging as individuals were at different stages of change.

Staffing Requirements and Training

The group requires at least two dedicated clinicians. At times, there are staff who are interested in attending some of the groups, but the consistent attendance of dedicated clinicians is absolutely necessary in order to support patients in their change. Dedicated clinicians can more easily recognize the progress that patients are making as well as times when their confidence wavers. The therapeutic relationship is paramount to building trust and confidence. Although it is important to challenge ideas, clinicians are allies in the change process. Groups need to be led by individuals who deliver both mental health and addiction treatment. Best practice guidelines have identified that this approach is most beneficial for individuals seeking support with concurrent disorders.

Program Evaluation

Questionnaires administered to participants and used in the evaluation of the program include the Readiness Ruler (Hesse, 2006; Miller, 1985), the Perceived Social Support Questionnaire (Zimet et al., 1990), the DTCQ-8 for Alcohol (Sklar & Turner, 1999), the DTCQ-8 for Drugs (Sklar & Turner, 1999), the Attitudes to Drug Use Questionnaire (Harmon, 1993), Change Assessment (Hasler et al., 2003), and Goal Setting Sheet (unpublished). Currently, a research study is ongoing to assess the effectiveness of this intervention using the Readiness Ruler.

Recommendations and Considerations of the SSMTP

Recommendations

Treatment of individuals with concurrent disorders has been known to be more challenging due to the impact of each of the disorders. Individuals participating in this group may have different baselines with respect to cognitive function (i.e., memory, processing, or attention), and therefore, the group needs to accommodate their needs, including repetition of the content. Accommodations are made for individuals who have cognitive difficulties by providing individual support between sessions to allow for repetition and rehearsal of content to enhance their learning experience. Some individuals may require repeating the entire program.

Special Considerations in the Forensic Population

Case management is critical for this particular population; identifying primary clinicians to work with an individual will provide consistency in the delivery of care. Integrating various aspects of the individual's care into a comprehensive treatment plan is best achieved and most effective when case management is provided in the context of a multidisciplinary team.

The forensic psychiatric population presents a variety of challenges in treatment and requires adaptation and flexibility. A challenge that often arises is the issue of mandated interventions. Individuals may deny or minimize the use and effects of alcohol/drugs and or mental health issues for a variety of reasons. However, mandated or involuntary interventions such as obtaining and monitoring urine samples for drug and alcohol use are necessary and justified where there is a finding of potential significant harm to others (Mueser et al., 2003). Individuals with concurrent disorders tend to have impairments that make it difficult for them to use cognitive behavioral strategies, and therefore, this group of individuals may benefit from pharmacological therapies that assist in the reduction of urges or cravings. Furthermore, because these individuals are mandated to complete the treatment, their stage of change is technically "suspended use". As such, they may experience huge oscillations in their commitment to change throughout the treatment. This can feel frustrating to the therapist delivering the treatment. We recommend revisiting conversations assessing commitment to change using a motivational interviewing approach when these oscillations occur.

Although a harm reduction approach has been identified as an effective way to attract and retain patients in substance abuse groups, this is very difficult to implement in forensic programs when patients are required to abstain absolutely from all intoxicants. Adopting this approach might be seen as "permitting" or encouraging individuals to breach the conditions of their disposition. However, there are occasions when this can be implemented as part of the recovery plan, as a trial per se, while the individual is still under supervision. There are times when a patient uses a substance and their mental status does not change; with appropriate monitoring and support, it may be determined that it is a low-risk substance for the individual. In this case, the team may be able to support the individual's goal of using the particular substance and put this forward for consideration in the review board's decision on disposition. However, there is a need to consider that it is not only the use of a substance but also the amount and chronicity of its use that can cause changes in mental status and therefore impact risk. It is best to work with the individual to evaluate how substances have affected them in the past, assess their current insight and available supports, and build self-confidence and efficacy to make changes. As an example, there have been individuals who have been permitted to use alcohol while under a disposition, since it is a legal substance. The team is able to obtain urine samples to monitor the use of other substances but is aware that the individual will use alcohol. It is imperative to have a robust discussion about low-risk guidelines, the amount of alcohol the individual uses, potential interactions with medications, and possible medical complications. Despite individuals being legally permitted to use, it is very useful to have collateral information from family or community support regarding their behavior. This information will assist the team in assessing risk and making meaningful long-term recommendations.

Another important consideration of the program is to include individuals who are in "suspended use". These individuals temporarily stop using while under the jurisdiction of the review board, only to initiate use again once sanctions are removed. It is imperative that these discussions occur, as they will support the individual's ability to consider change in a more robust and honest manner and improve insight into their pattern of substance use.

Next Steps

Currently, research studies are underway within the FPP to assess the effectiveness of the SSMTP through questionnaires utilized in program evaluation.

Conclusion

Substance use is a massive public mental health issue in forensic-correctional settings for several reasons. Notably, substance misuse is highly prevalent among forensic-correctional populations and has been identified as a crucial mediator of criminal behavior. Although challenging, addressing substance misuse is critical for mental well-being, risk management, and the promotion of recovery in these populations. There is a rapidly expanding body of research investigating innovative treatment modalities for substance use disorders among correctional and forensic populations. A few important points and lessons regarding innovative practices to treat and manage substance use in forensic-correctional settings are listed hereafter. First, evidence strongly suggests that structured, psychosocial treatment in longitudinal, continuous client–counsellor interventions for substance use disorders is beneficial in forensic and correctional populations. Such interventions (e.g., SSMTP discussed in this chapter) have been shown to decrease substance use, recidivism, aggression, symptom recovery, and treatment non-adherence. The SSMTP for substance use disorders developed for the FPP at St. Joseph's Healthcare Hamilton is a three-part program consisting of nearly 30 group sessions delivered in levels or modules, starting with understanding the impact of substance use and assessing motivation and commitment to change, and then focusing on identifying strategies to reduce substance use and, finally, relapse prevention. Various validated questionnaires are used to measure the effectiveness and benefits of the program and a research study is currently underway to evaluate the program. In forensic-correctional populations, case management for comprehensive care, the mandated nature of the treatment, and the feasibility of a harm reduction approach in relation to disposition conditions are important considerations when providing substance abuse treatment.

References

Al Marzooqi, S., El Sheikh, A., Al Shehhi, N., Al Mesmari, A., Al Zaabi, M., Haweel, A., Wang, J., Prat, S.S., Chaimowitz, G.A., & Olagunju, A.T. (Winter 2022). Forensic-Correctional Psychiatric Services in Abu Dhabi: Lessons From a Descriptive Analysis of the Attributes of a Sample of Service Users. *Psychiatr Danub*, *34*(4), 635–643. https://doi.org/10.24869/psyd.2022.635

Bioku, A.A., Alatishe, Y.A., Adeniran, J.O., Olagunju, T.O., Singhal, N., Mela, M., Bradford, J.M., Chaimowitz, G.A., & Olagunju, A.T. (2021). Psychiatric Morbidity among Incarcerated Individuals in an Underserved Region of Nigeria: Revisiting the Unmet Mental Health Needs in Correction Services. *J Health Care Poor Underserved*, *32*(1), 321–337. https://doi.org/10.1353/hpu.2021.0026

Campagnolo, D., Furimsky, I., & Chaimowitz, G.A (2019) Absconsion from forensic psychiatric institutions: a review of the literature. *Int J Risk Recov*, *2*(2), 36–50. doi:10.15173/ijrr.v2i2.3920.

Canada, H. (2001). *Best Practices: Concurrent Mental Health and Substance Use Disorders*. Ottawa, Ontario.

Chaimowitz, G., Moulden, H., Upfold, C., Mullally, K., & Mamak, M. (2022). The Ontario Forensic Mental Health System: A Population-based Review. *Can J Psychiatry*, *67*(6), 481–489. https://doi.org/10.1177/07067437211023103

Criminal Code (1985). Accessed on 30/01/2023 from: https://laws-lois.justice.gc.ca/eng/acts/c-46/

Crocker, A.G., Nicholls, T.L., Seto, M.C., Charette, Y., Côté, G., & Caulet, M. (2015). The National Trajectory Project of Individuals Found Not Criminally Responsible on Account of Mental Disorder in Canada. Part 2: The People Behind the Label. *Can J Psychiatry*, *60*(3), 106–116. https://doi.org/10.1177/070674371506000305

Degenhardt, L., Charlson, F., Ferrari, A., Santomauro, D., Erskine, H., Mantilla-Herrara, A.,… Vos, T. (2018). The Global Burden of Disease Attributable to Alcohol and Drug Use in 195 Countries and Territories, 1990–2016: A Systematic Analysis for the Global Burden of Disease Study 2016. *The Lancet Psychiatry*, *5*(12), 987–1012. https://doi.org/10.1016/S2215-0366(18)30337-7

Drake, R. (2006). *Treating Concurrent Disorders: Clinician's Manual*. Hazelden.

Drake, R. E., Mueser, K. T., Brunette, M. F., & McHugo, G. J. (2004). A Review of Treatments for People with Severe Mental Illnesses and Co-Occurring Substance Use Disorders. *Psychiatric Rehabilitation Journal*, *27*, 360–374. https://doi.org/10.2975/27.2004.360.374

Fazel, S., Gulati, G., Linsell, L., Geddes, J. R., & Grann, M. (2009). Schizophrenia and Violence: Systematic Review and Meta-Analysis. *PLOS Medicine*, *6*(8), e1000120. https://doi.org/10.1371/journal.pmed.1000120

Harmon, M. A. (1993). Reducing the Risk of Drug Involvement Among Early Adolescents: An Evaluation of Drug Abuse Resistance Education (DARE). *Eval Rev*, *17*, 221–239. https://doi.org/10.1177/0193841X9301700206

Hasler, G., Klaghofer, R., & Buddeberg, C. (2003). [The University of Rhode Island Change Assessment Scale (URICA)]. *Psychother Psychosom Med Psychol*, *53*, 406–411. https://doi.org/10.1055/s-2003-42172

Herie M. & Watkin-Merek L. (2006) *Structured Relaps Prevention: An Outpatient Counselling Approach (2nd Edition)*. Published by CAMH. Pages 1–286. ISBN: 9780888685179

Hesse M. (2006). The Readiness Ruler as a measure of readiness to change poly-drug use in drug abusers. *Harm Reduct J*, *3*, 3. https://doi.org/10.1186/1477-7517-3-3

Hodgins, S., & Côté, G. (1993). The Criminality of Mentally Disordered Offenders. *Crim Justice Behav*, *20*, 115–129. https://doi.org/10.1177/0093854893020002001

Hubble, M. A., Duncan, B. L., & Miller, S. D. (1999). Directing Attention to What Works. In *The Heart and Soul of Change: What Works in Therapy* (pp. 407–447). American Psychological Association. https://doi.org/10.1037/11132-013

Joe, G.W., Chastain, R.L., Marsh, K.L., & Simpson, D.D. (1990). Relapse. In *Opioid Addiction and Treatment: A 12-Year Follow-Up* (pp. 121–136) (D.D. Simpson and S.B, Sells, Eds). Robert E. Krieger Publishing Co.

Johnson, M.E., & Tran, D.X. (2020). Factors Associated with Substance Use Disorder Treatment Completion: A Cross-Sectional Analysis of Justice-Involved Adolescents. *Subst Abuse Treat Prev Policy*, 15(92). https://doi.org/10.1186/s13011-020-00332-z

Kivimies, K., Repo-Tiihonen, E., & Tiihonen, J. (2012). The Substance Use Among Forensic Psychiatric Patients. *Am J Drug Alcohol Abuse*, *38*(4), 273–277. https://doi.org/10.3109/00952990.2011.643972

McFadden, D., Prior, K., Miles, H., Hemraj, S., & Barrett, E. L. (2022). Genesis of Change: Substance Use Treatment for Forensic Patients with Mental Health Concerns. *Drug Alcohol Rev*, *41*(1), 256–259. https://doi.org/10.1111/dar.13344

McGovern, M. P., & Carroll, K. M. (2003). Evidence-Based Practices for Substance Use Disorders. *Psychiatr Clin North Am*, *26*(4), 991–1010. https://doi.org/10.1016/s0193-953x(03)00073-x

Miller, W. R. (1985). Motivation for Treatment: A Review with Special Emphasis on Alcoholism. *Psychological Bulletin*, *98*, 84–107. https://doi.org/10.1037/0033-2909.98.1.84

Minkoff, K. (2000). An Integrated Model for the Management of Co-Occurring Psychiatric and Substance Disorders in Managed-Care Systems. *Dis Manag Health Out*, *8*(5), 251–257. https://doi.org/10.2165/00115677-200008050-00001

Mooney, L., & Haglund, M. (2014). Treating Methamphetamine Abuse Disorder: Experience from Research and Practice. *Curr Psychiatr*, *13*(9), 36–42.

Moos R. H. (2007). Theory-Based Active Ingredients of Effective Treatments for Substance Use Disorders. *Drug Alcohol Depend*, *88*(2–3), 109–121. https://doi.org/10.1016/j.drugalcdep.2006.10.010

Mueser, K. T., Noordsy, D. L., Drake, R. E., & Fox, L. (2003). *Integrated Treatment for Dual Disorders: A Guide to Effective Practice*. The Guilford Press.

Mueser, K. T., Yarnold, P. R., Rosenberg, S. D., Swett, C., Jr., Miles, K. M., & Hill, D. (2000). Substance Use Disorder in Hospitalized Severely Mentally Ill Psychiatric Patients: Prevalence, Correlates, and Subgroups. *Schizophr Bull*, *26*(1), 179–192. https://doi.org/10.1093/oxfordjournals.schbul.a033438

Ogloff, J. R. P., Lemphers, A., & Dwyer, C. (2004). Dual Diagnosis in an Australian Forensic Psychiatric Hospital: Prevalence and Implications for Services. *Behav Sci Law*, *22*(4), 543–562. https://doi.org/10.1002/bsl.604

Olagunju, A.T., Bioku, A.A., Poluyi, C., Abdullahi, I., Olagunju, T.O., Alatishe, Y.A., Kolawole, O.F., Mela, M., Bradford, J.M.W., & Chaimowitz, G.A. (2022). Substance Use Disorders and Antisocial Personality Disorder among a Sample of Incarcerated Individuals with Inadequate Health Care: Implications for Correctional Mental-Behavioural Health and Addiction Services. *J Health Care Poor Underserved*, *33*(3), 1401–1418. https://doi.org/10.1353/hpu.2022.0120. PMID: 36245171.

Olagunju, A. T., Bouskill, S. L., Olagunju, T. O., Prat, S. S., Mamak, M., & Chaimowitz, G. A. (2022). Absconsion in Forensic Psychiatric Services: A Systematic Review of Literature. *CNS Spectr*, *27*(1), 46–57. https://doi.org/10.1017/s1092852920001881

Olagunju, A.T., Li, A., Palmer, A., & Chaimowitz, G.A. (2023). Animal-Assisted Intervention: "Paws for Wellness Program". In *Innovative Treatment Approaches in Forensic and Correctional Settings*. Ed: Zaph, P. & Siglag, M. Routledge Publishing, (In Press).

Olagunju, A.T., Oluwaniyi, S.O., Fadipe, B., Ogunnubi, O.P., Oni, O.D., Aina, O.F., & Chaimowitz, G.A. (May-June, 2018). Mental Health Services in Nigerian Prisons: Lessons from a Four-Year Review and the Literature. *Int J Law Psychiatry*, *58*, 79–86. https://doi.org/10.1016/j.ijlp.2018.03.004.

Olagunju, A.T., & Slavin-Stewart, C. (2023). *Medications for Treating Substance Use Disorders. Pocket Guide to Practical Psychopharmacology*. Ed: Macaluso, M. & Huntsinger, C. American Psychiatric Association Publishing. (In press)

Sklar, S. M., & Turner, N. E. (1999). A Brief Measure for the Assessment of Coping Self-efficacy Among Alcohol and Other Drug Users. *Addiction*, *94*(5), 723–729. https://doi.org/10.1046/j.1360-0443.1999.94572310.x

Slavin-Stewart, C., Minhas, M., Turna, J., Brasch, J., Olagunju, A. T., Chaimowitz, G., & MacKillop, J. (2022). Pharmacological Interventions for Alcohol Misuse in Correctional Settings: A Systematic Review. *Alcohol Clin Exp Res*, *46*(1), 13–24. https://doi.org/10.1111/acer.14751

Swartz, M.S., Swanson, J.W., Hiday, V.A., Borum, R., Wagner, H.R., & Burns, B.J. (1998). Violence and Severe Mental Illness: The Effects of Substance Abuse and Nonadherence to Medication. *Am J Psychiatry*, *155*(2), 226–231. https://doi.org/10.1176/ajp.155.2.226

Thekkumkara, S.N., Jagannathan, A., Muliyala, K.P., & Murthy, P. (2022). Psychosocial Interventions for Prisoners with Mental and Substance Use Disorders: A Systematic Review. *Indian J Psychol Med*, *44*(3), 211–217. https://doi.org/10.1177/02537176211061655

Velasquez, M.M., Crouch, C., Stephens, N. S., & DiClemente, C. C. (2015). *Group Treatment for Substance Abuse: A Stages-of-Change Therapy Manual (Second Edition)*. Published by Guildford Press. ISBN 9781462523405 (pages 1–308)

Zimet, G. D., Powell, S. S., Farley, G. K., Werkman, S., & Berkoff, K. A. (1990). Psychometric Characteristics of the Multidimensional Scale of Perceived Social Support. *J Pers Assess*, *55*(3–4), 610–617. https://doi.org/10.1080/00223891.1990.9674095

2 Integration of Eye Movement Desensitization and Reprocessing in a Prison-Based Therapeutic Community

Geraldine Akerman

Incarcerated individuals who apply to participate in a prison-based therapeutic community (TC) are generally seeking to address their offending behavior and contributing factors. This could include their relationships, beliefs, and emotional management. An important aspect of this can be a wish to address the impact of past trauma. The TC model has been applied at His Majesty's Prison (HMP) Grendon since it opened in 1962. HMP Grendon is a category B prison, which also takes those who have progressed to the lower security category, C.

The establishment functions as individual TCs each applying the accredited model. Each community has its own culture and traditions while applying the principles coined in 1960 by Robert Rapoport, "community as doctor." He described how the social environment was the agent of change, rather than any single intervention or mode of therapy within it. He wrote about the importance of all members, including staff, participating equally in decision-making ("democratization") and sharing responsibility for problem-solving, decision-making, and domestic arrangements. "Communalism," which involves each individual offering a unique contribution and perspective to the community, and "Permissiveness," or the need to tolerate each other's thoughts, words, and actions within boundaries and to have a shared responsibility, were also identified as key principles of treatment success. A fourth principle, "Reality Confrontation," involves residents providing feedback to others about the impact of unacceptable behavior on others. Accordingly, all interactions that occur in the TC are explored through a "culture of inquiry" to better understand their meaning and purpose. See Akerman (2019); Akerman and Shuker (2022); and Shuker and Sullivan (2010) for further details. It is a group-based, social learning model that relies on all the work undertaken being fed back into the core group.

The TC model offers a range of modalities to explore the past. For some, the traditional group sitting in a circle and talking can enable the emotions to be evoked. For others, participating in additional therapies such as

DOI: 10.4324/9781003360926-4

psychodrama, art therapy, and music therapy helps express emotions that are not yet fully expressed and processed. Some individuals find the memories complex, shameful, and difficult to process. The use of Eye Movement Desensitization and Reprocessing (EMDR) was introduced to offer an alternative way through which to revisit and come to terms with past experiences. There was much discussion with regard to the introduction of a one-to-one method into the TC, which is generally a group model. Consideration was given to the impact on how the work could be integrated into the frame of work being undertaken, including reduction of risk. A research program was built in to evaluate the impact of the additional resource on the journey everyone makes in therapy.

A TC strives to replicate everyday living as much as that is possible within the constraints of a prison. It generates countless therapeutic opportunities for the resident to acquire the skills that are needed to live in the outside world. Any small interaction can be considered in the therapy group to explore its meaning. Each day consists of therapy sessions, association time, and general daily tasks. Twice weekly community meetings (whole community, i.e., approximately forty residents and three or four staff) enable the administration of community living, exploring daily interactions, and assigning tasks, as well as allowing therapeutic discussion regarding relationships in the community. Three weekly therapy groups (eight residents and two staff) offer a more in-depth exploration of aspects of the residents' histories related to the current problems, often tracing back from presenting behavior through previous enactments to the basis of beliefs underpinning and leading to such acts. The work of the small group is fed back to the community by residents and staff to encourage them to process the dynamics at play. In addition, a range of creative therapies, such as art therapy, psychodrama, music therapy, and drama therapy (see Augustus & Jefferies, 2022), are utilized to use alternative ways of accessing underlying emotions, some of which may be pre-verbal and therefore not as responsive to talking therapy. All these interventions are group-based.

The progress each resident makes is dependent on a number of factors, such as their willingness to give and receive feedback, to explore their past trauma, and to be open to changing long-held attitudes. Also, who else is in the community at the time, their group, their relationship with staff, and the availability of interventions that meet their needs, to name a few variables. Many individuals continue to suffer from and have difficulty tolerating the repercussions of past traumatic experiences, and these can be triggered at times. The TC model offers the opportunity to explore these as they arise. However, for some, the symptoms are overwhelming and interfere with their ability to access the groups. Many have experienced adverse childhood experiences (ACEs), for instance, neglect, physical or sexual abuse, and being separated from their primary caregiver.

When residents arrive in Grendon, they complete several measures, including an initial interview about their past. Akerman and Geraghty (2016) reported that 50% report had previous acts of self-harm, 52% had experienced physical abuse, and 32% had a history of sexual abuse. Further, 69% report had a significant separation from their primary caregiver. Attachment theory tells us that if an individual's caregiver struggles to meet basic physical needs, it is difficult to develop feelings of safety and security. The individual will not feel able to develop the sense of safety required to explore the social world, as they will still be striving for their basic need to survive. This fundamentally affects their sense of self and how they view the world and the people in it. Research has shown that physical neglect is the greatest predictor of later difficulties, particularly in emotional recognition impairment across multiple patient groups (Rokita, Dauvermann, Mothersill et al., 2020). Speaking of these experiences and listening to the accounts of others' lives can also trigger long-repressed memories. It is often the first time these events are spoken of, and deep feelings of shame may be evoked (Kotova & Akerman, 2022). Those who have experienced ACEs can go through life being hyperalert to threats and triggered in a range of situations, so they constantly feel they are in a state of stress (Mothersill & Donohoe, 2016). This can hamper further disclosure and, thus, the fear of more dysregulation. Having seen this occur, the need for an intervention to help the individuals relieve the immediate symptoms to be able to access the TC intervention was clear. Discussions were held as to the feasibility of undertaking training in EMDR with fundholders in the establishment. In addition, with the senior management team, the Offender Personality Disorder (OPD) pathway (which is jointly funded by His Majesty's Prison Service, National Health Service England, and co-commissions work within the prison service), and colleagues in the TC.

Process of INTEGRATING EMDR

To develop a new intervention within a TC, by the very nature of its democratic style, agreement is sought from those providing funding. Prior to incorporating EMDR into the TC program at HMP Grendon, discussions were held with the senior management team, and concerns were raised regarding the use of a one-to-one intervention in the context of a program where group interventions are prioritized. The concern was that this may cause splitting of work and staff. The added value of an intervention that is well-researched and validated for those with traumatic histories was put forward. It was seen to complement the work of a TC, which is trauma--focused. There can be a range of views expressed, and a lack of understanding of a new intervention can cause anxiety and mistrust. An evidence-based case needs to be made for agreement to be achieved. In its history, the TC model has integrated many new interventions, with lesser and greater success. The most important principle is that the work will be incorporated into the matrix of the group, so each member of staff will communicate back to the staff team, and the resident will talk it over in their group. This prevents splitting off the work and one intervention from being seen as special or better than another. Examples such as the integration of psychodrama psychotherapy and art therapy (Augustus & Jefferies, 2022) and the fantasy modification program (Akerman, 2008) provide a path to follow.

There was much anxiety among those with a lack of understanding of EMDR that the introduction of EMDR to the program would lead the residents to become deeply unsettled and fragmented. Despite this, the OPD commissioners agreed to fund the training of the author. It was seen as important to ensure the staff and residents were informed as to how it worked and the possible outcome of allaying anxiety. Originally, the plan was to apply it to the enhanced assessment and preparation unit, where the author was employed at the time of training. However, the author then changed roles and was employed by the National Health Service as a psychologist, providing trauma support for those on the secondary care mental health team. This narrowed the range of people who qualified for the service with the author. To be deemed suitable for assessment for EMDR, the individual is first assessed by primary care mental health staff and needs to be deemed to be suffering from an enduring mental illness, post-traumatic stress disorder (PTSD), or complex PTSD. After more therapists trained in the use of EMDR, two pathways were provided to treatment, one being to the author as described, and the others could be referred to therapists who work on the wings. This made the service much more accessible, and as such, anyone in the prison could apply.

Trauma

Trauma can be described by the Diagnostic Statistical Manual of Mental Disorders (American Psychiatric Association, 2013). To qualify for such a diagnosis, several criteria need to be met. These involve the level of exposure the individual is exposed to and how it continues to impact them. The International Classification of Disorders (World Health Organisation, 2017) recognizes PTSD and complex PTSD. People experiencing complex PTSD would have the same re-experiencing, avoidance of stimuli, and sense of fear, but in addition, they would demonstrate emotion dysregulation, negative self-concept, and interpersonal disturbance. Such disturbances may encourage a resident to seek additional support through EMDR. It is like walking a tightrope and working with those who are suffering from such trauma. As a therapist, the goal is to help alleviate distress and not make things too unbearable for the client. Therefore, having another skill through which to do this is invaluable.

EMDR

EMDR is a therapy developed by Francine Shapiro (2018). She worked directly with war veterans and victims of abuse using EMDR. To date, its efficacy is widely known, and it is listed in the National Institute for Clinical Excellence[1] guidelines as a treatment of choice. It is based on the Adaptive Information Processing (AIP) model, whereby the individual experiences an event that induces humiliation, shame, fear, and guilt, and the event is not processed and the memory stored correctly. This would happen in an adaptive model by, for instance talking about what happened, being offered support, making sense of it, possibly dreaming about it, and the memory gradually fading and losing its intense impact. However, on some occasions, this does not happen, and the memory is stored in fragments of the smell, taste, sounds, etc., like pieces of a puzzle being stored separately that need to be put together. The memory can be triggered when something slightly similar happens, such that the individual thinks the same event is happening again, but they are not always aware of what has triggered the feelings and may often simply react.

When one of these is triggered, the individual can feel as though they are back in the event. EMDR helps trigger the memory and re-experience it in a safe way, thus allowing it to be stored in an adaptive way. It has now been shown that using bilateral stimulation (eye movements left to right, tapping left and right, listening to sounds in headphones in alternate ears) horizontally or diagonally can directly influence brain function so that traumatic memories are processed. This is thought to work by replicating the rapid eye movement, which happens naturally when we sleep. Thereafter, the distressing events can still be remembered, but the person is less likely to be troubled by them.

An EMDR Session

The first sessions would involve explaining to the resident how EMDR works, history-taking, and seeking understanding of what the presenting problem involves. A discussion would be had to consider the timing of the intervention, as well as other factors that may impact its efficacy. Some prefer to work with the most symptom-inducing event first. Others prefer to start with less intense incidents first. EMDR would not be undertaken if there were other stressors happening, such as the individual being physically unwell or undergoing intense work in their group. In a TC, such work would not be undertaken when the core therapy is not happening (for example, during therapy breaks in the Summer, Easter, and Christmas), as individuals would lack therapeutic support outside of sessions. Consideration would be given to what the resident wants to achieve, looking at what happened in the past, how it affects them now, and how that continues to impact them. Also, what do they hope for the future and if that is realistic? The resident is encouraged to revisit the memory as if they were on a train moving past it rather than in it, such that they are observing it from an increasing distance. A stop signal is also identified, which can be used at any time by the resident so that they remain in control of the session and do not repeat previous lack of control when things happen to them, but they cannot stop them.

The symptoms activated in the present may well link back to an earlier memory that has not yet been accessed. The presenting issue would be identified, and a plan would be developed as to the order in which the incidents may be addressed. The TC environment provides an ideal context in which to undertake the work, as the group structure provides the opportunity to further explore the newly recalled memories and their impact.

In the early sessions, a timeline of the past is developed. This is an important aspect for many reasons. It gives the resident the opportunity to develop a therapeutic alliance and helps them visualize how far removed they are from the events now. The line could be drawn up in five-year increments, and the resident talks about other events happening at that time. It is important to recall both positive and negative memories. World events include popular music of the time, holidays, and so forth. This can help build a sense of identity over time at a cellular level and integrate positive aspects of the past. If there is a traumatic experience, a resource can be introduced, for instance, someone to be with them. This could be a real or imagined person, or a superhero, comic character, etc. They may choose to have a variety of people with them: a wise person, a strong one, a brave one, and so forth. Consideration can be given to how old the individual was at that time. They may want different people as a young child or as a teenager, for instance. As they look at the timeline, they are reminded that these events were in the past, sometimes many years ago.

Once a plan for the order of work is devised, the next phase is to help develop a secure foundation from which to undertake the processing. Initially, this would involve practicing calming emotions when they occur by using guided imagery and emotional regulation. Bi-lateral stimulation can also be used in this phase; for instance, while the individual imagines a calming scene, they can alternately tap on their knees or thighs. Alternatively, they can use a butterfly hug, placing their thumbs on their breastbone and fluttering their fingers just beneath their collar bones, which is a soothing motion. The individual is encouraged to practice this daily in their own space to increase their sense of calm and well-being. This alone would have a calming and soothing impact and is useful as an intervention. Along with this, there is a range of techniques used to instil or evoke resources through which to equip the individual to undertake the work.

Only when these preparations are made would the desensitization begin. They would be reminded of their calm place so that the feelings evoked by them would be induced. In a session, the resident would identify which memory they wanted to process, and the worst part of it would be identified.

In an EMDR session, the therapist would sit at a slight diagonal to the client, known as passing ships if using hand movements, or they could use a light bar (a long strip light that pulsates from side to side), hand-held pulsators, headphones, drumsticks, etc., to simulate bi-lateral movement. A snapshot image of the event is identified, along with the thoughts and emotions associated with it, attributing a score as to the level of subjective disturbance (subjective units of distress, SUDs) it evokes. Consideration is given to where in the body it is experienced, often the stomach, chest, or throat. Thoughts about what the event evokes in the resident are identified. These generally relate to feeling responsible (I'm not good enough, I'm useless), action (I should have prevented it, I am weak), safety (fearing death, I cannot trust anyone), and power/choice/control (I am not in control, I cannot stand up for myself). The aim is to develop positive cognitions, such as that I am good enough, I could not have prevented it, I am safe, and I am in control. These cognitions are scored in relation to their strength. This is also scored as to its strength. It is hoped at the end of the session that the level of disturbance will be lower and the positive cognition will be integrated.

The resident then brings the memory to mind, repeats the negative words they associate with it, and begins the processing. After a set of eye movements, the resident is encouraged to describe what they notice. This could be remembering something they had not recalled previously, such as another person being present or what people in the scene were doing. The person is encouraged to repeat this process as they recall the memory. They may initially become distressed and experience the emotions they would have felt at the time, as it is pairing the senses together in the memory. This can also be felt by the therapist, so it may feel like nausea, intense fear, anger, and so forth, and both are processing the reaction together. The individual may even vomit and continue. This is a natural response to what they are experiencing, and so it is seen as a positive progression as they integrate what they are seeing, feeling, and experiencing, which they could not express when it happened previously. However, it is important to remind the resident that they are safe, whether it is old trauma, etc.

As the memory is processed, they notice symptoms decreasing, and once there are consecutive reports of no change, neutral or positive material, this indicates the end of that channel has been reached. If the processing seems to be stuck, other movements may be used, for instance, diagonal movements. The resident is then asked to return to the image they started with and what they notice. They can often have a much wider perspective and a noticeable lack of affect when describing it. They again score the level of their distress, and if it is not at zero, they may need to revisit aspects of the memory. However, it may not be zero if the individual thinks they may not stop having feelings about the event, for instance, grief at the death of a loved one. The resident then considers how true their positive cognition feels; for instance, they were too young to have done anything to stop the event, with the aim being that this is more valid for them. This positive cognition is integrated using slow bilateral stimulation. They then scan down their body from head to toe to see if there is any residual emotion, and if there is, it is processed with eye movements. The resident is reminded that they may experience new memories, or dreams, as the brain continues to process the memories after the session. In the next session, this is explored, and the extent of change is assessed.

To protect the confidentiality of those who have undertaken EMDR, no actual cases will be described. Instead, a composite example of a variety of clients is used to illustrate the process.

Mr W described how his mother sexually and physically abused him as a child. As a result, he was placed in the care of social services and in a children's home. In the home, he was sexually abused by the female care home leader, and although he reported, it no action was taken. He reported viewing others being abused too, and he felt alone and terrified. This led to him having hostile views of women and being sexualized and secretive. He was highly sexually preoccupied in the time leading up to his offence and held hostile, offence-supportive attitudes towards women. He committed several offences prior to his arrest. He had described how he was offended when he felt under stress from the threat of his previous life experiences coming to light. He served his sentence, returned to life in the outside community, got married, and had children, keeping his past secret. Later, a police officer came to the door to inform him they were investigating the abuse in the care home, thus exposing his secret past. He went on to commit a further sexual offence. Earlier in his time in the TC, he appeared sexually preoccupied as he spoke about sex frequently, using sexualized banter and telling sexual jokes. He also possessed a great deal of pornography. Mr W requested additional trauma work, having found it difficult to engage in therapy due to intrusive memories of his childhood.

A goal he set that was to be addressed in EMDR was to move away from the memories of the abuse by his mother and thus reduce his anger towards her. In sessions, he chose to focus on a less traumatic memory first to experience the process. He had worked hard to develop his calm place, a woodland on which he walked in the sunshine and heard birds singing, leaves whispering, dogs barking, and so forth. It is important to choose a place that is not associated with his past and may evoke other feelings. Therefore, an imaginary place will often work best. He worked on a memory of physical abuse in the care home. As he worked through the memory, the worst part of the memory was being alone when a master went to his bedroom. As is common, the memory demonstrates tunnel vision and not seeing things in the periphery. While working with the memory, he became aware that there were others in the dormitory, which helped challenge his negative cognition, "it's my fault, I could have prevented it," and he reached his positive cognition, "I was too young to stop it." He worked on his anger towards his mother, and although he was left with extreme sadness that she had treated him that way, he was able to process that with his group. He sought additional support to help manage his emotions, but acknowledged that he had carried this grief and anger throughout his life.

The Flash technique

There are a number of additional components that can be integrated with EMDR, for instance, the Flash Technique, in which the therapist will begin by asking the client to identify a traumatic memory. A principle underlying the Flash Technique is that unresolved traumatic memories are responsible for most non-organic symptoms. If the resident presents with a symptom not associated with a specific memory, the therapist will help them find the memory that seems to be generating the symptom. After this "target" memory has been identified, the therapist will ask the resident to turn his attention to another issue, for instance, a hobby. While continuing to focus on this distraction, the resident is asked to momentarily think about the painful memory in a flash, and blink three times quickly, then return to the discussion. Processing of the target memory is accomplished without the client consciously attending to the original disturbing memory. This can be particularly helpful if the memory is very shame-inducing. Research (e.g., Kotova & Akerman, 2022) shows that shame can be an extremely debilitating emotion and block being able to access and talk about traumatic events. This technique, and EMDR in general, does not require you to speak out loud about the memory, as once it is in mind, that is sufficient.

Havening

Another technique that can be incorporated is known as "havening" (see Ruden, 2019 for full explanation), which, in brief, enables a traumatic memory to be recalled and become labile, and the traumatic content decoded. Havening is known as a psychosensory technique as it uses sensory aspects to generate an electroceutical effect. Initially, the event is recalled, and as in traditional EMDR, the SUDs are generated on a scale of 0–10, with ten being the most distressed. Havening is then applied, which involves the individual closing their eyes and bringing the memory to mind. They then open and close their eyes, using the movements (see www.Havening.org), first gently massaging the eyebrows, then rubbing palms together, and then hugging upper arms and making circular movements from shoulders down to elbows. These movements are continued while the practitioner encourages the individual to remain calm, using guided imagery of a peaceful, calm scene. Then the individual is asked to hum a familiar tune while continuing the movements, which helps pair calm and peace with the movements while keeping the working memory activated for distraction. Then SUDs are assessed, and the process continues until they are at zero and the individual feels calm and relaxed. There may be evidence of other transient emotions, such as anger or sadness, but these will pass.

Dissociation

Dissociation is a disconnection between a person's thoughts, sensory experience, memory, and/or sense of identity, often occurring as a result of trauma. This is usually evident in EMDR by the resident being stuck or not continuing with the processing. On a mild level, dissociation is a common experience that many people recognize as a form of detachment from something that is emotionally stressful. On a more extreme level, it can cause difficulty functioning in everyday life and can create a loss of connection to a person's sense of self. Dissociation. When taking the individual's history in the initial stages of the intervention, a lot of the information may be compartmentalized or kept by different dissociative parts, especially at the beginning of treatment.

When therapists meet with individuals who have dissociated for the first time, the presenting parts may not be aware of the most relevant pieces of their history. There may be dissociation to a greater or lesser degree. It could be that the person tunes out briefly or can lose periods of time. The personality can be fragmented and not cohesive, such that the individual is not aware this is happening. That is why having background knowledge of the individual from their work in therapy is useful. Dissociative parts can withhold information, bring it forward unconsciously, or share it consciously, depending on many factors. Some of the dissociative parts stuck in trauma time are usually on alert during the history-taking and could be scanning the therapist for any danger signals (Mosquera, 2021). These various aspects of the individual can be addressed and spoken to in the preparation stages, acknowledging why they may have been developed in the first place as protection during difficult times as the individual was growing up. Informing the individual that they are not the only person this happens to and explaining the process as a natural way our brain protects us helps alleviate anxiety. EMDR therapists know that during the reprocessing phases of EMDR, the individual AIP system tends to flow spontaneously towards resolution and integration. In simple trauma cases that do not involve a dissociative disorder, the therapist's intervention is often minimal, and most blocking points will easily be resolved with brief interweaves. For example, a two-handed cognitive interweave is used when the resident is stuck, and it is a way of "nudging" the stuck AIP system so the person's brain can naturally move towards a resolution. The resident is asked to place one side of their stuck place or ambivalence in one hand and the other side in the other hand, letting the client choose which hand holds which side of the ambivalence. Most individuals seem to put the more adaptive part of the ambivalence on their more dominant side, right or left. Then the resident is encouraged to "Let your mind observe with curiosity. Notice what is in each of your hands, allow it to go back and forth, and when you are ready, tell me what you notice." Using bilateral stimulation, ask for what they notice in between each set. Residents generally experience the more positive adaptive side becoming stronger and the more disturbing negative side decreasing. This technique helps residents resolve conflicting feelings, emotions, thoughts, beliefs, and somatic symptoms. An example of a cognitive interweave would be asking, what would a child of that age usually do? Thus introducing the idea that the individual had limited options in their position at the time.

Using the standard EMDR protocol in complex trauma cases involving dissociative disorders will be more challenging and require a longer preparation phase, a well-defined structure, and gradual movement towards processing. Gradually introducing trauma processing or desensitization will help these residents remain within their window of tolerance, which will increase their capacity for effective processing.

Intervention Evaluation

As a new intervention, it is important to evaluate its efficacy. Each resident is asked to complete an evaluation form at the end of the sessions. Individuals' comments included reporting that they feel much lighter, as if a weight has been lifted off their shoulders, or that they can watch television or be in a group without fear that they will be triggered by what is happening. One commented on how he was told by staff and other residents that he was much less aggressive in his approach to others. Further research is required as more cases are processed.

Conclusion

Introducing a new treatment modality into an existing model can raise feelings of concern. To address this, it is important to make a sound case as to why there is a need for it, what the benefits will be, and how it will be integrated. All interventions need to be evidence-based and complementary to the existing model. It is also vital that there is an ongoing evaluation.

Note

1 NICE guidance provides best available evidence to develop recommendations that guide decisions in health, public health, and social care.

References

Akerman, G. (2008). The Development of a Fantasy Modification Programme for a Prison-Based Therapeutic Community. *International Journal of Therapeutic Communities, 29*, 180–188.

Akerman, G., & Shuker, R. (Eds) (2022) *Global Perspectives in Forensic Therapeutic Communities*. Taylor and Francis Group.

Akerman, G. (2019). Communal Living as the Agent of Change. In D. Polaschek, A. Day & C. Hollin (Eds.), (Chapter 37) *The Wiley International Handbook of Correctional Psychology*. Wiley Blackwell.

Akerman, G., & Geraghty, K.A. (2016). An Exploration of Clients' Experiences of Group Therapy. *Therapeutic Communities: The International Journal of Therapeutic Communities, 37*, 101–108. http://dx.doi.org/10.1108/TC-12-2015-0026

American Psychiatric Association, (2013). *Diagnostic and Statistical Manual of Mental Disorders (DSM 5)*. American Psychiatric Publication.

Augustus, J., & Jefferies, J. (2022). Evaluating the Efficacy of Core Creative Therapies within Therapeutic Communities at HMP Grendon. In G. Akerman & R. Shuker (Eds.), *Global Perspectives in Forensic Therapeutic Communities* (pp. 107–126). Taylor and Francis Group.

Kotova, A., & Akerman, G. (2022). Navigating Lateral Power and Re-balancing Power Inequalities – The Experiences of Men with Sexual Convictions and Histories of Sexual Abuse Serving Sentences in a Therapeutic Community. *Incarceration, 3*, 1–17. https://doi.org/10.1177/26326663221074263.

Mosquera, D. (2021). *Challenges in the Use of EMDR Therapy with Dissociative Disorders*. EMDR Association. GWT.2021.26.4.Mosquera.Challenges-in-EMDR-Therapy-and-Dissociation.pdf (emdria.org)

Mothersill, O., & Donohoe, G. (2016). Neural Effects of Social Environment Stress-An Activation Likelihood Estimation Meta-Analysis. Psychological *Medicine*, 46(10), 2015–2023.

Rapoport, R. (1960). *Community as Doctor: New Perspectives on a Therapeutic Community*. Tavistock Publishing.

Rokita, K.I., Dauvermann, M.R., Mothersill, D. et al., (2020). Childhood Trauma, Parental Bonding, and Social Cognition in Patients with Schizophrenia and Healthy Adults. *Journal of Clinical Psychology*, 77(1), 241–253.

Ruden, R.A. (2019). Harnessing Electroceuticals to Treat Disorders Arising from Traumatic Stress: Theoretical Considerations Using a Psychosensory Model. *Explore*, May/June, *15*(3) 222–229. https://doi.org/10.1016/j.explore.2018.05.005

Shapiro, F. (2018). *Eye Movement, Desensitisation and Reprocessing Therapy. Third Edition. Basic Procedures Protocols and Procedures*. Guildford Publications.

Sullivan, E., & Shuker, R. (Eds.) (2010). *Grendon and the Emergence of Forensic Therapeutic Communities: Developments in Research and Practice*. Wiley UK.

World Health Organisation (2017). *WHO. ICD-11 Clinical Descriptions and Diagnostic Guidelines for Mental and Behavioural Disorders*. 2018. https://gcp.network/en/private/icd-11- guidelines/disorder

3 Treating Individuals Who Commit Sexual Offenses

What To Do With Denial?

Liam E. Marshall, Zach Yeoman, and Kristina Shatokhina

Prevalence of Denial in Sex Offense Cases

Excuses, justifications, and minimization are normal human reactions to being caught doing something wrong (Maruna & Mann, 2006). Indeed, several positive outcomes are associated with externalizing as opposed to internalizing responsibility for one's negative actions. One of the most robust findings in cognitive psychology is that excuse-making for negative events is both healthy and beneficial (Greenwald, 1980; Bandura, 1989; Dodge, 1993; Seligman, 1991; Schlenker et al., 2001). People who externalize tend to be: better at coping with stress; less anxious; have higher self-esteem; and feel they have more control when similar things happen in the future (Wortman, 1976; Snyder et al., 1983). In contrast, people who internalize and/or accept full responsibility for their failings put themselves at risk of depression (Abramson et al., 1978).

Despite denial being an automatic reaction of healthy people, as Schlenker et al. (2001) articulated, denial is "universally condemned while being universally used." Denial is quite common among individuals who commit sexual crimes (Barbaree, 1991; Marshall, 1994; Maruna & Mann, 2006. Being labeled as someone who commits sexual offenses can translate to permanent excommunication from society. Faced with this possibility and the related shame and embarrassment, it is understandable that many alleged and convicted ICSOs do what many of us do when faced with dire consequences: act in our own self-interest by denying wrongdoing.

Why, then, do we expect ICSO to be any different? If an accused ICSO were to make a pre-adjudication admission, they could place themselves in an unfavorable legal position by providing self-incriminating information. ICSOs are subject to more restrictions and supervision than any other type of offender. Should they admit their actions or motives in treatment or to their legal supervisors, they are at risk of extending the length of their court-ordered treatment and incurring further loss of liberty. Despite the emphasis on the admission of guilt and offense-related sexual arousal

DOI: 10.4324/9781003360926-5

in traditional sex offense-specific treatment, the legal conditions put on ICSO further reinforce the choice to maintain one's innocence and deny offense-related arousals. And, of course, there are undoubtedly some ICSOs who are, in fact, innocent of the crimes for which they have been convicted.

Impact of Denial on Risk for Reoffense and Treatment

Beyond the moral outrage at those who refuse to take responsibility for their sexual crimes, there is also concern about the impact of denial on recidivism. Although proven repeatedly inaccurate, the public continues to believe that most ICSOs will reoffend. In reality, reoffense base rates are somewhere between 8% and 19% (Swinburne et al., 2012; Hanson et al., 2016). If engagement and successful completion of therapy lower recidivism (Gannon et al., 2019), then, presumably, denial increases their already (erroneously believed) high risk of reoffending. However, the Association for the Treatment and Prevention of Sexual Abuse Adult Practice Guidelines (ATSA, 2014) state the following:

> ...denial and minimization may impact the client's engagement in treatment, but... the influence of denial and minimization on sexual recidivism risk has not yet been clearly established and may vary among client groups.

In most research, denial has not been found to increase recidivism risk (Witt & Yeoman, 2018). Thinking about the impact of denial on sexual recidivism risk began to change with two large meta-analyses by Hanson and colleagues in 1998 and 2005. Their research found that neither denial nor admission was associated with recidivism (Hanson & Bussière, 1998; Hanson & Morton-Bourgon, 2005). However, those offenders, deniers or otherwise, who failed to complete treatment, were found to be at higher risk for reoffending than those who completed treatment, a finding later replicated by other research (Olver et al., 2011). More recent individual studies have attempted to clarify whether the relationship between denial and recidivism interacts with or is moderated by other factors:

> Nunes et al. (2007): Denial was associated with increased sexual recidivism among low-risk offenders and decreased recidivism among high-risk offenders. Post hoc analyses suggested that the risk item most responsible for the interaction was the "relationship to victims." For incest offenders, denial was associated with increased sexual recidivism, but denial was not associated with increased recidivism for offenders with unrelated victims.

Langton et al. (2008): When denial was defined as an either/or variable, there was no significant association with sexual recidivism. When denial was defined as a continuous variable, higher minimization levels predicted sexual recidivism among higher-risk offenders only when controlling for treatment completion status and psychopathic traits.

Harkins et al. (2010): Denial predicted decreased sexual recidivism among high-risk offenders. An opposite pattern was observed for the low-risk offenders in denial, although these differences were not significant. In terms of denial of risk, those who were denying they presented a future risk for offending (i.e., higher on denial of risk) were less likely to reoffend than those who reported seeing themselves as presenting an increased risk.

Looman (2014): The continuum of denial was coded and studied to see if different levels of denial increased risk. Their results were complex, indicating that for some but not all ICSO, some types of denial were associated with increased recidivism:

For moderate-risk offenders (based on the STATIC-99R), the sexual recidivism for men low on denial was higher than for other groups.

For high-risk offenders, denial was associated with increased sexual recidivism.

Men who denied the facts of their offense and denied sexual intent at pre-treatment were more likely to reoffend sexually. In contrast, men who denied victim impact and denied they were in denial were less likely to reoffend sexually.

Men who denied the facts of their offense and denied sexual intent at post-treatment were more likely to reoffend sexually, while men who denied grooming their victims were less likely to reoffend sexually.

Harkins et al. (2015): Lower levels of sexual recidivism were found for those who denied responsibility for their offense, independent of static risk. For specific offender types, denial of responsibility was not significantly associated with sexual or violent recidivism.

Updated literature reviews confirm what was already demonstrated: the common assumption that deniers are more likely to reoffend is not scientifically supported (Ware & Blagden, 2020).

Conflict Between Psychology and the Legal System

Given the current state of research on denial and recidivism, the continued overemphasis on the admission of guilt by the legal system is puzzling. This gap between state-of-the-art research findings and legal practice could be due to poor education. If professionals provide conflicting information to the legal system, confusion about how to approach the topic will abound. However, legal and mental health professionals' opinions and reactions to denial may also be attributable to philosophical differences between law and psychology. Scientific research is only one factor influencing legal decision-making. Laws are based on the morals and values of society. At the core of our community, and thus the legal system, is the assumption that individuals must accept responsibility for their actions before they can receive redemption. As social scientists, we know that this is a flawed premise. It only takes a cursory look at the research on ICSO desistance to see that many individuals who commit criminal acts simply stop doing so for various reasons other than acceptance of responsibility—for example, the decreased sexual drive and increased risk aversion associated with aging (Hanson & Bussière, 1998; Hanson, 2002; Barbaree et al., 2003).

It is clear that the philosophy of the legal system is in conflict with what we, and many others, have concluded from the body of research on denial. Denial cannot be assumed to increase the risk of reoffense for all individuals substantially. Yet, the legal system remains seemingly impervious to much of what social science offers in this regard. As a result, many people are placed in ICSO-specific treatment regardless of expert opinions to the contrary. What happens next depends on the expertise of the treatment provider and their knowledge about current best practices. A review of the history of Sexual Offender-Specific Therapy (SOST) will illuminate the foundations of this type of treatment and why many are still placed in highly confrontational treatment programs for years longer than is necessary.

A Brief History of Treatment for Individuals Who Commit Sexual Offenses

Traditional SOST typically requires the ICSO to admit culpability for offending prior to being allowed to enter treatment or demonstrate progress made in therapy. When this approach is pursued, therapy often becomes adversarial with no benefit to the ICSO and may even result in the ICSO telling the therapist what they believe the therapist wants to hear in order to be able to move forward. Building a strong therapeutic alliance is a far more effective strategy than a highly confrontational approach for facilitating change (Willis et al., 2013). Adversarial therapy also increases the likelihood of treatment dropout. ICSOs, then, would not get the therapeutic intervention they need, and some research suggests that treatment dropout increases the risk of reoffense (e.g., Olver et al., 2011).

Early Draconian Approaches

Years before the development of comprehensive treatment models for sexually violent behavior, efforts were made to constrain sexually deviant behavior. As described in a review by Laws and Marshall (2003), during these early years (the 1880s), these interventions primarily focused on homosexuality. The aim of treatment was to shift sexual interest away from young males and toward young females, and the approach was behavioral in nature. These behavioral interventions for homosexuality were, then, applied to those engaging in sexually violent behavior. Antisocial arousal was positioned as the central reason behind offenses against children, sexual violence against adult women, and other sexually violent offenses such as exhibitionism (Laws & Marshall, 2003). With time, however, it became evident that solely attempting to eliminate shameful sexual arousal was ineffective and that more comprehensive forms of treatment were necessary.

The Relapse Prevention Approach (RP; Pithers et al., 1983)

Following a call for more comprehensive forms of treatment, the relapse prevention (RP) approach was applied to the treatment of sexual violence and gained substantial popularity. When applied to a sexual offending context, ICSOs were taught to identify the thoughts and actions that led them to their initial sexual offense (the lapse) so that they could avoid these circumstances and stop themselves from reoffending (the relapse) (Pithers et al., 1983). These cognitions and behaviors are integrated into treatment using a cognitive-behavioral approach (Ward & Gannon, 2006). Through learning more effective coping mechanisms in high-risk situations and becoming better at problem solving, clients are purported to build their sense of self-efficacy, which leads to living a prosocial life (Barnett et al., 2014).

ICSOs who denied their offenses presented an immediate obstacle to treatment providers following an RP approach. If a client minimizes or categorically denies committing a sexual offense, how can they identify which situations are high-risk? Further, how can they evaluate their own personal characteristics to determine how they can change their tendencies to better cope in high-risk situations? As a result of these obstacles, ICSOs who deny their offenses were refused or removed from therapy. They may also have refused to participate in treatment or intellectualize throughout, regurgitating what they believe the treatment provider wants to hear rather than participating meaningfully.

The Self-regulation Model (SRM; Hudson et al., 1999; Ward et al., 1998) and the Good Lives Model (GLM; Ward & Stewart, 2003)

Researchers began to question whether the avoidance-based nature of RP was sufficient for rehabilitation. Within the RP framework, ICSOs learn strategies for avoiding and managing high-risk situations that make up a single pathway to offense—a relapse or sexual offense—and represent a failure to utilize these strategies (Ward & Gannon, 2006). However, this perspective was limiting, they reasoned, because ICSOs can also engage in active planning to engage in sex crimes. This idea formed the basis of the self-regulation model (SRM; Hudson et al., 1999; Ward et al., 1995).

According to this approach, multiple pathways to sexual offending exist; these pathways represent varying combinations of goals related to offending and ways of regulating sexually violent contact. Through the avoidant-passive pathway, the individual aims to avoid offending but lacks the skills to do so. Individuals in the avoidant-active pathway aim to avoid offense but use ineffective strategies to control deviant cognitions and fantasies. Those taking the approach-automatic pathway desire to sexually offend and do so in a poorly organized manner. Through the approach-explicit pathway, the individual desires to sexually offend and follows through on this with careful planning.

As did the developers of the SRM, Ward and Stewart emphasized that ICSOs are driven by goals. According to their Good Lives Model (GLM; Ward & Stewart, 2003), all people, including ICSOs, harbor meaningful goals that they strive to achieve, and they become drawn to sexual violence when they are unable to achieve these goals in prosocial ways. The authors proposed a set of 11 goals, which are called "Primary Goods": (1) Life; (2) Knowledge; (3) Excellence in Play; (4) Excellence in Work; (5) Agency; (6) Inner Peace; (7) Relatedness; (8) Community; (9) Spirituality; (10) Happiness; and (11) Creativity. Goods that are particularly relevant to sexual offending are Relatedness and Agency, with ICSOs struggling to connect with others and perhaps defining Agency in ways that are antisocial (Barnett & Wood, 2008). Through GLM-based treatment, ICSOs can learn to balance their Good prioritization and achieve their aims in ways that are not harmful. For instance, to achieve the Relatedness Good, they build a therapeutic alliance with their therapist and learn to repair social relationships. The GLM has been a key part of the greater movement toward strength-based approaches to treating ICSOs.

In identifying the factors that ICSOs should strive for in the future, Ward and colleagues acknowledged that the model could have done more to outline the etiological factors of sexual offenses and provide guidance with respect to treatment strategies (Ward & Gannon, 2006). Thus, in their (2006) paper, Ward and Gannon proposed a reformulated model—the

GLM—Comprehensive (GLM-C), which included the original Goods, etiological assumptions, and treatment implications. Treatment based on this reformulated model involves identifying criminogenic needs such as social difficulties and deviant arousal, determining the client's good prioritization, highlighting the link between goods and sexually abusive behaviors for that particular client, selecting a personally meaningful good that would serve as the focus of treatment, identifying the specific environment that the client would reside in upon release, and constructing a full treatment plan that allows the client to align their skills to their unique environment. In doing so, offense-specific goals are integrated with how the ICSO envisions building a meaningful life, integrating the two models.

The SRM and GLM were integrated into a comprehensive framework (Ward et al., 2006). This approach involves assessing the ICSO's good prioritization and offense-related goals, bringing to light the various pathways they have taken to offending and the interrelationship between the pathways and good prioritization. Through a cognitive-behavioral framework, clients learn to manage their risk factors and attain meaningful life goals.

Some elements of the SRM and GLM appear highly relevant to deniers because these interventions allow them to target other areas of their lives that are not necessarily explicitly tied to their offenses, such as repairing relationships. However, a key stage in treatment across both approaches involves exploring the ties between these life circumstances and sexual offending. Therefore, those who do not believe they have offended may deny or resist these interventions. It might even be suggested that guiding ICSOs through exploring meaningful areas of their lives and then tying these elements back to offending in a confrontational manner could appear manipulative to clients and harm the therapeutic alliance. In essence, those who deny the offenses of which they have been convicted may benefit from treatment if their denial is not aggressively confronted, and they may further make therapeutic gains in non-offense-related areas.

What Are We To Do?

Researchers, treatment providers, and policymakers have put forth various methods of managing ICSOs that deny.

Excluding Deniers from Treatment

One approach involves excluding ICSOs from treatment (Ware et al., 2015). In these scenarios, opportunities to target other risk factors are missed, and the ICSO re-enters the community without many of the necessary tools to rebuild prosocial lives. Further, in circumstances where the

ICSO could apply for earlier release, being untreated may result in them being incarcerated for a longer period of time than if they were to admit their convictions. Pressure from the judicial system to admit and the inability to gain earlier release may lead to the categorical denier ICSO having negative attitudes toward the judicial system when they are released, and this may increase the risk of future offending. Ware and colleagues (2015) highlight that ICSOs may benefit from treatment despite maintaining their denial.

Providing Deniers with Treatment Designed to Help Them Overcome Denial

A second approach involves targeting denial specifically, which can involve participating in pre-treatment designed to target their denial or addressing their denial as part of conventional programs. Pre-treatment approaches include face-saving exercises (Brake & Shannon, 1997), psychoeducational content (O'Donahue & Letourneau, 1993), cognitive restructuring (O'Donahue & Letourneau, 1993), and enhancing victim empathy (O'Donohue & Letourneau, 1993; Schlank & Shaw, 1996; Brake & Shannon, 1997). Ware and colleagues (2015) highlight that these interventions have been met with mixed results; across all of these programs, about 50% overcome their denial by treatment completion.

Take a Risk Management Approach to Treatment

Within conventional programs, it is also possible to include deniers in a way that avoids directly challenging their denial and, instead, establishes an effective alliance and addresses criminogenic targets. One such program is Marshall and colleagues' (1994) open-ended treatment group, in which ICSOs who admit their offenses work together with partial deniers and categorical deniers. Rather than confronting clients with the sexual offenses of which they have been convicted, these treatment providers aim to examine the circumstances that led to the accusation of a sexual crime, such as certain expressed attitudes and behaviors. Clients are told that even if they have not committed a sexual offense, they may still utilize these tools to address certain obstacles and avoid being accused again in the future. This approach has been found to result in successful outcomes, with over 85% of participants in the program fully admitting to the offense upon the treatment's end (Ware et al., 2015).

Setting Aside Denial: The Rockwood Psychotherapy & Consulting Program for ICSOs in Categorical Denial of Their Offending

The evidence reviewed above suggests that there may be no need to overcome denial in therapy for ICSOs. This led Marshall et al. (2001) to formulate an alternative approach to treating sexual offenders through categorical denial. It was, therefore, decided that we would design a program aimed exclusively at deniers that would set aside the issue of their denial but would focus on the criminogenic needs identified in extant literature. We eventually decided to use the same program we have described in many publications (e.g., Marshall et al., 2011) and apply it to these categorical deniers, except that we do not challenge their position on their responsibility for their offense.

We have now operated this program since the late 1990s and have had almost no refusals of our offer of treatment to the categorical deniers. We present the program to these men as an opportunity for them to learn the skills and attitudes necessary to avoid, in the future, placing themselves in a position where they could be falsely accused again. We tell them that, for the purposes of treatment, we will not challenge their view that they were falsely accused and convicted in the past. Laws (2002), in commenting on this approach, suggested that it adopted a clever tactic in dealing with denial:

> By making a simple promise and keeping to it, the therapists engage the clients in a programme they say they do not need, for a problem they say they do not have, to prevent another offence that they say they did not commit in the first place.
>
> (p. 187)

As outlined in greater detail in other publications (e.g., Marshall & Marshall, 2014), our general approach to treating men who have been sexually offended is grounded in positive psychology and adopts a motivational approach (Miller & Rollnick, 2002). The foundation of our treatment model is based on group processes and emphasizes the importance of therapist characteristics. Our approach is flexible and individualized for each client, and we emphasize the development of a trusting client-therapist relationship.

Our Categorical Deniers' Program was first implemented in 1998 at a medium-security prison in Ontario. A small but significant number of clients incarcerated at this institution were refusing treatment because they were categorically denying their offenses. One of the most immediately pressing issues was that these clients could not be moved to lower security or get parole due to their untreated status. Often, these men were seen as resistant and treated as such by other staff and by the Parole Board. However, some of them indicated they would be willing to participate in programming but would not agree to join a group in which they would be forced to admit their offenses. We ran approximately one Deniers' Program each year, consisting of eight to ten participants. The program is run on a 'closed' basis due to the lack of continuing numbers, which would be necessary for it to be run as a 'rolling' program.

Program Description

Although most of what we do in our Deniers' Program is a match for our primary program, we provide details here (albeit somewhat truncated) so that readers who are interested in implementing a deniers' program do not have to continually refer to our other sources. In designing this Categorical Deniers program, however, the primary program we gave to ICSOs served as our template, with the exception that we would not challenge any aspect of denial. We tell the clients that the treatment goal is to help them identify problems in their lives that led them to be falsely accused of sexual offending, perhaps by generating sufficient animosity in another person that led that person to deliberately accuse them of an offense they did not commit. This stated goal was aimed at motivating these men to fully participate in treatment. Consistent with our regular program, we address all dynamic risk factors that are relevant to sexual offending. The following represents an overview of the components.

Preparatory Sessions

At the outset, most categorical deniers present themselves as suspicious and distrustful of the intentions of the program. They tend to be focused on attempting to "retry" their case with every professional they meet, including the therapists. These clients frequently appear disinterested (e.g., sitting slumped over, falling asleep), engage in problematic group behavior (e.g., making inappropriate comments, whispering, giggling), or fail to engage meaningfully in session discussions. Due to the demonstrated value of our general preparatory program for readying offenders for treatment (see Marshall et al., 2008), we begin with two preparatory sessions for the deniers.

These sessions are motivational in nature and provide information about the behavior that will best contribute to the clients achieving their goals (i.e., early release). Group rules (confidentiality, participation, attendance, and respect) are discussed, and group members are encouraged to contribute to building group rules. Participants are also provided information about treatment, the nature of our final treatment reports, and the results and meanings of their risk assessments. We follow this with a group exercise, which addresses the clients' self-esteem. Although this is not an explicit dynamic risk factor, it is relevant to engaging clients and facilitates the attainment of other treatment targets such as relationships and lifestyle. As well, low self-esteem across various domains characterizes sexual offenders (Marshall et al., 1994; Fernandez et al., 1999). The domains where self-esteem deficits are evident include relationship functioning, physical appearance, academic and occupational performance, and social and sexual functioning.

The following sections address issues covered in our primary program. Here, we will briefly outline our strategies for addressing the various topics with categorical deniers.

Lead-up to Offending (aka Disclosure)

The first assignment the group members complete is their version of the circumstances surrounding the "accusation." When they present this, we make no effort to challenge their version of events, which gives us the opportunity to demonstrate that we are not trying to coerce them to admit to the offense. Instead, we focus on the themes we describe as immediate factors, such as the use of intoxicants, relationship problems, other ongoing stressors, and being in a situation where their behavior could be misconstrued. These are among the relevant proximal factors preceding the event that prompted the allegation.

As part of our attempt to identify more distal factors, we have the clients complete an autobiography between sessions, which they then present to the group. Clients are encouraged to include in this autobiography both problems and successes in their lives. The problem areas they identify help us to determine the specific issues to concentrate on during treatment. Their strengths are aspects we can utilize to encourage positive change. One particularly problematic, and reasonably common autobiography given by deniers, involves a presentation that reflects a "perfect" life. This type of client is one of the most challenging to work with, as he is not willing, at least initially, to acknowledge any problematic aspects of his life. In these cases, we provide direct feedback, emphasizing that it is important to identify problem areas so that we can offer help and demonstrate change. We reinforce successive approximations to a full account of background factors by initially encouraging any semblance of the behavior we want and subsequently reinforcing more elaborate accounts. If the client continues to insist he has no problems, we explain to him the consequences of continuing to present in this way, most importantly that this will limit our ability to provide a final report that will be favorably considered by the National Parole Board.

Categorical Deniers are required to examine the circumstances and their actions around the time of the accusation. The goal is to help them identify proximal factors that occurred at the time of the alleged event (e.g., anger, intoxication, perceived failures, and problems in relationships). These, plus the distal factors, are the criminogenic features we address during treatment. Clients are then asked to consider those factors that might place them at risk of being falsely accused again in the future (i.e., risk factors and awareness exercises). These factors will differ for each group member, although there might be similarities. These factors typically include: feeling depressed, lonely, isolated, or rejected; having casual sexual relationships, particularly when alcohol is involved; using the computer in an isolated area; and having unsupervised contact with minors. We assist clients in developing strategies for avoiding these issues, escaping from circumstances that might pose a threat, or providing someone with the opportunity to falsely accuse them. Although we do not emphasize these RP issues in our primary program, we find that this exercise with the deniers helps clarify for them situations that might place them at risk of being suspected or accused of offending.

Victim Harm

In discussing victim harm (the recognition of which is a prerequisite to victim empathy), we are careful to ensure that our clients do not think we are trying to trick them into admitting they committed the offense. To this end, the discussion focuses on the potential effects on the victims of other perpetrators. If any client becomes defensive about engaging in these discussions, we inform him that this topic is one of particular concern to the Parole Board. Each client is required to identify the effects of sexual abuse on the victims, both in the short and long term. The participants are informed that by understanding the effects of sexual abuse, they will be more sensitive to signs that it is happening, and this will help them avoid or withdraw from situations where abuse might be occurring so that no one can accuse them of offending.

Self-Management

Following the problem analysis, group members construct a self-management plan in which they design strategies and learn the behaviors necessary to enhance their lives. We focus on helping them build a positive and satisfying lifestyle based on the GLM, pointing out to the clients that this will decrease the likelihood of them being "falsely accused" again. Group members are required to set realistic and positive goals for themselves in several domains (particularly around education, work, leisure pursuits, and relationships). They are also asked to develop a support network consisting of family, friends, and organizations (e.g., John Howard Society, Salvation Army), and professionals (e.g., counselors). We encourage the development of approach rather than avoidance goals, as these are more motivating and easier to achieve. By emphasizing the development of skills, attitudes, and beliefs that are supportive of a positive and prosocial lifestyle, it is assumed that clients will be less likely to reoffend. In a collaborative and constructive manner, we work with each client to help him identify an individualized set of goals consistent with his interests and abilities. Next, we help our clients identify, develop, and practice the skills required to achieve their goals.

Outcome

We have now conducted two small-scale studies examining the utility of our approach to treating categorical deniers. In the first study (2005), we examined the 56 ($M = 8$ participants per year) men who had participated in the program from 1998 to mid-2005. We found that compared to the participants in our regular program, the Categorical Deniers: had fewer prior sexual offences; were more likely to offend against adult women; were more likely to target female victims; were more likely to have unrelated victims; and were overall lower risk to reoffend. One of the aims of the program was for the participants to be able to move to a lower-security institution or be released to the community after participation. Whereas greater than 95% of Categorical Deniers were held until the end of their sentence prior to the implementation of the program, in this examination, 47.5% of the participants in the Categorical Denier program were able to gain earlier release. Finally, of the 56 participants in mid-2005, 40 had been released for enough time to be able to examine the impact on recidivism. Although this is a small number of participants, it at least allowed us to see if the program was likely to have a positive effect in terms of reducing recidivism. The observed rate of reoffending among this group was 2.5%, compared to an expected rate of over 10% based on Static-99 estimates.

In our second examination of the efficacy of the Categorical Deniers program (2012), there were a total of 109 participants ($M = 7.79$ per year). In this examination, 74.4% of the participants had gained release prior to the end of their sentence, with some getting day parole prior to the statutory release date of 2/3rds of their sentence, which is when, unlike Categorical Deniers in the past, most offenders are released. Of these 109 participants, 100 had been released for enough time to be able to examine reoffending. These 100 participants had been released for an average of 3.47 years (SD = 2.26, Range 0.5 to 8.89 years) and evidenced a reoffence rate of, again, 2.5% versus an expected rate of reoffending based on Static-99R estimates of 13.5%.

Although the reduction in the number of victims of reoffenders ought to be justification enough for treatment programs for sexual offenders, in a recent paper (Marshall & Marshall, 2021), we examined the cost versus benefit of our regular treatment program and demonstrated that this program, after all costs of the program, saved the government over

$11 million over the time it ran in the Canadian Federal Prison Service. Applying the same formulas used in that examination shows that the Categorical Deniers program reductions in reoffending saved the government $1.85 million for every 100 participants.

Conclusions

Working with deniers has and continues to pose a problem for treatment providers. Often, these men have refused treatment or been barred from entering treatment. If they enter treatment, all too often they are removed from the program for failing to admit to the official version of their offense. We have developed a motivational approach that addresses the key issues that led to the accusation without directly dealing with the issue of their denial. This approach has effectively served to engage clients and allowed us to address issues relevant to risk. The program accepts clients who are in categorical denial but who express some interest in working towards a more favorable parole outcome or who express some interest in dealing with problems they have encountered in their life. Clearly, ICSOs who are in denial can be motivated to engage in effective treatment aimed at identifying and overcoming the problems in their lives that led them to offend, or, as they view it, led them to place themselves in a position where they could be successfully accused and convicted of sexual offending. We have conducted a tentative evaluation of the Deniers' Program that is described above. This evaluation strongly suggests that the program is effective in reducing long-term recidivism. The results indicate that the program is as effective as our regular program, which targets clients who admit to having been sexually offended.

References

Association for the Treatment and Prevention of Sexual Abuse (2014). Adult Practice Guidelines. https://www.atsa.com/

Bandura, A. (1989). Human agency in social cognitive theory. *American Psychologist*, *44*, 1175–1184.

Barbaree, H.E., Blanchard, R., & Langton, C.M. (2003). The development of sexual aggression through the life span. *Annals of the New York Academy of Science*, *989*, 59–71.

Barnett, G., & Wood, J. (2008) Agency, relatedness, inner peace and problem-solving in sexual offending: How sexual offenders prioritise and operationalise their Good Lives conceptions. *Sexual Abuse*, *20*(4), 444–465.

Barnett, G. D., Manderville-Norden, R., & Rakestrow, J. (2014). The good lives model or relapse prevention: What works better in facilitating change? *Sexual Abuse*, *26*(1), 3–33. https://doi.org/10.1177/1079063212474473

Brake, S. C., & Shannon, D. (1997). Using pretreatment to increase admission in sex offenders. In B. K. Schwartz & H. Cellini (Eds.), *The sex offender: New insights, treatment innovations and legal developments* (Vol II; pp. 5.1–5.16). Kingston, NJ: Civic Research Institute.

Dodge, K. A. (1993). Social-cognitive mechanisms in the development of conduct disorder and depression. *Annual Review of Psychology*, *44*, 559–584.

Fernandez, Y. M., Anderson, D., & Marshall, W. L. (1999). The relationship among empathy, cognitive distortions, and self-esteem in sexual offenders. In B. K. Schwartz (Ed.), *The Sex Offender: Theoretical Advances, Treating Special Populations and Legal Development* (pp. 4.1–4.13). Kingston, NJ: Civic Research Institute.

Gannon, T. A., Olver, M. E., Mallion, J. S., & James, M. (2019). Does specialized psychological treatment for offending reduce recidivism? A meta-analysis examining staff and program variables as predictors of treatment effectiveness. *Clinical Psychology Review*, *73*, 101752. https://doi.org/10.1016/j.cpr.2019.101752

Greenwald, A. G. (1980). The totalitarian ego: Fabrication and revision of personal history. *American Psychologist*, *35*, 603–618.

Hanson, R.K. (2002). Recidivism and age: Follow-up data from 4,673 sexual offenders. *Journal of Interpersonal Violence*, 17(10), 1046–1062.

Hanson, R. K., & Bussière, M. T. (1998). Predicting relapse: A meta-analysis of sexual offender recidivism studies. *Journal of Consulting and Clinical Psychology*, *66*(2), 348–362.

Hanson, R. K., & Morton-Bourgon, K. E. (2005). The characteristics of persistent sexual offenders: A meta-analysis of recidivism studies. *Journal of Consulting and Clinical Psychology*, *73*(6), 1154–1163. https://doi.org/10.1037/0022-006X.73.6.1154

Hanson, R. K., Thornton, D., Helmus, L.-M., & Babchishin, K. M. (2016). What sexual recidivism rates are associated with Static-99R and Static-2002R scores? *Sexual Abuse*, *28*(3), 40–54. https://doi.org/10.1177/1079063215574710

Harkins, L., Beech, A.R., & Goodwill, A.M. (2010). Examining the influence of denial, motivation, and risk on sexual recidivism sexual abuse. *A Journal of Research and Treatment*, *22*, 78–94.

Harkins, L., Howard, P., Barnett, G., Wakeling, H., & Miles, C. (2015). Relationships between denial, risk, and recidivism in sexual offenders. *Archives of Sexual Behavior*, *44*(1), 157–166.

Hudson, S. M., Ward, T., & McCormack, J. C. (1999). Offense pathways in sexual offenders. *Journal of Interpersonal Violence*, *14*(8), 779–798. https://doi.org/10.1177/088626099014008001

Langton, C. M., Barbaree, H. E., Harkins, L, Arenovich, T., Mcnamee, J., Peacock, E. J., et al. (2008). Denial and minimization among sex offenders: Post-treatment presentation and association with sexual recidivism. *Criminal Justice and Behavior*, *35*, 65–98.

Laws, D. R. (2002). Owning your own data: The management of denial. In M. McMurran (Ed.), *Motivating offenders to change: A guide to enhancing engagement in therapy* (pp. 173–192). Chichester: John Wiley & Sons, Ltd.

Laws, D. R., & Marshall, W. L. (2003). A brief history of behavioral and cognitive behavioral approaches to sexual offenders: Part 1. Early developments. *Sexual Abuse, 15*(2), 75–92. https://doi.org/10.1177/107906320301500201

Looman, J. (2014). Denial and recidivism among high-risk, treated sexual offenders. In B. Schwartz (Ed.) *The sexual predator: Legal, administrative, assessment and treatment concerns, Volume V (pp. 18-1–18-13)*. Kingston, NJ: Civic Research Institute.

Marshall, W. L. (June 1994). Treatment effects on denial and minimization in incarcerated sex offenders. *Behaviour Research and Therapy, 32*(5), 559–564. https://doi.org/10.1016/0005-7967(94)90145-7. PMID: 8042968.

Marshall, L., Marshall, W.L., Fernandez, Y., Malcolm, P.B., & Moulden, H.M. (2008). The Rockwood Preparatory Program for sexual offenders description and preliminary appraisal. *Sexual Abuse: A Journal of Research and Treatment*, 20, 25–42. 10.1177/1079063208314818.

Marshall, W. L., & Marshall, L. E. (2014). Psychological treatment of sex offenders: Recent innovations. *Psychiatric Clinics of North America, 37*, 163–171.

Marshall, W. L., Marshall, L. E., Serran, G. A., & O'Brien, M. D. (2011). *Rehabilitating sexual offenders: A strength-based approach*. Washington, DC: American Psychological Association.

Marshall, W. L., Thornton, D., Marshall, L. E., Fernandez, Y. M., & Mann, R. E. (2001). Treatment of sex offenders who are in categorical denial: A pilot project. *Sexual Abuse: A Journal of Research and Treatment, 14*, 205–215.

Maruna, S., & Mann, R. E. (2006). A fundamental attribution error? Rethinking cognitive distortions. Legal and *Criminological Psychology, 11*, 155–177.

Miller, W. R., & Rollnick, S. (2002). *Motivational interviewing: Preparing people for change* (2nd ed.). New York: The Guilford Press.

Nunes, K. L., Hanson, R. K., Firestone, P., Moulden, H. M., Greenberg, D. M., & Bradford, J. M. (2007). Denial predicts recidivism for some offenders. *Sexual Abuse, 19*, 91–105.

O'Donohue, W., & Letourneau, E. (March-April 1993) A brief group treatment for the modification of denial in child sexual abusers: outcome and follow-up. *Child Abuse & Neglect*, 17(2), 299–304. https://doi.org/10.1016/0145-2134(93)90049-b. PMID: 8472182.

Olver, M. E., Stockdale, K. C., & Wormith, J. S. (2011). A meta-analysis of predictors of offender treatment attrition and its relationship to recidivism. *Journal of Consulting and Clinical Psychology, 79*(1), 6–21. https://doi.org/10.1037/a0022200

Pithers, W. D., Marques, J. K., Gibat, C. C., & Marlatt, G. A. (1983). Relapse prevention with sexual aggressives: A self-control model of treatment and maintenance of change. In J. G Greer & I. R. Stuart (Eds.), *The sexual aggressor: Current perspectives on treatment* (pp. 214–239). New York: Van Nostrand Reinhold.

Schlank, A. M., & Shaw, T. (1996). Treating sexual offenders who deny their guilt: A pilot study. *Sexual Abuse, 8*(1), 17–23. https://doi.org/10.1177/107906329600800103

Schlenker, B. R., Pontari, B. A., & Christopher, A. N. (2001). Excuses and character: Personal and social implications of excuses. *Personality and Social Psychology Review, 5*, 15–32.

Seligman, M. E. P. (1991). *Learned optimism*. New York: Knopf.

Snyder, C. R., Higgins, R. L., & Stucky, R. J. (1983). *Excuses: Masquerades in search of grace*. New York: Wiley.

Swinburne Romine, R. E., Miner, M. H., Poulin, D., Dwyer, S. M., & Berg, D. (2012). Predicting reoffense for community-based sexual offenders: An analysis of 30 years of data. *Sexual Abuse*, *24*(5), 501–514. https://doi.org/10.1177/1079063212446514

Ward, T., Hudson, S.M., & Keenan, T. (1998). A self-regulation model of the sexual offense process. *Sex Abuse*, *10*, 141–157. https://doi.org/10.1023/A:1022071516644

Ward, T. & Stewart, C. A. (2003). The treatment of sex offenders: Risk management and good lives. *Professional Psychology: Research and Practice*, *34*, 353–360.

Ward, T., & Gannon, T. A. (2006). Rehabilitation, etiology, and self-regulation: The comprehensive good lives model of treatment for sexual offenders. *Aggression and Violent Behavior*, *11*(1), 77–94.
https://doi.org/10.1016/j.avb.2005.06.001

Ward, T., Yates, P.M., & Long, C.A. (2006). *The Self-Regulation Model of the Offence and Relapse Process, Volume II: Treatment*. Victoria, BC: Pacific Psychological Assessment Corporation. Available at www.pacific-psych.com

Ware, J., & Blagden, N. (2020). Men with sexual convictions and denial. *Current Psychiatry Reports*. 22. https://doi.org/10.1007/s11920-020-01174-z.

Ware, J., Marshall, W., & Marshall, L. (2015). Categorical denial in convicted sex offenders: The concept, its meaning, and its implication for risk and treatment. *Aggression and Violent Behavior*, *25*, 215–226. https://doi.org/10.1016/j.avb.2015.08.003

Willis, G.M., Prescott, D.S., & Yates, P.M. (2013). The Good Lives Model (GLM) in theory and practice. *Sexual Abuse in Australia and New Zealand: An Interdisciplinary Journal*, *5*, 3–9.

Witt, P.H. & Yeoman, Z. (2018). Denial among sex offenders: Does it make a difference? *Sex Offender Law Report*, *19*, 81–96.

Wortman, C. B. (1976). Casual attributions and personal control. In J. H. Harvey, W. Ickes, & R. F. Kidd (Eds.), *New directions in attribution research* (Vol. 1, pp. 23–52). Hillsdale, NJ: Erlbaum.

4 The Eye with Which We Behold Ourselves

Group Poetry Therapy in a Forensic Psychiatric Center

Paul S. Saks

There is a healing power in poetry, for through the act of creative expression, one can give voice to things that might otherwise go unsaid in ordinary syntactic communication. The writing and discussion of poetry can create a protective screen that encourages the expression of material laden with affect in a form that is less threatening than direct verbalization, allowing for it to be processed, managed, and integrated into the self. Cognitions associated with experiences of trauma, for example, can take form as feelings of nameless dread; the technique of poetic expression allows for the organization and naming of such formless experiences, allowing both the writer of original material and the readers of others' work to begin to create some sense of understanding that can eventually lead to a capacity to bear witness and give name to previously intolerable experiences (Saks, 2007). The title of this chapter, taken from Shelley's "Hymn of Apollo (1820)," alludes to the ability of poetry to aid us in seeing things in ourselves that might otherwise be inscrutable, rendering even the most profane of things beautiful: "I am the eye with which the Universe Beholds itself, and knows it is divine..." It speaks to the possibility that, despite the adverse experiences through which we survived, there is always a spark of light within that can be accessed through the art of creative expression.

When conducted in a group format, the reading and creation of poems is a way to create cohesion, encourage a sense of normalcy related to experiences of mental illness, and encourage participation from even the most withdrawn and isolated of members. Specifically, when working with forensic populations, clinicians can be faced with guardedness and an unwillingness to honestly and meaningfully disclose feelings or personal experiences. In such populations, feelings that are not acknowledged can become the basis of projections and externalized violence. Furthermore, in environments in which treatment tends to be focused on "instant offenses" and risk mitigation, poetry can help individuals reconnect (or perhaps connect for the first time) to beauty, joy, love, and hope. It can help teach that vulnerability is

DOI: 10.4324/9781003360926-6

not weakness and that the pen can be mightier than the sword. It can inspire those who may have come to believe that they are only capable of destruction to engage in the act of creation. Poetry can inspire the blooming of metaphoric flowers between the stretches of razor wire and humanize a population that much of the world has written off as monsters. It allows for its members to rise to the occasion, as for one hour a week they are seen as poets and not criminals and "mental patients." Based upon this writer's twenty years of experience with poetry therapy, this chapter will discuss how such groups can be structured and successfully run in institutional settings with forensic populations. The chapter will reference the beautifully written work created by the extraordinary individuals with whom this writer has worked.

There Is Nothing New Under the Sun: Historical Antecedents of Modern Poetry Therapy

Poetry Therapy, as defined by Mazza (2017), is "the use of language, symbol, and story in therapeutic, educational, and community-building capacities (p. 3)." Though he initially denied that poetry was therapeutic, W.H. Auden added that the purpose of all writing was to "enable people to enjoy life or a little better to endure it" (Morrison, 1985). Poetry has been referenced as an intervention to ease psychological pain for almost as long as humanity has had the capacity to communicate. Spells, incantations, songs, and chants are employed as the traditional therapeutic tools of priests, shamans, and other healers (Blinderman, 1985). In his anthology of Native American writings, Astrov (1962) asserts that it is not herbs or potions that possess the curative power in many cultures, but the words that the healer says over them. Ancient Egyptian physicians wrote verses on pieces of parchment and dissolved them in potions to be consumed by their afflicted charges (Nunn, 2002). In the Old Testament, David sang Psalms to soothe the ravages of divine madness inflicted upon King Saul (Bhayro, 2004). In the mythos of Ancient Greece, Apollo was the deity of numerous natural and human experiences, including the sun, art, music, poetry, dance, archery, prophesy, and healing; his son Asclepius was the mythic forbear of all physicians, who learned the mechanics of medicine from his guardian Chiron and the art of healing from his divine father (Hamilton, 1987). This connection alludes to a complicated intuitive connection between mind and body long before modernity delineated such distinctions, as well as an implied belief that physicians are the healers of the corporeal form, while poets are the healers of the soul. In Poetics, Aristotle acknowledged the insights and universal truth contained in poetry, as well as the power of poetic catharsis in emotional healing (Weller & Golden, 1993; Mazza, 2017). Soranus of Ephesus, a physician who practiced in the Later Roman Empire, recommended interventions such as the watching of comedies to ease depression and tragedies to aid with mania (Gerdtz, 1994).

Use of the arts, and poetry in particular, as instruments of healing were cornerstone principles of the "Moral Treatments" of 18th and 19th century practitioners such as Benjamin Rush and Thomas Kirkbride; though the former also used "medical" treatments that are now considered barbaric, both advocated for the compassionate treatment of the mentally ill, including active engagement in the arts (Whitaker, 2019). For Freud, the symbolism of poetry was born in the unconscious and shared commonalities with dreams and fantasies. (Freud, 1953). While he never explicitly discussed the writing of poetry as an analytic technique, many of his ideas were set into the narrative frameworks of poets and writers such as Sophocles, Aeschylus, Shakespeare, and Ipsen.

In the 1920s, Smiley Blandon and Eli Grieffer recommended the use of poetry as a tool and used the term *poetry therapy* (Blanton, 1960). A crucial part of their work involved the interaction between therapist and patient, particularly when applied to those with serious mental illness. By the 1960s, several clinicians were advocating for the use of poetry in clinical practice including Pearson (1965), Leedy (1969, 1973, 1985), Lerner (1978), Hynes and Hynes-Berry (2012), and Chavis (2012). Mazza discusses the use of poetry therapy both as a general tool (2017) and with specific populations, including substance users (1979), adolescents (1981, 1991a), geriatric populations (1988), survivors of domestic abuse (1991b), and survivors of trauma (2012). Jones (1985), Edgar et al. (1985), and Saks (2019) discuss using poetry therapy with psychotic and psychiatric inpatients. Rubin (1974), Cellini and Young (1976), and Barkley (1985) discuss the use of bibliotherapy and poetry therapy with forensic populations.

Though This Be Madness, Yet There Is Method In't: The Theory and Practice of Poetry Therapy

There are several ways in which poetry can be introduced and integrated into therapeutic interventions. Mazza (2017) breaks these down into what he calls the RES model, wherein published works are introduced (the receptive/prescriptive component), patients are encouraged to write original material (the expressive/creative component), and the use of metaphors and rituals in therapy (the symbolic component). Hynes and Hynes-Berry (2012) discuss the different processes of reading bibliotherapy, wherein the act of reading in and of itself can have therapeutic potential, and interactive bibliotherapy in which the "triad of participant-literature-facilitator" encourages "confrontation with genuine feelings (2012)." They go on to discuss the fourfold therapeutic process of recognition, examination, juxtaposition, and self-application when introducing works of literature into the therapeutic process.

Focusing on the terminology set forth by Mazza (2017), all three of his components can be integrated into an ongoing poetry group. In such a group, particularly with inpatient, forensic populations, structure is crucial; it can serve as a ritualistic component while creating a meaningful, clinically relevant flow and at times aiding disorganized individuals to create a stronger sense of internal and cognitive cohesion. However, there should also be an element of flexibility, in that the leader and, to some extent, members should be able to focus on pressing matters should they arise. As is the case in most therapeutic groups (e.g., Rutan et al., 2007; Yalom, 2020), the leader should begin by establishing agreed-upon group ground rules so that the therapeutic space may feel safe from both internal and external threats while increasing a sense of individual commitment and ownership. It is important to have a discussion on confidentiality with a mind to the challenges that the environment of a forensic institution can have on individual privacy.

The inherent paradox of being a clinician in a forensic setting is the dual commitment to both treating and advocating for the humanity of the patients while being tasked with safeguarding the community from potentially dangerous individuals (O'Donohue & Levensky, 2004). It is strongly recommended that the leader of a poetry group be transparent about this, acknowledging that while every effort will be taken to protect individual privacy, notes will be written, progress will be assessed, and material that the patients perceive as damaging to their cases could end up being added to their records. From this writer's experience, these factors do not diminish the desire to participate in discussions and the creation of poetry. For individuals who have lost faith in a system that many believe is heavily stacked against them, honesty on the part of the clinician can help the group become a trusted space where feelings are shared. It should also be stressed that patients must protect each other's confidentiality, as members might speak of intense feelings, past traumas, and details of their instant offenses. Other rules can be left for the members to develop and deal with, including not interrupting, taking turns, attending regularly, coming on time, and other issues related to individual respect and safety.

The Expressive Phase I: Using Original Material

This writer has found that a basic structure that has proven to be effective involves dividing an hour-long group into four components. The first and perhaps the most important and productive section is the sharing of original material, the expressive/creative factor in poetry therapy. When groups are run by this writer, all members are encouraged to write in their "off hours" and are invited to share any original material at the start of the group; for the time that they are in the group, all of the members are poets, and they will be respected as such. They are also encouraged to employ writing as a coping skill, thinking about and translating their feelings into words as an alternative to acting-act behaviors. Freedom and creativity, including the use of expletives and violent themes, are allowed, though it must be explained that specific threats or violence that target individuals are not to be tolerated. Furthermore, it is important to add that there are times and places that are appropriate for the expression of intense and colorful language; a poetry group is appropriate while court hearings are not.

Patients often join espousing an interest in poetry but lack the confidence to share their original material. Some do not consider the raps and songs they write to be in the same category as poetry, and early groups will often include discussions about the definition and broad fluidity of poetry. This writer has used poems about poetry such as "Introduction to Poetry" by Billy Collins, "The Poem Wants a Drink" by Karen Glenn, "Poetry" by Pablo Neruda, "Some Like Poetry" by Wislawa Szymborska, and "On Writing Poetry" by C.J. Hecht. With support from the leader and members, most patients will eventually begin to bring in and share their own material. Some have been writing poetry (openly or secretly) and relish the chance to have an audience where their work is taken seriously, while others pen their first poems. Many individuals, after lifetimes of being forced to focus on their limitations, relish the creation of a space that is about possibility, support, and encouragement.

After listening to the poems, the leader can offer positive, constructive feedback and encourage a discussion about the impact of the work, modeling for the members how to receive a poem. The group leader can ask questions of the presenter, such as, "What do you think you were trying to say with that?" or "How were you feeling when you wrote that, and how did it feel to read it?" or "What would you like the group to know about your poem?" Again, this is often the starting point for discussion and the sharing of feelings from all members; the poems will often speak to shared experiences or capture feelings that other members have been struggling to put into words. This writer has shared his own original poems to model and normalize the expression of feelings through writing; of course, one must be conscious of the appropriateness of disclosing personal details. For example, on the week of Valentine's Day, the theme was "What does it mean to love?" and this writer shared an original poem written for his infant daughter.

Without disclosing facts about his family, the writer was able to convey feelings about his daughter, love within the constraints of appropriate boundaries, and the complex mix of joy and sadness that can accompany loving attachment. The poem had a tremendous impact upon the group, moving one member, whose instant offense has separated him from his children, to tears; he initiated a difficult but productive discussion about love and loss. Other members talked about mourning lives and relationships that were denied to them by the vicissitudes of their mental illness. There is always a potential risk associated with personal disclosures to forensic patients, and thought must be given to the protection of personal details. Generally, this writer is comfortable sharing disclosures about feelings without revealing contextual details.

A clinical case example for the efficacy of expressive/creative interventions can be seen through Curtis, a patient who spent the better part of 25 years in psychiatric institutions. When he met this writer on the forensic unit of a civil facility, Curtis had recently been deemed appropriate for a less secure level of care. He had grown accustomed to the rigid routines of a secure facility and, fearing change, was hesitant to leave. Artistic and creative, he was extremely reluctant to produce anything new and was extremely emotionally constrained. He presented with haughty, intellectual arrogance and was dismissive of his peers, whom he often described as "low functioning". As a result, he was not popular with his peers. Beneath the mask, he concealed a history of trauma, intense feelings of grief for his lost potential, and shame about his sexual orientation (he identified as a gay man). When he first joined the group, he would insist upon reading long passages from writers such as Baudelaire, highjacking the group to the frustration of this writer and the other members. There was a sadistic component to keeping the group in symbolic bondage and a narcissistic lack of empathy for the other members. He refused to share his own material, citing a fear that, in the past, doing so had been used "against him".

Several weeks into the group, and after much encouragement from this writer, Curtis proudly announced that he had written something (his first poem in years) and wished to read it aloud. His motivation partly came from a narcissistic desire to show that he was more skilled than his peers, coupled with a genuine desire to be known by others. He composed a soulful and elegant lament about the time he had spent on Rikers' Island, repeating a refrain that stated, "Just don't end up at Rikers 'cause Rikers will break your heart'."

The powerful emotions and beautiful language resonated with the other members and inspired a discussion about the dehumanizing experience of incarceration. He was touched by the positive reception and support his poem received. As the weeks progressed, Curtis began to show a willingness to relinquish control, to be genuinely vulnerable, and to tap into immense experiences of pain and trauma. Curtis initiated the process of humanizing himself to his peers while enabling him to be more comfortable, allowing the genuine man beneath the obnoxious façade to be seen and known. Within several weeks, a creative floodgate opened, and Curtis prolifically put forth multiple poems a week, bravely exploring themes such as mental illness, being queer, and trauma. He was able to tap into the experience of feeling relegated to the role of eternal "other", not belonging in a world in which he had been persistently rejected. He wrote, for example, that society expects everyone to conform, "...expecting all to go along, and all else in insane."

Over time, Curtis began to show interest in the poetry of his peers and tried to mentor newer group members. The evolution of the way in which Curtis interacted with the world began in the poetry group; becoming more comfortable in his own skin allowed Curtis to more meaningfully engage with others and aided in the path to his discharge. Tragically, several months after being discharged, Curtis died in the early days of the pandemic.

The Receptive Phase and Expressive Phase 2

Once all members who are willing to share their original work have done so, the leader can begin the second, receptive/prescriptive phase, in which selected poetry focusing on a specific theme or topic is introduced. Much thought must be put into selecting works to feature in the group, as poetry can have a powerful, affectively evocative effect on the members. Leedy (1985), in his collection of essays on poetry therapy, likens the choice of poetry in therapy to the isoprinciple in music therapy, namely that in the latter, selecting a song that "has the same feeling as the mood or mental tempo of the patient has proved a valuable tool (Leedy, 1985, p. 82)." Hynes and Hynes-Berry (2012) discuss how the criteria by which poems are chosen must strike a balance between the literary merits of the work and its potential value as a therapeutic tool. They discuss specifics, such as making sure that chosen poems are manageable in length, conveying experiences and emotions that are universal, and conveying some sense of hope. Chavis (2011) states that care should be taken to avoid works that glorify suicide or convey "unrelenting despair" (Chavis, 2011, p. 42). She ultimately suggests keeping an open mind and allowing oneself to consider one's own and other people's evolving reactions to poems. Mazza (2017) includes sixteen questions that a poetry therapist should ask themselves of a poem before choosing it; these include "What is your personal reaction," "Does the poem relate to what is going on in your life," and

"Is there a particular line or image that has specific significance for you?" (Mazza, 2017, p. 204).

When working with forensic populations, hope is a crucial element to consider for individuals facing decades, if not lifetimes, of institutional confinement within the drab walls of a psychiatric facility. Works such as "Invictus" by William Ernest Henley and "Mother to Son" by Langston Hughes do not sugarcoat adversity and tragedy but speak to the capacity of the spirit to endure and find hope in the face of despair. Furthermore, one should not necessarily avoid works that are dark or deal with loss and grief; encountering such intense feelings in a poem can be a way to confront, find commonality of experience, and ultimately process effects that are often left unspoken. This writer, for example, has on many occasions used the work of Sylvia Plath, who referred to the traumas and intense rage that led to her suicide. Poems such as "Lady Lazarus" are filled with disturbing imagery that evokes the tortures of the Holocaust, set in the context of the perceived horrors of her own mental health treatment. As difficult as the poem may be, when read and shared within a group, members can begin to put words to their own experiences related to the traumas of being mentally ill. Rather than act out or project nameless feelings, group members can discuss such experiences and perhaps even come to create something meaningful. Another difficult work with particular resonance for a forensic group is "Hard Rock Returns to Prison from the Hospital for the Criminal Insane" by Etheridge Knight. The poem employs racially charged language and concludes with the heartbreaking lobotomy of the protagonist, powerfully speaking to the unique experiences of environments that have features of both treatment centers and prisons.

The process by which the poems are read is an important element of facilitating group cohesion and creating a safe therapeutic space. It is helpful to invite individual patients (usually beginning with those who did not share new material) to read a stanza aloud for the group; sharing a poem in this way allows for collaboration and sets the stage for other creative endeavors. The reading is then followed by a led discussion.

This writer often designs groups that focus on a particular theme. One such central subject can be holidays or seasonal occurrences, with curated poems that resonate with the emotional experiences of the group members. Care and sensitivity must be taken in selecting these poems and songs, for holidays can be emotionally evocative and potentially triggering for members who have past histories of familial traumas or are separated from their families and loved ones. Specific thematic groups include Christmas, in which this writer has used works such as "Christmas Bells" by Henry Wadsworth, which speaks to the possibility of rediscovering joy and hope even in the darkest of times, and the lyrics to "White Christmas"

(Berlin), which speak to the bittersweet nostalgia of longing for more joyful times and places far away. Furthermore, an exploration of a seemingly well-known song can be particularly powerful. In one group, a member who had been institutionalized for the better part of 40 years was able to speak about the dysfunctional realities of a family that took great pains to create a pastiche of American suburban bliss and how this great disparity led to his mental illness and ultimately his instant offense.

Groups can feature the works of a single poet, including both didactic and clinical components. This writer will often choose poets whose struggles are likely shared by members of the group. The poets that this writer has successfully used include the already-discussed Sylvia Plath and Robert Frost. W.H. Auden, Rainer Maria Rilke, Lennon and McCarthy, William Shakespeare, Shel Silverstein, Langston Hughes, Billy Collins, Maya Angelou, John Clare, and a particular favorite of this writer, William Blake. When using a poem such as "The Tyger" (1977), which asks a string of unanswerable, existential questions, a therapy group can discuss themes such as the fine line between creative genius and madness (Jamison, 1996) and consider why a benevolent god allows evil in the world. The "Poison Tree" is also an effective poem to use with forensic populations, as it can be looked at as a metaphor for the self-destructive path of seeking revenge with hateful violence.

Finally, a group can use curated poems by several writers focusing on a specific theme. Three effective themes that this writer has used in his forensic groups are "masks", "mirrors", and "haiku." For the former, a handout was prepared with the poems, "We Wear the Mask" (Paul Laurence Dunbar), "The Mask of Evil" (Berthold Brecht), O Make Me a Mask (Dylan Thomas), and The Mask (William Butler Yeats). These poems tend to resonate deeply with many forensic patients, in that the theme of needing to hide one's feelings and true nature beneath the veneer of social acceptability characterizes many of their journeys through life and the legal system. The discussion is then followed up with a second expressive phase; a handout with a large, blank mask is distributed, and the members are encouraged to write a poem inside the boundaries of the mask. They are also invited to draw the features of this mask if they so desire.

For "Mirrors," the handout can include works such as "Mirror" by Sylvia Plath, "Mirrors" by Elizabeth Jennings, "A Crack in the Mirror" by Ben Gieske, and "A Hand Mirror" by Walt Whitman. Such poems can evoke feelings and experiences of being confronted with the reality of how one is perceived in the world and how this differs from inner experience; such dissonance is a mechanism of many psychotic disorders. This writer has created a worksheet with the prompt, "I look in the mirror and see," which includes a small foil mirror.

Finally, a popular group involves an exploration of Haiku. After reading the classics by Bassho, the members are invited to write their three-line poem. Such an exercise imposes the need for structure on individuals who may experience inner disorganization and fragmentation. It encourages them to express a variety of feelings through nature-related metaphors. The brevity of Haiku forces the writer to choose every word carefully, so one can be precise about the expression of feelings.

"If What Began Will End": Final Thoughts

This chapter scratches the surface of the ways in which poetry can be utilized as a therapeutic tool when working with the justice involved mentally ill. Poetry can be the means by which the unspeakable becomes expressed, lending voice to individuals in an underserved population. The reading and discussion of resonant works of literary art can speak to a connection of human experience for those who are disconnected metaphorically by their mental illness and the often-horrific crimes they committed, and literally by the wire fences that define their daily existence. The gift of poetry is its ability to convey the feelings that most define our humanity; this can restore dignity and respect to those who have been written off as inhuman. This chapter offers, but some suggest, uses of poetry therapy; its scope and potential to heal are limited only by the creativity, imagination, and passion of the practitioner who uses it.

References

Astrov, M. (Ed.) (1962). *American Indian Prose and Poetry: An Anthology*. New York: Capricorn.

Barkley, B.J. (1985). Poetry in a cage: Therapy in a correctional setting. In J.J. Leedy (Ed.). *Poetry as Healer: Mending the Troubled Mind* (pp. 135–149). New York: The Vanguard Press.

Bhayro. S. (2004). The madness of King Saul. *Archiv fur Orientforschung*, 50, 285–292.

Blake, W. (1977). *Songs of Innocence and Experience: Shewing the Two Contrary States of the Human Soul, 1789–1794*. Oxford: Oxford University Press.

Blanton, S. (1960). *The Healing Power of Poetry Therapy*. New York: Crowell.

Blinderman, A.A. (1985). Shamans, witch doctors, medicine men and poetry. In J.J. Leedy (Ed.). *Poetry as Healer: Mending the Troubled Mind* (pp. 40–56). New York: The Vanguard Press.

Cellini, H.R., & Young, O. (1976). Bibliotherapy in institutions. *Transactional Analysis Journal*, 6(4), 407–409.

Chavis, G.G. (2011). *Poetry and Story Therapy: The Healing Power of Creative Expression*. London: Jessica Kingsley Publishers.

Edgar, K.E., Hazley, R., & Levit, H. (1985). Poetry therapy with hospitalized schizophrenics. In J.J. Leedy (Ed.). *Poetry as Healer: Mending the Troubled Mind* (pp. 184–192). New York: The Vanguard Press.

Freud, S. (1953). The relation of the poet to day-dreaming. In J. Riviere, trans., *Collected Papers of Sigmind Freid*, Vol.4. New York: Hogarth Press, 24–28.

Gerdtz, J. (1994). Mental illness and the Roman physician: The legacy of Soranus of Ephesus. *Hospital & Community Psychiatry*, 45(5), 485–487.

Hamilton, E. (2012). *Mythology*. New York: Little, Brown and Company

Hynes, A.M., & Hynes-Berry. M. (2012). *Biblio/Poetry Therapy: The Interactive Process: A Handbook*. St. Cloud, Minnesota: North Star Press.

Jamison, K.R. (1996) *Touched with Fire: Manic-Depressive Illness and the Artistic Temperament*. New York: Free Press.

Jones, R.E. (1985). Treatment of a psychotic inpatient by poetry therapy. In J.J. Leedy (Ed.). *Poetry as Healer: Mending the Troubled Mind* (pp. 175–183). New York: The Vanguard Press.

Leedy, J.J. (1969). The healing power of poetry. In J.J. Leedy (Ed.) *Poetry Therapy: The Use of Poetry in the Treatment of Emotional Disorders* (pp. 11–13). Philadelphia: Lippincott.

Leedy, J.J. (1973). *Poetry the Healer*. Philadelphia: Lippincott.

Leedy, J.J. (Ed.) (1985). Principals of poetry therapy. In *Poetry as Healer: Mending the Troubled Mind* (pp. 82–88). New York: The Vanguard Press.

Lerner, A. (Ed.). (1978). *Poetry in the Therapeutic Experience*. New York: Pergamon Press.

Mazza, N. (1979). Poetry: a therapeutic tool in the early stages of alcohol treatment. *Journal of Studies on Alcohol*, 40(1), 123–128.

Mazza, N. (1981). The use of poetry in treating the troubled adolescent. *Adolescence*, 16(62), 403–408.

Mazza, N. (1991a). Adolescence: Crisis and loss. In A. Lerner & U. Mahlendorf (Eds.) *Life Guidance Through Literature* (pp. 110–121). New York: Plenum Press.

Mazza, N. (1991b). When victims become survivors: Poetry and battered women. In S.M. Deats & L.T. Linker (Eds.) *The Aching Hearth: Family Violence in Life and Literature* (pp. 33–50). New York: Plenum Press.

Mazza, N. (2017). *Poetry Therapy: Theory and Practice*. New York: Routledge.

Morrison, M.R. (1985). In defense of poetry therapy. In *Poetry as Healer: Mending the Troubled Mind* (pp. 82–88). New York: The Vanguard Press.

Nunn, J.F. (2002) *Ancient Egyptian Medicine*. Oklahoma City: University of Oklahoma Press.

O'Donohue, W., & Levensky, E. (Ed.) (2004). *Handbook of Forensic Psychology*. San Diego: Elsevier.

Pearson, L. (Ed). (1965). *The Use of Written Communications in Psychotherapy*. Springfield, IL: Charles C. Thomas.

Rubin, R. (April 1974). Prison Libraries: Focus on service to the ex-advantaged. *Catholic Library World*, 45, 438–440.

Rutan, J.S., Stone, W.N., & Shay. J.J. (2007). *Psychodynamic Group Psychotherapy*. New York. The Guildford Press.

Saks, P. (Winter 2007). Aftermath: The implicit processes of integrating traumatic experience in the poetry of Siegfried Sassoon. *Journal of the American Academy of Psychoanalysis and Dynamic Psychiatry*, 35(4), 591–604.

Saks, P. (2019). Listening to the music of the mind: The uses of psychological assessment in the diagnosis of psychotic disorders in a state psychiatric center. In Siglag, M., & Grinshpoon, A. (Ed.). *Clinical Psychology in the Mental Health Inpatient Setting*. New York: Routledge.

Shelley, P.B. (1820). "Hymn of Apollo." *Public Domain Poetry*. https://www.public-domain-poetry.com/percy-bysshe-shelley/hymn-of-apollo-31418.

Weller, P., & Golden, L.G. (1993). Catharsis. In A. Preminger & T.V.F. Brogan (Eds.) *Encyclopedia of Poetry and Poetics* (pp. 175–176). Princeton, NJ: Princeton University Press.

Whitaker, R. (2019). *Mad in America*. New York: Basic Books.

Yalom, I.D., & Leszcz, M. (2020). *The Theory and Practice of Group Psychotherapy*, 6th Edition. New York: Basic Books.

5 Averting Harm, Deferring Danger, or Providing a Path to Safety? Treatment of an Aggressive, Psychotic Young Man in a Forensic Psychiatric Hospital

Michael Siglag

Introduction

Forensic psychiatric hospitals possess specialized physical designs, administrative policies, and highly trained staff, all aimed at maintaining safety and control. But they are also facilities where treatment addressing mental health issues and behavioral problems is an important part of the mission (Chaimowitz, 2018). The effort to treat individuals in such a setting requires navigating the physical environment, being attuned to systemic issues relevant to administrative goals and staff priorities, working with staff who may prioritize safety over treatment, and dealing with numerous therapeutic challenges posed when carrying out treatment.

A window into the complexity of treatment in such an environment is provided in this chapter. The treatment approach presented involves the utilization of multiple theoretical models and therapeutic tools and approaches (Davies, Howells, & Jones, 2007), as well as efforts to deal with numerous organizational variables. Treatment issues are addressed that are shared by many patients in forensic hospital settings, including emotional dysregulation, psychological regression, physical aggression, and social isolation (Barnao & Ward, 2015). Treatment progress is far from linear and includes episodes of failed treatment interventions, missed treatment opportunities, and withdrawal from treatment engagement.

Names and personal information have been disguised to protect confidentiality. Although the person described here is a composite of many individuals treated in a forensic psychiatric hospital setting, aspects of the history, the treatment setting, and system parameters will most likely seem familiar to many who have treated individuals in such settings.

DOI: 10.4324/9781003360926-7

Treatment

Tamir was a young man admitted to a forensic psychiatric hospital when he was 19 years old. Despite his youth, he had been treated in several other mental health facilities before arriving at this one.

Based on historical information documented in his medical chart, substance use and psychiatric problems began when he was approximately 11 years old. Around that time, his parents divorced. Tamir stayed with his mother.

Over a period of years, beginning in early adolescence, Tamir's behavior problems became increasingly problematic. His behavior progressed from erratic, irrational, and asocial to aggressive and dangerous. There were periods in his life when he was able to function adequately. He attended high school episodically. Since age 12 or 13, however, he has had episodes that led to mental health treatment. Treatment settings progressed from outpatient office appointments to residential youth programs. During early adolescence, there were instances when Tamir was reportedly victimized by other patients in some programs and facilities. When Tamir's mother became aware of these situations, she removed him from those facilities. Late in his teens, Tamir was admitted to a psychiatric unit in a general hospital following an incident of aggressive behavior toward police officers in the town where he lived with his family. After a period of treatment, he was not considered stable enough for discharge and was transferred to a state psychiatric hospital. In the state hospital, he continued to engage in violent behavior, assaulting staff and other patients. Ultimately, his aggression toward staff and other patients in the civil facility led to his transfer to a higher-security forensic hospital.

I first encountered Tamir in the forensic hospital. Due to repeated episodes of aggressive behavior during his two-year admission, he spent most of his time contained in a small cell-like room. Several therapists of various disciplines had been seriously injured by him when he was allowed to come out of his room and meet with them on the unit. When I met him, he was rarely willing to come out of his room, even when given the opportunity. When he did come out of his room, he was usually held in restraints or shackles that restricted his movement. When he met with clinical staff, or the full treatment team, he often remained in his room with security personnel standing in his doorway for the protection of other staff and patients.

Competing pressures to ensure protection and to provide treatment pose a dilemma in such settings (Chaimowitz, 2018). Tamir was contained and separated from his family and from the broader community, housed in a locked unit in a secure forensic hospital. But even within the hospital, others were perceived as safer when this young man was contained in his room or wore physical restraints when out of his room. He was seen as extremely dangerous. He displayed seemingly unpredictable episodes of explosive aggressiveness as well as periods of intense emotional distress and disturbance.

My first encounters with Tamir took place on a unit that served as the men's admissions unit and the crisis unit, where patients from other hospital units within the forensic hospital were transferred when they were regressing or considered behaviorally unmanageable. In other words, these were the most unstable, violent, and, at times, self-injurious individuals in the forensic hospital. Following evaluation and a brief period of treatment, primarily medication, many patients showed some degree of improvement and moved on to less acute units. Some quickly returned to jail or prison after completing court-ordered evaluations or interventions. Others remained on the unit for extended periods of time.

Tamir had remained on this unit for a period of years. He was seen as psychotic, aggressive, unpredictable, and dangerous. Despite treatment efforts by some experienced therapists, he not only had failed to improve but possibly had gotten worse since his admission.

When I began working with Tamir, he was 20 years old. Most of Tamir's daily interactions were with medical security officers, those most directly responsible for maintaining safety in the hospital. As front-line staff, these staff members usually bore the brunt of violent and aggressive patient interactions. If, based on their observations and often well-honed knowledge of the patients, security staff perceived a patient as displaying signs that they were likely to harm someone, they often contained them in their room. This intervention was seen by many – security staff, as well as administrators and clinical staff – as the best way to keep potential victims safe.

Even when Tamir was allowed out of his room, he wore shackles on his legs to slow him down from possible attempts to assault staff or other patients. However, despite these preventive measures, on several occasions, he had succeeded in assaulting and seriously hurting staff, other patients, and even family members during visits.

Although the restrictions enforced by medical security staff were sometimes seen as excessive by clinical staff, such restrictions were not necessarily challenged. Security staff decisions were generally upheld.

Clinical treatment team functions and roles were similar to those in many clinical/hospital settings. A program coordinator addressed administrative questions and managed steps being taken on each patient's behalf. Social workers facilitated interactions with family members and often took the lead in communicating with patients about their treatment progress, progress to less restrictive units, and eventual discharge from the hospital. Psychiatrists addressed crises, wrote evaluations and medical orders, and prescribed medication. Nursing staff monitored behavior, administered medication, and implemented most medical orders. Psychologists carried out evaluations and provided individual and group therapy interventions.

Rehabilitation staff provided a range of therapy interventions in modalities that included music, art, vocational skills, computers, physical activity, and more.

When I first met Tamir, when team members, including myself, approached him, he frequently would not respond. When he did respond, he was usually hostile, and what he said was often incomprehensible. An underlying theme in his communication was sometimes evident, however. That theme was that he wanted to be released from his room and from the hospital.

Physically, he did not appear imposing. He was about 5′9″ tall and appeared wiry and muscular. He was disheveled, generally dressed in a dirty-looking t-shirt and a pair of sweatpants. Occasionally, he appeared calm and would smile. More often, he presented himself as angry, agitated, and threatening. He was regarded with extreme caution by all staff.

On my rounds with the treatment team and in my encounters with him through the door of his room, the perceptions others had of Tamir impressed me as understandable. His communication was difficult to comprehend. He was often clearly angry, yelling and banging on his door.

Despite concerns for my own and others' personal safety, I wondered if some of his threatening behavior, apparent anger, and seeming confusion was being exacerbated by his long confinement. On the ward, through a scratched plexiglass window, Tamir could see medical security staff, nursing staff, and other clinicians or team members when they came to provide medication or to see him and other patients on the unit. There was a television on the unit that seemed to be on continuously. He could also see some of the other men housed on the unit, many of whom were equally distraught, confused, threatening, and/or violent.

Interactions with patients by team members, nursing staff, and rehabilitation therapists were limited and typically short and purposeful, e.g., twice-per-week rounds in which the clinical team did a brief check-in with each patient. Throughout the week, psychiatrists met with patients primarily to address immediate behavioral or medication issues or regarding competency or sanity evaluations. Nurses provided prescribed medications. A social worker might speak with patients about family, legal, or other issues. If a psychological evaluation needed to be carried out, the psychologist would work with the patient to carry out the evaluation.

The medical security staff maintained close control. Some were friendly and made efforts to engage patients in various ways, including sometimes bringing in much-appreciated food from the outside world. Most of Tamir's limited interactions were through the plexiglass windows and a port in his door that was used to pass his food trays through. He rarely went to the section of the hospital where rehabilitation groups were held. Some rehabilitation staff attempted to meet with him through his door on the unit, often with the door open and medical security staff closely monitoring the interactions.

When I began attempting to work with Tamir in therapy, my initial goal was to establish the foundations of a therapeutic relationship (Barnao & Ward, 2015; Shepherd et al., 2016). For treatment to be successful, I saw it as necessary for him to see me as someone who was interested and willing to listen to whatever he was willing to communicate about (Karon & Vandenbos 1981; Messer & Wampold, 2002; Shedler & Gnaulati, 2020), and in nearly whatever manner he chose to communicate.

One thing I had been able to understand from my observations and limited interactions with Tamir so far was that he wanted more freedom. A paradox was that on occasions when he was provided more freedom, he often behaved in ways that quickly led back to greater containment. I wanted to convey to him that I wanted to help him gain increased freedom, but that I also valued safety, both for him and for myself and others. I spoke to him about this hope and let him know that I did not want to keep him contained in his cell and deprive him of freedom. I wanted to help generate hope that obtaining more freedom was possible. I also wanted to convey an understanding of what was necessary in order for him to be granted more freedom. Part of what I hoped to successfully communicate was that behaving in a non-aggressive manner would help him attain more freedom. I didn't know at that point whether he would be interested in or trusting of such a message from me. Nor did I know whether he was capable of altering his behavior if he did understand and trust my message. I didn't know if he had the emotional resources or the capacity to develop and utilize strategies and internal control over his behavior that might enable him to interact in a less aggressive manner and to sustain less aggressive behavior.

I understood that there were both known and unknown obstacles ahead. For example, I knew that Tamir's understanding and his ability to comprehend and act on whatever understanding he might possess were compromised by psychosis, as well as the cognitive impact of past drug and alcohol use and possibly other factors. I also knew that if I sought to provide Tamir with increased freedom, I would be working against aspects of well-established hospital culture, particularly the degree to which physical containment was used to maintain safety.

Working within this culture, I developed a behavioral tool that I hoped might be productive in this case. I called it a Progress Plan. In this setting, full-fledged behavioral plans were difficult to implement, and not seen as viable even by many of my clinical colleagues. But I found that a Progress Plan, which was essentially a simplified version of a behavior plan, was more palatable to most. The plan specified concrete benefits to be afforded to the patient when they fulfilled specified behavioral expectations. These benefits were a combination of increasing freedoms, lessening restrictions, and the provision of limited but potentially valued incentives or reinforcers that could easily be provided and were acceptable in the stark environment of the unit in which these patients resided. Unlike behavior plans that allowed for unique rewards for individual patients, everything offered within the Progress Plan was potentially available to any patient on the unit.

While the progress plans that I developed for Tamir and other men on the unit provided seemingly limited incentives, within the context of this unit, the incentives were significant. Most importantly, both patients and staff understood that these incentives were steps to greater things, such as transfer to a less restrictive unit with increased freedom and a step to potential discharge to a non-forensic state hospital, where discharge to the community was more possible.

Utilizing ideas borrowed from a Cognitive Behavioral Therapy (CBT) model used for psychotic patients (Chang et al., 2014), motivational interviewing (Silverstein, 2010), my understanding of good therapeutic practice (Beck et al., 2009; Hussain, Mia & Rose, 2020), and also guided by the emphasis on establishing a therapeutic relationship that my training and work using psychodynamic models taught me (Karon & Vandenbos 1981; Messer & Wampold, 2002; Shedler, 2010; Rosenbaum et al., 2012), I began my work with Tamir. I worked diligently to figure out what Tamir wanted, what might motivate him to engage with me, and what might lead to some change in his behavior. I made efforts to speak with him several times per week, sometimes with his door closed and sometimes open with medical security staff standing nearby or next to me. At times, I spoke with him through his food port (Kupers, 2022; Obegi, & Canning, 2022). Sometimes he rejected me, and sometimes he engaged with me in a minimal way. At other times, he spoke with me in a more understandable manner. I found that he liked my wrist watch, an old hand-wound watch that had been handed down to me. Tamir recognized that it was an item of some quality, or at least an interesting curiosity worthy of some of his attention. If so, maybe I was too.

I developed a Progress Plan that included several behavioral steps for Tamir to demonstrate in order to begin coming out of his room. Working within the hospital's culture at that time, but also extending its limits, I identified and outlined specific behavioral steps that demonstrated safety, cooperation, and the willingness and ability to interact without becoming aggressive. Security staff were initially clearly skeptical of this process. At times, when it was time for one of our sessions, the medical security staff member assigned to assist me would disappear on a break. Some clinical team members were skeptical as well, although they expressed approval of the concrete behaviors and steps that were identified. Significant, for the success of my therapeutic approach, the program coordinator was supportive. As the administrative leader of the team, her support was crucial.

Within a few weeks of initiating the progress plan, and despite staff resistance and skepticism, Tamir eventually did what he needed to do in order to be allowed to come out of his room for therapeutic phone contact with me. This was arranged in a way that security staff supported. The interaction was similar to a prison contact, in which Tamir and I would be able to see each other but would speak by phone. We spoke on the phone for about 20 minutes, face-to-face and about 2 feet apart, but with a plexiglass barrier between us.

Although it did not seem obvious at the time, it soon became clear that this was a significant breakthrough. Once our phone session took place, some of the staff resistance lessened. With clinical staff's agreement and security staff's facilitation, Tamir and I next began meeting face-to-face with no physical barrier at one of the tables on the unit, where patients ate their meals. Medical security officers stood and sat close by. At times, we met with a medical security officer sitting at the table in between us, ready to respond if Tamir became aggressive.

Tamir was able to engage in occasionally meaningful, brief discussions, mostly about his desire to leave the hospital and sometimes about his family. I also spoke with him about why I was meeting with him and how continuing to be safe could lead to more freedom. We did that for several weeks. A couple of weeks increased to a couple of months. Our discussions were usually superficial and limited in scope, but we were communicating, and Tamir was not behaving aggressively toward me.

What appeared to be a promising trend did not last, however. Tamir's progress at that time ended fairly abruptly around his 21st birthday. He began insisting that, since he was 21 years old, he should be able to do whatever he wanted. What he said he wanted to do was leave the hospital and join a branch of the United States military. He had somehow obtained what appeared to be a military service application.

He began to refuse to meet with me, indicating that he was joining the military and that since he was now legally an adult, he could do whatever he wanted. He became increasingly angry and agitated, and he would bang on his door when the treatment team came to do rounds. He refused to meet with me, indicating that he had done what had been asked of him and that he should now be allowed to leave the hospital and carry out his plans.

My efforts to speak with him over the subsequent weeks were met with further anger and agitation. Efforts to emotionally empathize and provide reality-based responses were fruitless. He was not receptive to being told that he had been progressing and that if he continued his past behavior, it could lead to more freedom and even lead to discharge. He wanted immediate results, which to him meant immediate discharge.

Tamir had shown that he could respond to the behavioral expectations placed on him. He had been spending time outside of his room. He had not been aggressive toward me. He also appeared to be capable of forming some level of attachment when that attachment related to his wishes. He knew that speaking and meeting with me were related to his discharge from the hospital, something he wanted. However, his understanding of the complex process needed to accomplish discharge and his ability or willingness to engage in a long-term plan toward that end were limited.

Had he not turned 21 at that particular time, maybe we would have made more progress. While the therapeutic work I had done with him provided some evidence that he had the potential to progress further, he refused to see or speak with me further, as he was not immediately getting discharged despite doing what he had been asked to do. In his view, meeting with me had no further purpose and was therefore of no further interest to him.

I was not able to wait out his rejection and see if he might re-engage with me in therapy. Soon after he consistently refused to meet with me, I left that unit for another assignment. Other therapists would be assigned to work with him.

For the next several years, Tamir remained on that unit. He reverted to his previous behavior. He assaulted several therapists who had made efforts to work with him. He returned to spending most of his time in the cell-like setting that was his room.

Four years later, however, after I had left employment at the hospital and was working privately, I received communication from the new hospital administrator. A new administrative team had taken charge of the hospital. They had a strong interest in increasing treatment provision in the forensic hospital and were implementing more active treatment modalities. They had reached out to me to see if I would work with Tamir again and serve as a consultant to the team on the unit where I used to work.

The new administrative team's effort to increase the provision of hospital treatment was motivated by many factors. Implementation of increased treatment opportunities in the forensic hospital was consistent with their own prior work in other settings and with efforts that were taking place nationwide in other settings (Shepherd, Doyle, Sanders, & Shaw, 2016). SAMHSA's trainings on trauma-informed care and treatment were an additional influence. There were also various legal pressures on the hospital to provide more treatment and decrease containment. For example, the hospital was being required to reduce the amount of time patients were secluded in their rooms and to reduce or eliminate some more extreme restrictions.

In Tamir's case, he also had involved family members advocating for him. His family was putting increased pressure on the hospital to provide a pathway to discharge and was working with a private lawyer and communicating with the prosecutor from the county where Tamir had lived prior to his hospitalization. During my previous work with Tamir, the progress Tamir had made was known both to hospital staff and to Tamir's parents.

From the beginning of my involvement in this new treatment effort, I recognized that the multiple factors contributing to my renewed involvement with Tamir's treatment meant that it was likely that resources and attention would be focused on this case. I knew that administrative and staff support of this effort could increase the likelihood of a more successful therapeutic process and outcome. However, I also knew that it was possible that the goal of bringing me in was to create a perception, i.e., to demonstrate that treatment efforts were being made. If that was a primary goal, it was also a concern that support might fall short of what was needed for a successful outcome. While a successful outcome might be seen as desirable, if it was a demonstration of the effort that was the goal, not the outcome for the patient, adequate resources might not be provided or sustained. Numerous factors and motivations could influence how this renewed effort might evolve (Shur, 1994). Knowing this, but also knowing the administrator who had reached out to me, I perceived a genuine intention to provide the support that would be needed for a successful process and outcome.

My goal was to help Tamir and help his team work with him. The treatment team now working with him consisted of a different group of people than those I'd worked with before. I did not know their attitudes or investment in this process, or how they might react to my renewed presence.

A good first step to restarting this process was a demonstration of support from administrative staff. The team directly treating Tamir needed to know that their investment in this effort was as important, if not more so, than my work with him, and that they remained centrally involved in Tamir's treatment. A planning meeting with all available staff involved in Tamir's treatment would be a venue to convey these important messages to the team. The location and content of the meeting were important and would communicate a message to the team and unit staff. The meeting was set in the unit's treatment team room, their turf.

Those present included the hospital CEO, Clinical Director, clinical and medical treatment team members, nursing staff representing each shift, key medical security staff, and myself. The primary agenda of the meeting was to explain the plan for reviving Tamir's treatment and to discuss the hopes for this enhanced treatment effort. The agenda included discussing both how we were going to approach this therapeutic effort and the importance of the team's involvement.

After introductions and some comments by the administrators present, I took the lead in the discussion, explaining my past involvement with Tamir and why I had been asked to work with him now. I described the work Tamir and I had done together when I worked on the unit and what we had accomplished in the past. I explained how it had ended and some of the immediate and potential obstacles I saw ahead. I emphasized that this would need to be a team effort, especially as I would only be present in the hospital for limited times each week as a consultant and would not be present to follow through or see what was happening when I wasn't there. I asked clinical team members and medical security staff for their input and opinions, solicited their understanding of Tamir's background and behaviors, and sought input. I asked for their perspectives on making this effort productive and effective. We spoke about communication with the family, including the importance of sharing significant family communication.

All staff present at the meeting, including medical security officers who were present, provided valuable input and information. For example, a member of the nursing staff suggested that the best time to attempt to meet with Tamir was in the afternoon. A medical security staff member reported that some of what Tamir spoke about in his presence seemed to relate to some kind of past traumatic experience. I felt hopeful, as the level of communication suggested that the team members would be invested in and willing to help with this treatment. They appeared to accept and welcome my being part of the treatment process.

Following the meeting, I went onto the unit and spoke with Tamir himself. It was not clear whether or not he recognized me. He was neither hostile nor particularly responsive, but he indicated that he recognized me. I explained who I was, why I was there, and reminded him of some of what we had done in the past. He appeared disengaged and somewhat unimpressed, but he didn't overtly reject the idea that I would come back to speak with him again. I did my best to respond to him in a way that was attuned to his reaction to me, which was fairly neutral, and to not put much pressure on this interaction. I indicated that I would be coming back to meet with him and that I would see him again the following week.

I was hopeful about our next meeting but was also realistic. This was a tenuous reunion, and I knew that things could go in any number of directions when we met again.

I began meeting with Tamir twice weekly. Following the recommendation of members of the treatment team, I initially approached Tamir during the afternoon hours, when it was felt that he would be most receptive. Sometimes he was responsive to my efforts to meet with him during these afternoon times, other times not. It was not unusual for him to be sleeping in his room when I came. Efforts by medical security officers to awaken him had varied results.

During this phase of treatment, which lasted several weeks, he began coming out of his room to meet with me sporadically. Each time I met with him, I reminded him who I was, why I was there, and conveyed to him that I was hoping to help him get out of his room more and down to "Rehab," which was where most of the hospital's therapies and activities were offered. I described some concrete goals, telling him that the treatment team at the hospital and the judge who was overseeing his case wanted to see him come out of his room, go to "Rehab," be with other people more, behave in a safe way, and not hurt other people. I again tried to explain that this could lead to discharge, which I understood to be one of Tamir's goals. I conveyed my understanding that this had been his goal when we had met before and that this was how that goal could be achieved.

To many staff, and perhaps to Tamir, the idea that he could and would take the steps I was suggesting may have seemed like a remote possibility. I was hopeful that we could get back on the trajectory we had begun when I worked with Tamir several years ago. But I knew that, after all this time, that might not happen. I was also concerned that the idea that Tamir would behave more safely and would then actually be discharged seemed implausible to many hospital staff members and to Tamir himself. I knew that some staff wondered why we were really doing this and whether the investment being put into this case was primarily a response to legal pressures, to demonstrate to the court that efforts were being made.

As we began to work together again, it was evident that Tamir continued to struggle with active psychosis and, at times, had difficulty managing his extreme anger. However, he also appeared to understand what I was suggesting and demonstrated some trust by making efforts consistent with those suggestions. He began agreeing to come out of his room more consistently. After steps paralleling what we had done before, he soon began accompanying me, with a contingent of medical security officers, to the "Rehab" wing of the hospital.

On those therapeutic walks to rehab, he could be smiling and pleased, silent and troubled, or seemingly passive. His emotional expression could change in a moment. Initially, we spent much time in the gym or a classroom where he could be logged onto a computer and listen to music or play chess. Most of the time, he sat with headphones on, selecting songs to listen to and appearing to enjoy the music. It was hard at times for him to make the transition from listening to music to disengaging and returning to the unit. On one occasion, we obtained a set of headphones from the Rehab Library to help with the transition. He was able to listen to music on those headphones all the way back to the unit.

Eventually, at the suggestion of medical staff officers, I began approaching Tamir during the morning instead. Security staff suggested that if Tamir started the day meeting with me, it would help provide him with some structure for his day. When I started meeting him during the morning hours, he began coming out of his room to meet me more consistently and was more interactive. He began to be ready to come out of his room more consistently and showed more interest in going to the rehabilitation wing of the hospital, at times directly asking to go to "Rehab" when that choice was presented to him as one of the options for each session.

With this consistency, medical security officers and clinical rehabilitation staff began greeting him, smiling, and telling him they were glad to see him, and chatting with him about other positive encounters they had experienced with him over recent years. They mentioned food they had provided him, which he appeared to recall. Tamir would sometimes stop at the doors of certain staff members to say hello. He began returning to the unit more easily. Medical security staff also sometimes began independently bringing him to the rehab wing on occasions when I was not seeing him for therapy.

As time passed, however, some problems arose. At times, he began to appear agitated in the "Rehab" wing. He occasionally behaved aggressively, sometimes after being provoked and other times without apparent provocation. Though concerning, these situations did not escalate as medical security staff monitored him closely and quickly stepped in to physically contain Tamir when necessary. On one occasion, when he was listening to music on the computer, it was reported that a female patient took the headphones off his head. He responded by striking out at her. One time, Tamir charged another patient with a basketball, throwing it at him. On one occasion, another patient threw Tamir down onto the gym floor after Tamir had charged him with a basketball and threw the ball at him. While each situation was contained, Tamir's behavior could easily have escalated further. Such situations could have become more dangerous to other patients, to Tamir, and to the staff who intervened. On one occasion, Tamir ran up the stairs of the gym bleachers, where another male patient was sitting. Tamir pulled his pants down and made a sexual proposition. When the other patient calmly declined, Tamir closed his pants back up and ran back down the stairs without becoming aggressive. He was escorted back to the unit. He did not become physically aggressive, and some staff, recognizing his restraint, praised him for that aspect of his behavior.

While his verbal communication remained limited and the meaning of his behavior was not always clear, it seemed that through his behaviors, Tamir was communicating about some of his wishes and impulses and the pressure he felt to satisfy his impulses, even in such awkward ways. A therapeutic goal at that point became to try to better understand his needs and work on his ability to communicate such needs in safer and more socially acceptable ways.

Once, after being brought back to the unit and saying goodbye for the day, I returned with a rehab staff member who had accompanied us that day and wanted to also say goodbye to him. My attention during that session had been divided between Tamir and the rehabilitation staff member who accompanied us. When we approached his door, which security staff had opened, Tamir came charging out of his room in what appeared to be an aggressive manner. When I backed off and tried to move away without overtly running from him, he took a swing at me, catching the corner of my cheek. He knocked my glasses off, but it caused little other damage.

Efforts to discuss incidents with Tamir led to mixed results. The week after he struck me, during our scheduled session, I asked him what had been happening with him the previous week and why he had charged and swung at me. He denied remembering what happened. I asked whether he had been mad or upset, if I had said something to him or done something that day that he didn't like. He didn't acknowledge anything I suggested and offered no explanation. Later, I was told that he had asked a security staff member who worked closely with him why I had run away from him, suggesting that he felt rejected by me. Perhaps feeling rejected was something he wasn't ready to speak directly about. I suspected that my divided attention that day bothered him. He did speak about the incident in which the headphones were grabbed off his head by the other patient. It was clear that bothered him. He was conveying how hurt and angry he felt when he perceived rejection and insensitivity. We were able to speak about that.

On one occasion, when he was both more agitated and more talkative than usual, he sat on the floor in an alcove on the unit and spoke with me and a security staff member he knew and trusted. He initiated discussion about his sexual orientation and wishes. The security staff member and I gave supportive feedback. We spoke about how difficult it must be for him in this environment, for many reasons, to acknowledge his wish for physical affection and sexual contact, and how difficult it was to get that contact in a safe way, if at all, considering where he was. I considered whether he was experiencing affection for me and whether his apparent anger when he struck me was in part a transferential response to me, as someone who was being kind to him and trying to gain his trust. Beyond that, was his reaction to me in part sexual? Was this therapy awakening complex sexual urges he had difficulty verbalizing in a setting where there were no safe ways of fulfilling such urges with others?

Tamir's behavior indicated that his sexual wishes and frustrations were becoming more pressured. While on the unit, he began spending extended time in his room masturbating. He went through a period where he would not shower or take care of his hygiene.

Also around this time, for the first time in years, a discharge plan was taking shape. During a court hearing he had attended, he was told he was going to be able to be discharged to an agency out of the state. For that to happen, several things still needed to be accomplished by the state's attorney, his family's attorney, the hospital, and the agency where he would be discharged.

I wondered whether this situation replicated anything Tamir had experienced before. Was this the first time, or one of a series of times in his life, when he was told that if he did what was asked, he would get something he wanted? While he expressed wanting more freedom, did he have fears or doubts about what he would encounter or how he would handle that freedom? How much self-awareness regarding his own functioning did he have after so many years in the hospital? Did he recognize the support he would need to succeed outside of the hospital? Would he accept support that might feel intrusive? Could he meet community expectations? What would life outside the hospital once again be like for him?

On one occasion, when we spoke about discharge as a real possibility, he appeared to be more lucid in his recognition of the situation he was in. He asked to come out of his room to take a shower. In the midst of the effort to shave, wash, etc., he saw himself in the distorted metal mirror and became extremely upset. He was bereft, wailing loudly about his state. What was wrong with him? What had happened to him? He knew his family had enough financial resources so that, under different circumstances, he would have a good life available to him. He was despairing about what had happened to his body and mind, including his ability to function properly sexually, a side effect of the medication he was taking. He threw clothes and other objects and aggressively pushed a laundry cart around the unit. He did no damage to anyone or anything except a shower curtain, but his pain was palpable. When one of the medical security officers who had been a consistent and caring support for him helped bring him back to his room, Tamir went willingly, while asking this man why he was his friend and how he could care about him.

After this took place, and subsequently during our meetings, Tamir became more withdrawn during our interactions. He showed less interest in going to the "Rehab" wing, often staying in his room and isolating himself. At times, he would come out of his room to meet with me. But often, he remained in his room, preoccupied with his attempts to obtain sexual relief through masturbation. Although I continued to speak with him, he became less verbally communicative. I often felt that I was speaking to him instead of with him.

When we met, I sometimes described steps and efforts being made to discharge him and assured him that discharge efforts were continuing and were genuine. I wondered if he no longer believed that the plan for his discharge was real. Might he believe that it was never truly real or that it had fallen through, and that once again his efforts had been for naught and were not worth continuing? Perhaps he was anticipating and preparing for disappointment. After his despair came to the surface, I also wondered if he continued to respond to the perception he had of himself and of his current life that he had conveyed on the day that he looked in the distorted mirror on the ward. Did he see himself as too damaged to be able to have a life like he had envisioned? I also wondered if, despite the apparent persistence of his wish to leave the hospital, he experienced some ambivalence about being separated from the few people in this setting with whom he may have felt some attachment. My observations suggested that this primarily included the security officer who had stood by him and remained encouraging, and perhaps myself to a lesser degree.

In fact, the plans for discharge were becoming more uncertain. Before discharge plans were solidified, restrictions associated with COVID began. Questions arose about the agency where Tamir was supposed to be discharged. While questions about the appropriateness of the targeted agency had been raised by hospital personnel, to some extent those questions had been addressed – at least from a legal perspective. In court hearings, Tamir's judge communicated that he was satisfied with the appropriateness and adequacy of the discharge plan for the facility. Now, however, questions arose concerning whether the agency, which was newly opening, was actually ready to open and if it was prepared to accept Tamir. Now that discharge seemed more imminent, practical questions and obstacles were arising. Tamir's mother contacted me to help identify a possible alternative agency. With coronavirus restrictions, Tamir was spending much time in his room, and fewer therapeutic activities were available to him. The discharge plan that seemed imminent appeared to be dissolving.

This uncertainty cleared during the height of the initial phase of COVID restrictions. Ultimately, the agency identified for discharge was able to take Tamir. Some concerns about the logistics of the discharge plan persisted, but despite these concerns, Tamir was discharged. Tamir's next therapeutic steps were in the hands of a new agency.

Conclusion

The course of therapy described here was neither linear, with a clear progression, nor complete. In settings such as the forensic psychiatric hospital in which this treatment took place, this is not unusual. Yet, despite such limitations, therapeutic work in forensic settings is both important and needed. Looking at Tamir's progression over the course of therapy, there were several important ways in which Tamir responded to the intensified treatment regimen initiated and supported by administrative staff and carried out through collaboration with the team, medical security staff, and others. While continued treatment was clearly indicated, Tamir demonstrated improvement in social interactions and expression of aggression in some concrete ways.

Key problems initially identified, as with many individuals treated in such settings, were Tamir's social isolation and aggression. The concrete goals of therapy included working to help him safely come out of his room regularly after years of isolation and extremely limited interaction with other people. After spending literally years of his life in a small cell in a forensic hospital while manifesting continual and treatment-resistant psychiatric disturbance, Tamir had limited interpersonal skills and means of communicating or coping. He often became aggressive when he was allowed out of his room. Over the course of treatment, he began to come out of his room more regularly. He became able to modulate his aggressive responses to a degree, though not consistently. He began going to the rehabilitation wing of the hospital and interacting more safely, although he was clearly very troubled and provocative at times. On the few occasions during the concluding period of his hospitalization when he became aggressive, he did not hurt anyone. His aggression had become directed more at objects than people. When he did direct his aggression at others, his intent appeared to be less to hurt them than to physically express something that was distressing him, to attempt to satisfy urges, or to vent his frustration about a need that was not being met.

In the rehabilitation wing, he had begun to engage in a range of activities, including playing ping pong, shooting baskets, playing electronic chess, playing cards, and playing songs on the computer. While this was a limited range of activities, it was a significantly expanded array of activities for him. His engagement grew out of his own interests and was continuing to expand. He also interacted with some hospital staff members but remained unable to participate in group activities and social interaction.

Before he was discharged, he was progressing in his ability to communicate effectively. At times, he was able to communicate coherently about complex feelings and sensitive issues. He occasionally demonstrated the ability to speak about important issues which contributed to his being so troubled.

During treatment, some of the personal issues he struggled with became clearer, although some of those issues couldn't be easily addressed. For example, when it became apparent that he was coping with feelings regarding his ability to fulfill urges for intimacy and sexual expression, his ability to speak about these feelings was limited.

In addition, while he appeared to have become more lucid and more able at times to express himself more clearly, he was still continuing to struggle with psychosis. His psychosis and limited ability to communicate clearly were obstacles to further progress, impacting his mental status and behavior.

His active psychosis interfered with cognition. He had difficulties thinking rationally, remembering and verbalizing his personal feelings and reactions, improving his social and problem-solving skills, and applying the problem-solving skills he may have possessed to social and interpersonal situations. Yet it appeared that he understood that the efforts that were being made and the expectations of him that were being made were intended to help him gain his freedom. Inconsistently and with difficulty, he had responded to behavioral expectations consistent with this goal. He also displayed the capacity for interpersonal connections with staff members and demonstrated indications of interpersonal bonds, including a therapeutic bond.

In Tamir's case, family and legal forces were active and both provided support and added pressure, contributing to the extra resources put into Tamir's treatment and discharge. In a fair system, every patient and every individual would have the same opportunities and chances for support.

Tamir's opportunity to make more progress within the forensic hospital setting ended with his discharge from that setting. Taking more time to help Tamir articulate and handle emotions that were emerging more distinctly could have benefited him. It was hoped and expected, based on discharge planning, that his treatment in another facility would include the opportunity to build on his progress.

The course forward for this young man included much that was undetermined. This chapter describes a degree of success and improvement. An aftercare plan was in place to build upon that progress. However, how available resources would be applied to help Tamir and how he would respond to efforts to help him continue his progress were uncertain.

While the trajectory and specific implementation of therapy described here are unique, this is a composite case. The work described here provides several insights relevant to the work done with many individuals in such settings:

- The balance between treatment provision and minimization of risk can significantly impact the mental health of individuals housed and treated in forensic-correctional facilities. Physical containment of individuals in order to establish and maintain a desired degree of safety can be a primary approach in such settings. However, extreme and/or prolonged containment as a primary strategy, particularly with people suffering emotional distress or disturbance, can significantly isolate an individual and may prolong and exacerbate their mental health problems and symptoms. While establishing a safe environment is an important condition for psychological treatment, overemphasizing risk containment can make treatment goals more difficult to achieve. Some potential problems with years of relative physical isolation are evidenced in Tamir's case. These include deterioration of social and communication skills, deepening of symptoms such as psychosis and depression, and increasing the possibility that decline in psychological and interpersonal functioning may be harder to reverse (Reiter et al., 2020). Developmental issues are a consideration as well. For example, Tamir entered the facility as a socially underdeveloped adolescent.

- An individual's presentation in forensic and correctional settings may reflect a combination of iatrogenic and underlying problems. If conditions promoting iatrogenic problems can be lessened, underlying psychological problems exacerbated by incarceration may become clearer and potentially more accessible to treatment. For Tamir, after steps were initiated to facilitate him leaving his room more frequently, he became less isolated and began behaving less aggressively. He was able to begin communicating in a more rational manner at times. A number of unique psychological issues began to become clearer and more able to be addressed in therapy (Livingston, 2016; Hussain, Mia & Rose, 2020).
- Efforts to provide treatment addressing the psychological and behavioral problems of individuals with complex and significant disturbances in a forensic-correctional setting can have systemic benefits (Chang et al., 2014). Effective treatment addressing individuals' problems can make a facility less dangerous, both for individuals held in such settings and for all of those with whom they interact. Tamir began to come out of his room and interact in a safer manner. Rather than being seen as an individual with little hope of making progress, he began to be seen as someone who could improve and make progress. Staff's shift in perspective concerning Tamir's ability to progress was conveyed directly to Tamir and also began to be extended to several other patients who had seemed equally unresponsive or resistant to therapeutic interventions.
- Once an individual is housed in a highly secure environment, achieving a transition to a less secure environment can be difficult and complex (Barnao & Ward, 2015; Barnao et al., 2016; Livingston, 2016; Shepherd et al., 2016). Multiple factors, including the severity of the individual's behavior and mental health issues, perceived risk of the individual, available family and legal supports, financial resources, and other factors, come into play. Tamir spent years contained and isolated before engaging in a therapeutic plan that helped him progress.
- Mental health treatment can play an important role in facilitating transitions for those with problems responsive to such treatment (McIntosh et al., 2021). Tamir made progress and was less aggressive and dangerous when discharged from the forensic hospital. He had an agency willing to provide support and treatment for him upon discharge, and a

discharge plan considered acceptable by legal and mental health authorities advocating for him. Earlier therapeutic engagement and a more extended course of therapy may have helped Tamir progress sooner and reach a greater level of stability.

- While multiple factors contributed to Tamir's progress during the course of treatment described here, individual therapy can be a key and organizing treatment factor in forensic-correctional settings. A transtheoretical approach to individual therapy, especially when provided in conjunction with other effective therapy approaches, can provide individuals with concrete benefits and reinforce an individual's hope for improvement, as can consistency in the provision of therapy despite contraindications and risks (Hemming et al. 2020; Kingston et al., 2018; Shedler et al., 2021, Shepherd et al., 2002). The individual therapy approach utilized with Tamir was theoretically grounded but flexible. This included psychodynamic factors, in which central factors were attention to the importance of the therapeutic relationship and an awareness of the multiple levels of psychological significance of Tamir's actions and communications. Developing and utilizing behavioral tools such as the "progress plan" was important as well. While theory was rarely made explicit during therapy, this case incorporated psychosocial, cognitive-behavioral, psychoanalytic, systemic, and other models.
- Systemic factors within forensic-correctional facilities can both pose obstacles and facilitate treatment. Managing those factors plays a major role in treatment success (Rice & Rutan, 1987; Livingston, 2016). This includes recognizing the importance of administrative and treatment team support and working collaboratively with therapeutic staff as well as security staff where possible. In Tamir's case, such support and engagement were crucial. External systemic factors play an important role as well. The hospital, as part of a broader state treatment system, was adopting a greater understanding of psychological and behavioral disturbances and an awareness of how these problems are best treated in a hospital setting. Key administrators adopted a federally supported trauma-recovery-based model and treatment interventions consistent with that model.
- Hope is an essential therapeutic factor (Messer & Wampold, 2002). When therapy began, the idea that Tamir would improve enough to be discharged was inconceivable to many who had known him for a period of years. It was considered highly dangerous to even allow him to leave his room. The therapeutic gains that did occur and Tamir's safe and incident-free discharge were considered positive results for Tamir, the hospital, and his family and hopefully provided guidelines for future success with other patients.

References

Barnao, M., & Ward. T. (2015). Sailing uncharted seas without a compass: A review of interventions in forensic mental health. *Aggression and Violent Behavior*, 22, 77–86.

Barnao, M., Ward, T., & Robertson, P. (2016). The good lives model: A new paradigm for forensic mental health, psychiatry. *Psychology and Law*, 23(2), 288–301. https://doi.org/10.1080/13218719.2015.1054923

Beck, A.T., Rector N.A., Stolar, N., & Grant, P. (2009). *Schizophrenia Cognitive Theory, Research, and Therapy*. New York: The Guilford Press.

Chang, N.A., Grant, P.M., Luther, L. et al. (2014). Effects of a recovery-oriented cognitive therapy training program on inpatient staff attitudes and incidents of seclusion and restraint. *Community Mental Health Journal*, 50, 415. https://doi.org/10.1007/s10597-013-9675-6

Chaimowitz, G. (2018). Balancing risk and recovery. *International Journal of Risk Recovery*, 1(1), 1–3. https://doi.org/10.15173/ijrr.v1i1.3356

Davies, J., Howells, K., & Jones, L. (2007) Evaluating innovative treatments in forensic mental health: A role for single case methodology? *The Journal of Forensic Psychiatry & Psychology*, 18(3), 353–367, https://doi.org/10.1080/14789940701443173

Hemming, L., Bhatti, P., Shaw, J., Haddock, G., & Pratt, D. (2020). Words don't come easy: How male prisoners' difficulties identifying and discussing feelings relate to suicide and violence. *Frontiers in Psychiatry*, 11, 581390. https://doi.org/10.3389/fpsyt.2020.581390

Hussain, S., Mia, A., & Rose, J. (2020) Men's experiences of engaging in psychological therapy in a forensic mental health setting, *The Journal of Forensic Psychiatry & Psychology*, 31(3), 409–431. https://doi.org/10.1080/14789949.2020.1752286

Karon, B.P., & Vandenbos, G.R. (1981). *Psychotherapy of Schizophrenia Treatment of Choice*. New York: Jason Aronson.

Kingston, D.A., Olver, M.E., McDonald J., & Cameron C. (2018). A randomised controlled trial of a cognitive skills programme for offenders with mental illness. *Criminal Behaviour and Mental Health*, 28, 369–382. https://doi.org/10.1002/cbm.2077

Kupers, T. (Spring 2022) The cell-front interview. *Correctional Mental Health Report*, 23(4), 77–78.

Livingston, J. D. (2016). What does success look like in the forensic mental health system? Perspectives of service users and service providers. *International Journal of Offender Therapy and Comparative Criminology*, 1–21. https://doi.org/10.1177/0306624X16639973

Messer, S.B., & Wampold, B.E. (2002). Let's face facts: Common factors are more potent than specific therapy ingredients. *Clinical Psychology: Science and Practice*, 9(1), 21–25.

McIntosh, L.G., Janes, S., O'Rourke, S., Lindsay D.G., & Thomson, L.D.G. (2021) Effectiveness of psychological and psychosocial interventions for forensic mental health inpatients: A meta-analysis. *Aggression and Violent Behavior*, 58, 101551, ISSN 1359–1789. https://doi.org/10.1016/j.avb.2021.101551

Obegi, J. H., & Canning, R. D. (2022). The cell-front interview revisited. *Correctional Health Care Report,* 23(4), 81, 97–98.

Reiter, K., Ventura, J., Lovell, D., Augustine, D., Barragan, M., Blair, T., Chesnut, K., Dashtgard, P., Gonzalez, G., Pifer, N., & Strong, J. (2020). Psychological distress in solitary confinement: Symptoms, severity, and prevalence in the United States, 2017–2018. *American Journal of Public Health*, 110, S56, S62. https://doi.org/10.2105/AJPH.2019.305375

Rice, C. A. & Rutan, J. S. (1987). *Inpatient Group Psychotherapy A Psychodynamic Perspective.* New York: Macmillan Publishing Company.

Rosenbaum, B., Harder, S., Knudsen, P., Koster, A., Lindhardt, A., Lajer, M. Valbak, K., & Winther, G. (2012) Supportive psychodynamic psychotherapy versus treatment as usual for first-episode psychosis: Two-year outcome. *Psychiatry: Interpersonal & Biological Processes*, 75(4), 331–41.

Shedler J. (2010). The efficacy of psychodynamic psychotherapy. *The American Psychologist*, 65(2), 98–109. https://doi.org/10.1037/a0018378

Shedler, J. & Gnaulati, E. (March/April 2020). The tyranny of time: How long does effective therapy really take? *Psychotherapy Networker.*

Shepherd A., Doyle M., Sanders C., & Shaw J. (2016). Personal recovery within forensic settings – Systematic review and meta-synthesis of qualitative methods studies. *Criminal Behaviour and Mental Health*, 26(1), 59–75.

Shur, R. (1994). *Countertransference Enactment, How Institutions and Therapists Actualize Primitive Internal Worlds.* Northvale, N.J.: Jason Aronson, Inc.

Silverstein, S.M. (September 2010). Bridging the gap between extrinsic and intrinsic motivation in the cognitive remediation of Schizophrenia. *Schizophrenia Bulletin*, 36(5), 949–956. https://doi.org/10.1093/schbul/sbp160

Part II

Programmatic Approaches

6 Specialized Transitional Inpatient Care in Re-entry for Justice-Involved Persons with Serious Mental Illness[1]

Benjamin A. Rubin and Merrill Rotter

Introduction

It is well established by the government, and researchers estimate that a sizable percentage of individuals incarcerated in state prisons in the United States suffer from mental health problems (Maruschak, Bronson, & Alper, 2021) or serious mental illness (SMI; Prins, 2014). In turn, a significant percentage of adults hospitalized in state psychiatric centers or public mental health clinics are estimated to have been involved with the criminal justice system at some point in their lives (Ehntholt et al., 2022). Prevalence rates for criminal justice involvement among consumers of public mental health programs range from 25% to 75% (Bonfine, Wilson, & Munetz, 2020). In one study, 64% of individuals screened at a New York City urban psychiatric center had both a diagnosis of mental illness and a history of criminal justice involvement (West et al., 2015).

The overlap between criminal justice involvement broadly, violent crime specifically and mental illness is complex. Active symptoms of serious mental illness account for criminality and violence in only a small percentage of individuals with criminal justice contact. More often, the risk of re-arrest is related to so-called criminogenic risk factors, including past history of criminal justice contact and patterns of antisocial personality, thought and behavior, and not related to mental illness, even among individuals with diagnosed serious mental illness (Skeem et al., 2014). There is a need to address both the overrepresentation of individuals with serious mental illness in the criminal justice system and the corresponding significant percentage of individuals with histories of criminal justice involvement in community treatment programs, especially those with violence risk. But the complicated relationship between serious mental illness, violence and criminality requires more than just traditional mental health-focused assessment and interventions.

The intensive treatment unit (ITU) is a specialized 20-bed, all-male treatment unit housed in a civil psychiatric center. It was initiated by the New

DOI: 10.4324/9781003360926-9

York State Office of Mental Health (NYSOMH) to address the complex needs of individuals released from prison as they transition into the community. Patients admitted to the ITU suffer from serious mental illnesses. In addition, they possess an aggregate of risk factors for violence and criminal recidivism unrelated to acute psychotic or affective illness. The ITU is designed to treat patients' symptoms of SMI and begin to address characterological traits associated with violence and criminality.

In this chapter, we review the components of the ITU, the literature on the needs targeted by ITU interventions and the evidence base for those specialized interventions. We begin by describing New York State's (NYS) prison-based mental health services and re-entry planning.

New York State Prison Mental Health Services

Per NYS statute (Corrections Law [CL] §401–§402), the mental health treatment needs of persons in NYS prison are managed under a collaborative relationship between the Department of Corrections and Community Supervision (DOCCS) and NYSOMH. NYSOMH oversees a Joint Commission-certified continuum of care for individuals in state prisons. At its highest level of intensity sits a central inpatient hospital. Satellite programs located throughout the NYS prison system provide varied types and intensities of treatment services, including intake screenings, psychiatric assessments, 24-hour mental health care, counseling, and psychotropic medication management (Beck and Maruschak, 2001). NYSOMH also conducts pre-release planning for persons with identified mental health treatment needs. A percentage of these individuals are referred directly for inpatient psychiatric admission.

As of January 1, 2021, 24.3% (n = 8385) of individuals in DOCCS custody were on the NYSOMH caseload, receiving services. Around 11.7% of the total population (n = 4051) were identified as suffering from major mental illness. Around 75% of DOCCS inmates (n = 25417) did not require or receive NYSOMH services (NYS Corrections and Community Supervision, 2022).

As of August 1, 2001, personality disorders among prisoners on the NYSOMH caseload were approximately three times as common as found in NYSOMH's civil psychiatric centers. The most prevalent subtypes in the incarcerated sample were antisocial, followed by borderline. Patients suffering from personality disorder were distinguished by longer lengths of stay and greater numbers of inpatient admissions (Rotter et. Al., 2002).

Post-release Hospitalization Procedures

Pre-release planning for persons with SMI constitutes a basic, necessary and constitutionally mandated service (Appelbaum, 2020). NYSOMH operates specialized re-entry programs, such as the Community Orientation and Reentry Program at Sing Sing Correctional Facility. Additional re-entry units are geographically spread to be available in key locations throughout NYS. Discharge services include treatment referrals, case management, benefit applications, and supportive housing. The scope of services depends on the severity of the individual's illness.

If, upon reaching the date of release, an incarcerated individual is mentally ill and in need of inpatient care and treatment, a hospital director or superintendent of a correctional facility is able to apply for involuntary admission to a state hospital pursuant to the same civil Mental Hygiene Law (MHL) standard governing individuals in the community.

The statutory standard for civil mental health commitment is a mental illness for which inpatient care and treatment are necessary and a lack of capacity to appreciate the need for such care and treatment. The individual must also pose a substantial threat of harm to themselves or others. This may include the inability to manage essential needs such as food, clothing and shelter or the danger associated with repeated medication noncompliance. The last criterion is often the basis for post-release hospitalization (including the ITU), when the individual is symptomatically stable, but there is a historical pattern that suggests likely non-adherence to treatment, with consequent decompensation and dangerousness.

The Intensive Treatment Unit

The ITU is a 20-bed all-male treatment unit housed in a civil psychiatric center. The program is intended for individuals released from the DOCCS who would otherwise require civil psychiatric commitment due to SMI and who, unrelated to symptoms of their SMI, concurrently demonstrate elevated risk of violence and re-arrest. Unit staff include a multidisciplinary team of psychiatry, psychology, social work, rehabilitation services and direct care psychiatric aides. The team is led by an administrative treatment team leader. The unit emphasizes a high staff-to-patient ratio. ITU programming is organized around the psychiatric recovery model, with an additional focus on risk factors for violent recidivism.

ITU Admissions Criteria, Process, and Procedure

To be admitted to the ITU, an individual scheduled for release from prison must meet MHL criteria for admission to a civil psychiatric hospital. Additionally, his record will reflect a pattern of antisocial behavior, violence and personality traits that indicate an elevated risk for future violent recidivism. Personality disorders, most frequently antisocial or borderline types, are common and consistent with admissions criteria. Due to programmatic limitations, individuals with a significant intellectual disability or a history of sexual offending are ineligible for admission. Because the

ITU is a specialized treatment program, referrals are accepted across NYS, regardless of county of origin.

Individuals who appear to meet ITU criteria are flagged by NYSOMH pre-release service planning. The case is then reviewed for suitability. Admissions decisions are based on a review of records and results from the COMPAS pre-release criminogenic risk assessment.

The COMPAS assessment yields three overall risk scales, including failure to appear for a pretrial hearing, recidivism (i.e., arrest for an offense) and violence (i.e., re-arrest for a violent offense). The tool also yields scores for criminogenic risk-related treatment needs. Risk scale scores are derived by a proprietary algorithm. They are intended to be predictive, discriminating between offenders who are more or less likely to recidivate (Equivant, 2019). Need scales are not predictive but rather descriptive of the offender. The tool has been validated in multiple studies and is in use in multiple states at different junctures in the criminal justice process (e.g., Pinals et al., 2021). In the ITU context, COMPAS scores are not determinative but rather help identify individuals who have the inclusion criteria of higher risk and non-SMI-based recidivism needs (e.g., antisocial attitudes).

On the date of release, the individual is transported by DOCCS staff directly from the correctional facility to the ITU. Once having arrived at the psychiatric center, the newly admitted patient receives a full multidisciplinary intake evaluation, including psychiatric, nursing, and medical assessments. After completing the admissions assessments and being deemed safe to do so, the patient is transferred to the ITU.

ITU Treatment: Psychiatric Stabilization

On arrival, new patients are oriented to the ITU setting and introduced to peers and unit staff. The patient and treatment team have an initial meeting to identify a preliminary list of goals and objectives, methods to achieve those goals, anticipated discharge setting, and service needs. With that information in hand, the team formulates a schedule of groups and individual services to help the patient achieve his goals.

Patients transferred from DOCCS sometimes exhibit overt symptoms such as delusions, hallucinations and/or highly labile mood. During the first three to six weeks post-admission, staff work individually with each patient to achieve psychiatric and behavioral stability. In some cases, there are diagnostic questions, complex medication needs or a lack of treatment engagement. Consultation with senior clinical staff or, if needed, a court order for medication over objection are available strategies to address these barriers. If needed, this initial treatment phase may be extended.

ITU: Assessing and Addressing Violence Risk

Reduction of long-term violence risk is a primary treatment goal for all ITU patients. While most individuals with serious mental illness are not violent, there is a small but incremental risk associated with serious mental illness (Swanson et al., 1990). In the seminal MacArthur Foundation study of violence and mental illness, 1,000 individuals released to the community following involuntary psychiatric inpatient hospitalization were followed for one year; approximately 25% had an episode of violence (Steadman et al., 1998). Rolin and colleagues' 2019 review of 373 young adults enrolled in 10 OnTrackNY (a specialized NYS treatment service for individuals exhibiting first episode non-affective psychosis) clinics from October 2013 to August 2016 found that 24.6% (n = 90) exhibited violent behavior, ideation or intent in the 90 days prior to intake (Rolin et al., 2019).

However, even in a population with serious mental illness, violence is often not directly related to the symptoms of the diagnosed disorder. In studies of crimes committed by individuals with SMI, the symptoms of SMI accounted for less than 10% of the offenses. (Steadman et al., 1998). Other contributors, including substance use and community-based factors, may be more relevant (Steadman et al., 1998; Skeem et al., 2016).

ITU clients are specifically referred because of a history of violence, and they are screened as having a violence risk unrelated to their serious mental illness. Therefore, a comprehensive risk assessment for violence is necessary to ensure that all relevant risk factors are accounted for and targeted in treatment. The most widely accepted violence risk assessment for individuals with SMI is the HCR-20, a structured professional judgment instrument normed and designed for individuals with SMI (Douglas et al., 2013; Singh et al., 2014). It has been used with civil and forensic psychiatric patients to predict violence and inform treatment (de Vogel et al., 2022). It includes 20 empirically supported risk factors for violence organized into categories of historical, current, and problems with future planning.

A typical ITU violence risk assessment involves an intensive record review and a wide-ranging patient interview. Unit psychologists are supported in this effort by doctoral-level graduate students. As they develop experience and skills, trainees compose increasingly larger portions of the risk assessment. Team members also contribute to their professional areas of expertise. For example, the unit psychiatrist may provide information about the patient's psychiatric functioning, and a social worker may share knowledge about the patient's psychosocial history.

The initial assessment is completed within 30 days of admission, and the team develops a formulation about the critical factors driving violence risk. Subsequent treatment efforts address these relevant variables, including relationship issues, antisocial attitudes, and trauma history, that may play a role in violent reoffending. In consultation with hospital administration and forensic psychologists, the team routinely refines and enhances the violence risk formulation. Ultimately, risk assessment informs a risk management plan, or individualized service plan, crafted for each patient before discharge.

Treatment is multimodal and individualized to address the unique personal, psychiatric and risk profiles of each patient. Psychiatric oversight and intervention enhance the 'patient's overall well-being while mitigating symptoms of mental illness that elevate the risk of violence. Individual therapy with the unit psychologist empowers patients to work through personal issues, receive individualized feedback, and increase their emotional well-being. Therapy also addresses personal risk factors such as trauma history and problems with relationships.

All ITU clients participate in Aggression Replacement Therapy (ART). ART proposes three elements to violence: behavioral, affective and moral. A three-pronged treatment approach addresses each in turn. Social skills education and role-playing teach participants pro-social behavior. Anger management is used to develop more adaptive responses to emotional arousal. Finally, group discussion of social situations serves as a forum to promote mature moral reasoning.

ART has been implemented in the NYS prison system, as well as in the English and Welsh Departments of Probation. ART was available in the Swedish Department of Prisons and Probation from 2000 to 2010. Large-scale studies of ART in Sweden found minimal effectiveness in reducing general offending (Lardén et al., 2018). However, a smaller-scale study in England and Wales demonstrated a lower reconviction rate for ART treatment completers (Hatcher et al., 2008). A commissioned review of treatments for violent adults sponsored by the United Kingdom Ministry of Justice included ART as one of the other interventions that taught cognitive skills, anger control involved role playing, and were more effective than those that did not (Jolliffe & Farrington, 2007). It has also been found that ART non-completers pose a heightened risk of reconviction (Brännström et al., 2016).

ART was chosen, in part, because it is known to many ITU patients from their time in the NYS prison system. The familiarity of the group provides patients with a sense of comfort and an opportunity to review important skills. The cognitive skills and pro-social behavior modeling of ART are also relevant for addressing antisocial traits associated with the risk of re-arrest.

ITU: Assessing and Addressing Risk of Recidivism

As with the risk of violence, the risk of re-arrest or recidivism in individuals with serious mental illness is more complicated than originally thought (Peterson et al. 2010). Proponents of the "criminalization hypothesis" assume that the overrepresentation of individuals with serious mental illness in the criminal justice system is the result of "deinstitutionalization" and the downsizing of state hospital systems across the United States. Theoretically, individuals with significant community behavioral challenges are left in the community without access to hospital-based institutional support and with exposure to criminal sanctions for behaviors that they struggle to manage. In other words, their symptoms were "criminalized." However, traditional mental health treatment has not sufficed in addressing the risk of criminal recidivism for most clients (Skeem, Manchak, & Peterson, 2011). A more holistic, re-arrest-focused approach was needed. Forensic mental health professionals turned to the literature on recidivism risk management for individuals without SMI, i.e., the Risk, Needs, Responsivity Model.

In 1990, Andrews and Bonta proposed the RNR model, which has become the primary, evidence-based paradigm for addressing offender behavior (Skeem, Steadman, & Manchak, 2015). Programs adhering to RNR principles have demonstrated empirical evidence of their effectiveness in reducing criminal recidivism (Andrews & Bonta, 2010).

"Risk" speaks to the issue of who receives treatment and at what intensity. Individuals who pose the highest risk of criminal recidivism are matched to the highest-intensity treatments. Similarly, individuals who pose a low risk are matched to lower-intensity treatments. High-intensity treatments increase recidivism risk when mismatched to individuals of otherwise low risk (Bonta & Andrews, 2007). A risk focus on treatment includes a commitment to thorough risk assessment. Specific RNR risk assessment tools include the Level of Service Inventories (Andrews & Bonta, 1995) and the COMPAS (which, as described above, is completed prior to client referral for ITU services).

"Need," in this context, refers to treatment targets directly related to the risk of re-arrest. Criminogenic needs are variables that, when changed, correspondingly alter recidivism risk. There are four empirically derived primary treatment targets or criminogenic needs, including antisocial attitudes, antisocial associates, antisocial personalities and a history of antisocial behavior. A second, empirically derived set of factors impact risk to a lesser extent and include family circumstances, social or work issues, leisure or recreation issues and substance abuse. Criminal thinking is also recognized as an important contributor to recidivism risk (Gross & Morgan, 2013).

"Responsivity" is about the "how" of treatment. RNR literature delineates various kinds of responsivity, including general responsivity and specific responsivity. General responsivity refers to variables that enhance the receptiveness of broad groups to a treatment approach. A cognitive-behavioral orientation and assigning homework are examples of general responsivity factors. Specific responsivity covers factors unique to the individual that impact his/her receptivity to treatment. Mental illness is classified in the RNR literature as a specific responsivity factor, that is, for an individual to benefit maximally from an RNR-need-focused intervention (e.g., substance use treatment), the mental illness must be addressed (even if it is not a direct driver of criminal behavior).

In the past 15 years, researchers have demonstrated the relevance of RNR (both in terms of prediction and risk management) for individuals with SMI (Bonta, Blais, & Wilson, 2014). In NYS, the same criminogenic needs were found to equally predict recidivism among persons released from prison, with or without SMI. Psychiatric diagnosis, history of psychiatric hospitalization and intensity of mental health need while in prison did not differentiate between those clients who returned to prison and those who did not, nor did these psychiatric factors add to the predictive validity of criminogenic factors (Hall et al., 2012).

The broad implication of RNR theory is that the standard clinical focus of treatment for mental illness is insufficient to reduce criminal recidivism in the SMI population. The RNR literature recommends cognitive-behavioral therapy (CBT) due to its structure and process, to which offenders are generally responsive. However, in working with offenders, it is necessary to adapt the content of CBT by overtly targeting antisocial attitudes, such as self-serving rationalization, minimization and lack of empathy, and helping clients develop more pro-social problem-solving skills. Clients with SMI may also be prone to antisocial attitudes. In 2009, Carr et al. found a high level of criminal thinking styles in a state hospital sample. A high level of criminal thinking or antisocial attitudes was also found among incarcerated individuals with SMI (Wolff et al., 2011).

Several offender-specific CBT approaches have demonstrated effectiveness in recidivism reduction (Rotter & Carr, 2011). ART is a CBT intervention that is based on the RNR model. In addition, ITU clients complete Interactive Journaling (IJ), working through two manualized CBT-based journals focused specifically on antisocial attitudes such as rationalization, self-serving justification and externalization, as well as values such as integrity, honesty and empathy (The Change Companies, n.d.). IJ is used in re-entry programs across NYS. It has been used in drug treatment settings, jails, and youth services programs. As a structured journaling program, IJ provides topics and prompts for direct respondent writing. Written samples then serve as a springboard for guided discussion in therapeutic groups. The interactive aspect of journaling is theorized to increase patient engagement and enhance outcomes. A 2014 review of the published evidence base indicated that available data were favorable regarding IJ's efficacy to enhance participant knowledge, improve antisocial attitudes and reduce recidivism rates (Miller, 2014).

The responsivity principle also encompasses the qualities of treatment providers and the treatment setting. Treatment is most effective when provided by skilled and experienced staff within a framework of fidelity to the RNR model. Providers are meant to possess strong interpersonal and relationship skills. Rote adherence or repetition of treatment manuals is insufficient. Thus, a critical aspect of the ITU milieu is the individualized, non-judgmental approach that maximizes the opportunity for a trusting, therapeutic alliance.

ITU: Addressing Re-entry Readaptation

Individuals who have experienced incarceration and are later admitted to a standard psychiatric admissions unit may behave in ways that were adaptive in prison but are then misunderstood by providers who are unfamiliar with the prison culture. For example, being hypervigilant is an adaptive survival skill in a prison setting that may be misread as paranoia by an untrained clinician. To that end, all staff on the ITU receive specialized training, "Sensitizing Providers to the effect of Correctional Institutionalization on Treatment and Risk Management" (SPECTRM; Rotter, 2005). The training alerts staff to the behaviors and attitudes associated with prison culture, which can, if not addressed properly, interfere with the development of the therapeutic alliance that is the basis for any other productive clinical work (Rotter et al., 2011).

The third manualized intervention delivered to all ITU clients is SPECTRM's Reentry After Prison (RAP) group. RAP follows a cognitive-behavioral and psychoeducational treatment model specifically focused on the traumatic and enduring experience of incarceration. It is intended for formerly incarcerated individuals with SMI. Patients learn about the ways they have, sometimes unknowingly, adapted to life in prison and consider alternatives to promote healthy collaboration with clinical treatment and more successful community re-entry.

The RAP program was first implemented in a civil psychiatric ward in 1998. Approximately half of the ward's patients had a history of incarceration. Preliminary data indicated that disciplinary incidents were less frequent following program implementation than beforehand. This held true when controlling for demographic factors, diagnostic variables and violence risk as measured by the HCR 20 (Rotter et al., 2005). In 2002, the RAP program was implemented in two New York City homeless shelters. The shelters, one for men and one for women, housed single adults who were homeless and suffering from SMI. Qualitative data was obtained through interviews. Due to a small sample size, no statistical analysis was conducted. Participants who completed the program reported a greater sense of trust in peers and staff than those who had not completed the program. Male participants said that they found the experience of speaking about their time in jail or prison to be helpful (Rotter et al., 2005).

Typical Course of Treatment

ITU treatment may be usefully distinguished into three phases. The first phase of treatment emphasizes assessment and psychiatric stabilization. The second phase is the treatment phase. Patients participate in psychiatric medication management and psychotherapeutic treatments targeting co-occurring mental illness and behavior associated with criminal-legal contact. They attend groups (described above), participate in the therapeutic milieu and meet for individual therapy.

Throughout hospitalization, the team and patient work together to identify appropriate community services and secure them before discharge. The team also makes an initial determination about whether outpatient civil commitment is appropriate and warranted. In the latter phase of hospitalization, the primary focus is shoring up details of the service plan and ensuring a patient's readiness for community re-entry.

Continued supervision and support post-discharge is often useful. To that end, outpatient civil commitment, or Assisted Outpatient Treatment (AOT), is a common feature of ITU discharge plans. Individuals at heightened risk for violence and medication non-adherence may be eligible for AOT. An AOT application to the court includes an individualized service plan with mental health treatment, case management and therapeutic residential services. In designing and implementing AOT treatment plans, NYSOMH collaborates with local mental health authorities. Once an AOT order is issued, it provides a legal avenue to arrange for an emergency evaluation at a hospital in the event of medication noncompliance or worsening of symptoms.

Given the risk concerns associated with the ITU clients, administrative oversight and support for the clinical team are critical (Resnick & Saxton, 2019). Approximately one month before scheduled discharge, the treatment team applies to hospital administration for a pre-discharge review. In preparation, the team submits an updated HCR 20 risk assessment, an updated psychiatric evaluation and a preliminary individualized service plan. The review is conducted by a designee of the hospital clinical director, such as a director of psychiatry, medical director or director of hospital forensic services. The pre-discharge review serves as a final check to ensure that risk factors have been identified, treated to the extent reasonable, and accounted for in the individualized service plan. It also provides an opportunity to consult with the treatment team, learn from success, and plan or make small adjustments as needed.

System and Administrative Supports

ITU clients cross multiple systems, primarily mental health and criminal justice, but also social services and substance use. Consequently, the mental health and criminal justice systems need to work together in providing their care. It begins with a referral system that requires functional, prison-based collaboration between the NYS DOCCS and NYSOMH. And it extends through discharge planning that requires continued collaboration with NYS DOCCS, which is tasked with parole supervision both while the client is on the ITU and when he is released to the community. While on hospital grounds, ITU patients under post-release supervision can meet with a parole officer. An assigned officer visits the hospital on a scheduled basis, meeting with all patients on the caseload. Parole visits in the hospital offer a useful opportunity to assess a patient's readiness for return to post-release supervision in the community. A patient unable to meet calmly with parole in the hospital is unlikely to do so successfully in the community. Parole is also an important source of collateral information. Parole partners with the hospital to identify appropriate discharge services. Rarely, when there are behaviors of serious concern while inpatient, the hospital may consult with parole about the necessity for increased supervision or other legal consequences.

Within NYSOMH, the forensic and civil divisions communicate to identify appropriate clients for the ITU and to support those clients post-hospitalization with community-based forensic services, for example, specialized intensive case management. In addition, housing, medical care, substance use treatment services, employment and education are all part of a complex picture. Through collaboration between the various systems, justice-involved clients with SMI are supported as their risks and needs span those multiple systems. The NYSOMH central office plays a key role in helping to ensure that these connections are made, particularly since the single ITU serves the entire NYS, including regions very far from the unit itself. For example, a history of incarceration may be a barrier to obtaining appropriate housing and employment. With a more expansive reach than the individual hospital, NYSOMH is effective in identifying and securing appropriate services statewide. If a patient is discharged to NYSOMH-supervised mental health housing, NYSOMH facilitates and coordinates between the sending and receiving facilities.

Model ITU Case Example

The following represents a typical ITU individual and his course of treatment. Names, details and identifying information are fictitious or aggregated from various individual cases.

As a young adult, John lived on the streets of New York City. He moved through various homeless shelters and sometimes slept on the street. Early in his 20s, John had first been diagnosed with schizoaffective disorder after being picked up by police on the streets. He was disheveled and yelled unintelligibly at passersby. After a brief period of stabilization on psychiatric medication, John returned to the shelter system and city streets. Over the next two to three years, he repeated the cycle of symptom worsening, admission to City Hospital, stabilization on medication and eventual noncompliance, precipitating the return of psychiatric symptoms. When he had the money to do so, John smoked cigarettes and used marijuana.

John's criminal history included illegal possession of a firearm and multiple misdemeanor-level assault charges for fighting. He was an active member of a local gang. Once, he assaulted a peer with a knife at his homeless shelter, causing a severe injury and eventually leading to the victim's death. After being found unfit to proceed, he was admitted to a state forensic hospital for the restoration of competency. Psychiatric medication and psychoeducational groups were effective in helping him regain competency, and he returned to jail to proceed with his charges.

After sentencing, John arrived in NYS's prison reception center, where he was identified as an individual suffering from SMI. At that time, his case was opened with NYSOMH corrections-based operations. His adjustment to prison was difficult and marked by multiple instances of disruptive behavior. He received many disciplinary sanctions ("tickets") for disobeying orders, lewd conduct and fighting with staff and peers.

John spent periods of incarceration in specialized mental health prison units when his symptoms worsened to the point that he was no longer safe for the general population. On one occasion, his symptoms were such that he posed an imminent danger to himself and others. He was involuntarily committed to a two-month inpatient hospitalization.

John eventually began taking medication consistently. He was able to maintain behavioral control. He kept to himself, stayed away from other prisoners, and focused on finishing his prison sentence. He was conditionally released from prison under post-release supervision but was unsuccessful due to violating the conditions of parole by using drugs, failing to comply with prescribed psychiatric medication and missing appointments.

John was returned to prison and subsequently referred by NYSOMH prison services for ITU admission. The review of his referral packet was noteworthy for the violence associated with his initial offense, the multiple disciplinary infractions that John incurred while incarcerated, and his unsuccessful period of supervision after his first release. Most relevant, with reference to the ITU admission, was the course of these events and his clinical condition when the incidents occurred. While, as noted above, John did have one psychiatric hospitalization, most of the violent incidents in the community and in prison were not associated with a period of psychotic or affective decompensation. Rather, they appeared to reflect a need for services to address his predisposition to impulsivity and his resorting to violence too frequently as a coping strategy.

On release, John was transported directly from the prison to the civil psychiatric center where the ITU is housed. John arrived at the hospital in a confrontational state, complaining that he had been scheduled for release but was instead being confined against his wishes. He begrudgingly participated in initial evaluations with a psychiatrist, nurse and medical specialists in a very limited fashion.

During the first two weeks of admission, John was reluctant to participate in treatment. His mood was belligerent, and his anger often escalated quickly and intensely, leading him to lash out violently at peers. The team asked John for permission to contact his family for additional information and to support John. However, he declined to sign a release authorizing communication.

The ITU team tried various strategies to engage John in treatment. Direct care staff developed a warm, supportive relationship with John. They shared with him their experience seeing patients who had succeeded with the ITU program. Together, they discussed what choices would best serve John's interest in gaining his freedom. Clinical staff listened to John's stories about prison and complaints about his fellow patients. They validated John's feelings about the hospital environment and his ongoing lack of freedom. They worked with him to find alternative ways to manage his frustration. They also spent time getting to know John and working with him to identify experiences in the community (e.g. enjoying a cup of coffee or going to the pizza shop) that he found motivating. The team's efforts were moderately successful. However, John continued to insist that medication was not a necessary part of this treatment. Consequently, he remained irritable and symptomatic.

After a couple of weeks, John began to voluntarily comply with the prescribed psychotropic medications. He was prescribed antipsychotic and mood-stabilizing medications, which he began to take regularly. His speech was increasingly coherent, his mood calmer and he was able to interact with unit staff and peers. He was mistrustful and suspicious, but not overtly paranoid.

John entered the structured treatment, ITU-specific intervention phase of hospitalization. He spoke with the unit psychologist about previous episodes of violence. He was interviewed at length about his offense history, disciplinary incidents in prison and the circumstances surrounding those events. Putting together the information gleaned from John and observations from John's violent behavior during the first part of his stay in the ICU, the team developed a formulation of John's violence risk.

John's antisocial personality style had an outsized influence on his violent behavior. Interactions with peers were aggressive and marked by attempts to intimidate or cow others into respect. He believed that it was always necessary to be ready with a violent response should he be challenged or disrespected. When actively symptomatic, he was increasingly irritable and likely to perceive disrespect from others. He was also less able to respond in productive or adaptive ways.

John began attending the treatment groups described above, targeting his history of aggression (ART), antisocial attitudes (IJ) and adaptation to the clinical milieu (RAP). He was scheduled for ART to address anger, poor social problem solving and antisocial attitudes.

In planning for discharge, the team understood that medication adherence and psychiatric symptoms worsened in an unstable living environment. Overall, the evidence suggested that John needed support to manage his financial needs and assistance with medication administration. The team strongly recommended that he consider transferring to supervised mental health housing upon discharge from the hospital.

John's individualized service plan included specialized housing, forensic case management, mental health treatment at a local state-operated clinic and an intake for substance abuse services. After applying to the court for outpatient commitment, the team notified the hospital's administration that John would be approaching his discharge date. A pre-discharge review was scheduled with the hospital's director of forensic services.

Two weeks before discharge, the ITU team met virtually with the receiving housing provider and mental health clinic team. They discussed John's identified risk factors for violence. John had the opportunity to speak with the psychiatrist who would be treating him in the community. The ITU team encouraged receiving providers to work with him to develop pro-social interests and positive activities that would keep him busy and engaged in the community.

On the day of discharge, John was transported directly to the local parole office, where he met with the new parole officer with whom he would be working. From there, he was transported to his residence. A follow-up call three days later revealed that he was still in the residence and had begun work with his outpatient treatment providers.

Implementation Considerations

On the surface, there is an apparent tension when targeting both mental illness and criminal recidivism. However, the two elements share a common basis in a strength-based, problem-solving recovery model as applied to justice-involved clients with SMI. The ITU approach is necessarily broad and accounts for both short-term and long-term violence risks posed by its patients. It is understood to be in the best interests of community safety and the patient who wishes to remain at liberty.

Therapeutic alliance is a significant predictor of treatment success and recidivism reduction (Scanlon, Hirsch, & Morgan, 2022). Therefore, it is especially important that staff are invested in the unit's mission of treating mental illness and criminal recidivism. The ITU has been fortunate to employ staff members with a positive mindset and strong ability to connect with a challenging group of patients. As staff are promoted or move on, it is necessary to recruit new staff to replace them. Training, supervision and a culture of teamwork have all been effective means to support staff.

Staff competence is critical. ITU staff receive specialized training to equip them to deal with the unique needs of the patient population. Along with all NYSOMH inpatient staff, they receive two full days of training in managing behavioral crises. In addition, ITU staff complete training modules about the criminal-legal system, the principles of RNR, violence risk assessment and the SPECTRM approach to re-entry support. Internet-based training has been helpful in cutting down on time and training expenses.

Staff have developed familiarity with typical social patterns on the unit and maintain heightened vigilance for behaviors or interactions that pose a risk of escalation. Certain patient behaviors and social strategies may be more common in correctional settings but less so in psychiatric hospitals. These include trading, carrying contraband, debt collecting and financial wheeling and dealing.

Some clients present with high-frequency disruptive or violent behavior. While this tends to be rare, individualized behavior planning has been effective to address the difficulty. Behavioral treatment approaches can be challenging to implement since there are necessary limitations in identifying rewards and incentives. Opportunities for greater liberty, such as unescorted walks outside the buildings, are not possible due to the risk issues for which the client was admitted to the ITU.

Patients with prominent traits of borderline personality disorder or more severe psychopathic features present a particular difficulty from the standpoint of behavior management and treatment engagement. To meet the needs of these patients, there is a focused effort within the ITU team to maintain a consistent approach. This is important so that the patient and team share a common understanding and work together in a collaborative treatment process. In parallel, there are administrative mechanisms, such as morning meetings, to promote ongoing communication between teams and upper-level clinical administration about the needs and progress of patients. The result is that staff members at multiple levels are involved in dialogue, identifying individualized patient goals and working together to promote the best outcomes. In some instances, case consultation with senior clinicians is a helpful tool to fine-tune treatment strategies for more challenging cases.

Program Demographics and Outcome Data

In 2020, NYSOMH analyzed data comparing clients discharged from the ITU between 2015 and 2019 (n = 135) with a cohort of individuals who were discharged from a civil state psychiatric center after having been involuntarily hospitalized upon release from prison (n = 135). ITU and control clients were matched on age, gender, race and resident county. In terms of demographics, ITU and matched control groups did not differ in terms of marital status, high school grad status, trauma diagnosis or length of stay (LOS).

Since all ITU clients are male, only male controls were studied. The mean age for the whole cohort was 38.7; 64.4% were Non-Hispanic Black, 22.2% Hispanic and 10.4% Non-Hispanic White. Around 79% of the ITU clients were diagnosed with a schizophrenia spectrum disorder, 68.2% had a substance use disorder, 23.3% were given the diagnosis of antisocial personality disorder and only a handful of clients had an affective illness. Around 81% had graduated high school. Around 85% were never married.

Compared to the matched control group, the ITU group had a higher percentage of clients with a diagnosis of SUD, schizophrenia and antisocial personality disorder. The ITU group was more geographically diverse (58.5% from New York City) compared to the matched control group (96%). Preadmission arrest data showed that ITU clients had a lower number of arrests preadmission as well as a lower percentage of any arrests (7.4%), compared to clients in the matched control group (65.1%). This difference in arrest history likely reflects that the control group had more time at risk in the community than the ITU subjects, most of whom had been incarcerated during the preadmission study period.

Post-treatment, both groups had lower rates of recidivism than previously reported outcomes for individuals with SMI released from NYS prison (50% at three years; Hall et al., 2012). ITU clients had a much lower percentage of any arrests (n = 11.1%) in the one-year post-treatment period compared to matched control clients (n = 21.4%). The groups did not differ, though, in the frequency of violent arrests one-year post treatment. The rate of arrest for any offense in the ITU sample one year after discharge was lower than that of the matched control sample.

In summary, preliminary follow-up data suggest that ITU clients have a lower rate of one-year recidivism relative to clients who are civilly committed upon release to a general psychiatric unit. This is particularly noteworthy since ITU clients are targeted for ITU services precisely because of their higher risk profile. The next steps in ITU outcome evaluation will focus on identifying predictors of success within the ITU population.

Future Directions

There are clients who present unique re-entry behavioral challenges but who are not served well by the ITU interventions. These include clients with cognitive challenges and a predisposition to impulsive self-harm. Modifications of the ITU curriculum, behavioral treatment planning, and more specific intellectual disability or trauma-focused treatments – either on the ITU or with additional specialized units – would allow for even more robust availability of services and supports for clients reentering the community with behavioral health issues.

In the meantime, the ITU is a model for more welcoming and holistic care. It offers staff the competence and confidence to work in a caring and understanding manner with clients whose behavior can be off-putting or frightening. And it is a model that sees an individual's risks for criminally dangerous behavior as an appropriate and manageable target for mental health intervention. This holds true even when they are more associated with social, characterological and traumatic features of the individual's history. The net result is a broad consideration of patient needs as opposed to only addressing the traditional, narrowly focused psychotic or affective symptoms – an approach that supports both successful client re-entry and community safety.

Note

1 The authors want to thank Eric Frimpong, NYS Office of Mental Health, for his assistance in the outcome evaluation and data analysis.

References

Andrews, D. A., & Bonta, J. (1995). *The level of service inventory–revised*. Toronto, Canada: Multi-Health Systems.

Andrews, D. A., & Bonta, J. (2010). Rehabilitating criminal justice policy and practice. *Psychology, Public Policy, and Law*, *16*(1), 39–55. https://doi.org/10.1037/a0018362

Appelbaum, P. S. (2020). Discharge planning in correctional facilities: A constitutional right? *Psychiatric Services (Washington, D.C.)*, *71*(4), 409–411. https://doi.org/10.1176/appi.ps.202000084

Beck, A. J., & Maruschak, L. M. (2001). *Mental health treatment in state prisons, 2000*. (Bureau of Justice Statistics, NCJ 188215). Washington, DC: National Criminal Justice Reference Service.

Bonfine, N., Wilson, A. B., & Munetz, M. R. (2020). Meeting the needs of justice-involved people with serious mental illness within community behavioral health systems. *Psychiatric Services*, *71*(4), 355–363. https://doi.org/10.1176/appi.ps.201900453

Bonta, J., & Andrews, D. A., (2007). *Risk-need-responsivity model for offender assessment and rehabilitation*. (Public Safety Canada). https://www.publicsafety.gc.ca/cnt/rsrcs/pblctns/rsk-nd-rspnsvty/index-en.aspx

Bonta, J., Blais, J., & Wilson, H. A. (2014). A theoretically informed meta-analysis of the risk for general and violent recidivism for mentally disordered offenders. *Aggression and Violent Behavior*, *19*(3), 278–287. https://doi.org/10.1016/j.avb.2014.04.014

Brännström, L., Kaunitz, C., Andershed, A.-K., South, S., & Smedslund, G. (2016). Aggression replacement training (ART) for reducing antisocial behavior in adolescents and adults: A systematic review. *Aggression and Violent Behavior*, *27*, 30–41. https://doi.org/10.1016/j.avb.2016.02.006

Carr, W. A., Rosenfeld, B., Magyar, M., & Rotter, M. (2009). An exploration of criminal thinking styles among civil psychiatric patients. *Criminal Behaviour and Mental Health: CBMH*, *19*(5), 334–346. https://doi.org/10.1002/cbm.749

de Vogel, V., De Beuf, T., Shepherd, S., & Schneider, R. D. (2022). Violence risk assessment with the HCR-20^{V3} in legal contexts: A critical reflection. *Journal of Personality Assessment*, *104*(2), 252–264. https://doi.org/10.1080/00223891.2021.2021925

Douglas, K. S., Hart, S. D., Webster, C. D., & Belfrage, H. (2013). *HCR-20V3: Assessing risk of violence – User guide*. Burnaby, Canada: Mental Health, Law, and Policy Institute, Simon Fraser University.

Ehntholt, A., Frimpong, E. Y., Compton, M. T., Rowan, G. A., Ferdousi, W., Swetnam, H., Chaudhry, S., Radigan, M., Smith, T. E., & Rotter, M. (2022). Prevalence and correlates of four social determinants in a statewide survey of licensed mental health services. *Psychiatric Services (Washington, D.C.)*, *73*(11), 1282–1285. https://doi.org/10.1176/appi.ps.202100380

Equivant. (2019). *Practitioner's guide to COMPAS Core*. https://www.equivant.com/wp-content/uploads/Practitioners-Guide-to-COMPAS-Core-040419.pdf

Gross, N. R., & Morgan, R. D. (2013). Understanding persons with mental illness who are and are not criminal justice involved: A comparison of criminal thinking and psychiatric symptoms. *Law and Human Behavior*, *37*(3), 175–186. https://doi.org/10.1037/lhb0000013

Hall, D. L., Miraglia, R. P., Lee, L. W., Chard-Wierschem, D., & Sawyer, D. (2012). Predictors of general and violent recidivism among SMI prisoners returning to communities in New York State. *The Journal of the American Academy of Psychiatry and the Law*, *40*(2), 221–231.

Hatcher, R. M., Palmer, E. J., McGuire, J., Hounsome, J. C., Bilby, C. A. L., & Hollin, C. R. (2008). Aggression replacement training with adult male offenders within community settings: A reconviction analysis. *Journal of Forensic Psychiatry & Psychology*, *19*(4), 517–532. https://doi.org/10.1080/14789940801936407

Jolliffe, D., & Farrington, D. P. (2007). *A systematic review of the national and international evidence on the effectiveness of interventions with violent offenders*. London, UK: Ministry of Justice. https://www.crim.cam.ac.uk/sites/www.crim.cam.ac.uk/files/violmoj.pdf

Lardén, M., Nordén, E., Forsman, M., & Långström, N. (2018). Effectiveness of aggression replacement training in reducing criminal recidivism among convicted adult offenders. *Criminal Behaviour and Mental Health: CBMH*, *28*(6), 476–491. https://doi.org/10.1002/cbm.2092

Maruschak, L. M., Bronson, J., Alper, M. (2021). *Indicators of mental health problems reported by prisoners: survey of prison inmates, 2016*. (Bureau of Justice Statistics, NCJ 252643). Washington, DC: National Criminal Justice Reference Service.

Miller, W. R. (2014). Interactive journaling as a clinical tool. *Journal of Mental Health Counseling*, *36*(1), 31–42. https://doi.org/10.17744/mehc.36.1.0k5v52l12540w218

New York State Corrections and Community Supervision. (2022). *Under Custody report: Profile of under Custody population as of January 1, 2021*. https://doccs.ny.gov/system/files/documents/2022/04/under-custody-report-for-2021.pdf

Peterson, J., Skeem, J. L., Hart, E., Vidal, S., & Keith, F. (2010). Analyzing offense patterns as a function of mental illness to test the criminalization hypothesis. *Psychiatric Services (Washington, D.C.)*, *61*(12), 1217–1222. https://doi.org/10.1176/ps.2010.61.12.1217

Pinals, D. A., Gaba, A., Shaffer, P. M., Andre, M. A., & Smelson, D. A. (2021). Risk-need-responsivity and its application in behavioral health settings: A feasibility study of a treatment planning support tool. *Behavioral Sciences & The Law*, *39*(1), 44–64. https://doi.org/10.1002/bsl.2499

Prins, S. J. (2014). Prevalence of mental illnesses in US State prisons: a systematic review. *Psychiatric Services (Washington, D.C.)*, *65*(7), 862–872. https://doi.org/10.1176/appi.ps.201300166

Resnick, P., & Saxton, A. (2019). Malpractice liability due to patient violence. *Focus (American Psychiatric Publishing)*, *17*(4), 343–348. https://doi.org/10.1176/appi.focus.20190022

Rolin, S. A., Marino, L. A., Pope, L. G., Compton, M. T., Lee, R. J., Rosenfeld, B., Rotter, M., Nossel, I., & Dixon, L. (2019). Recent violence and legal involvement among young adults with early psychosis enrolled in coordinated specialty care. *Early Intervention in Psychiatry*, *13*(4), 832–840. https://doi.org/10.1111/eip.12675

Rotter, M., & Carr, W. A. (2011). Targeting criminal recidivism in mentally ill offenders: Structured clinical approaches. *Community Mental Health Journal*, *47*(6), 723–726. https://doi.org/10.1007/s10597-011-9391-z

Rotter, M., Carr, W. A., Magyar, M., & Rosenfeld, B. (2011). From incarceration to community care: Structured assessment of correctional adaptation. *The Journal of the American Academy of Psychiatry and the Law*, *39*(1), 72–77.

Rotter, M., McQuistion, H. L., Broner, N., Steinbacher, M., & Glazer, W. M. (Ed.). (2005). The impact of the "Incarceration Culture" on reentry for adults with mental illness: A training and group treatment model. *Psychiatric Services*, *56*(3), 265–267. https://doi.org/10.1176/appi.ps.56.3.265

Rotter, M., Way, B., Steinbacher, M., Sawyer, D., & Smith, H. (2002). Personality disorders in prison: Aren't they all antisocial? *Psychiatric Quarterly*, *73*(4), 337–349. https://doi.org/10.1023/A:1020468117930

Scanlon, F., Hirsch, S., & Morgan, R. D. (2022). The relation between the working alliance on mental illness and criminal thinking among justice-involved people with co-occurring mental illness and substance use disorders. *Journal of Consulting and Clinical Psychology*, *90*(3), 282–288. https://doi.org/10.1037/ccp0000719

Singh, J. P., Desmarais, S. L., Hurducas, C., Arbach-Lucioni, K., Condemarin, C., Dean, K., Doyle, M., Folino, J. O., Godoy-Cervera, V., Grann, M., Ho, R. M. Y., Large, M. M., Nielsen, L. H., Pham, T. H., Rebocho, M. F., Reeves, K. A., Rettenberger, M., de Ruiter, C., Seewald, K., & Otto, R. K. (2014). International perspectives on the practical application of violence risk assessment: A global survey of 44 countries. *International Journal of Forensic Mental Health*, *13*(3), 193–206. https://doi.org/10.1080/14999013.2014.922141

Skeem, J., Kennealy, P., Monahan, J., Peterson, J., & Appelbaum, P. (2016). Psychosis uncommonly and inconsistently precedes violence among high-risk individuals. *Clinical Psychological Science*, *4*(1), 40–49. https://doi.org/10.1177/2167702615575879

Skeem, J. L., Manchak, S., & Peterson, J. K. (2011). Correctional policy for offenders with mental illness: Creating a new paradigm for recidivism reduction. *Law and Human Behavior*, *35*(2), 110–126. https://doi.org/10.1007/s10979-010-9223-7

Skeem, J. L., Steadman, H. J., & Manchak, S. M. (2015). Applicability of the risk-need-responsivity model to persons with mental illness involved in the criminal justice system. *Psychiatric Services (Washington, D.C.)*, *66*(9), 916–922. https://doi.org/10.1176/appi.ps.201400448

Skeem, J. L., Winter, E., Kennealy, P. J., Louden, J. E., & Tatar, J. R., 2nd (2014). Offenders with mental illness have criminogenic needs, too: Toward recidivism reduction. *Law and Human Behavior*, *38*(3), 212–224. https://doi.org/10.1037/lhb0000054

Steadman, H. J., Mulvey, E. P., Monahan, J., Robbins, P. C., Appelbaum, P. S., Grisso, T., Roth, L. H., & Silver, E. (1998). Violence by people discharged from acute psychiatric inpatient facilities and by others in the same neighborhoods. *Archives of General Psychiatry*, *55*(5), 393–401. https://doi.org/10.1001/archpsyc.55.5.393

Swanson, J. W., Holzer, C. E., Ganju, V. K., & Jono, R. T. (1990). Violence and psychiatric disorder in the community: Evidence from the epidemiologic catchment area surveys. *Hospital and Community Psychiatry*, *41*, 761–770.

The Change Companies (n.d.) *The courage to change*. Carson City, NV: Author.

West, M. L., Vayshenker, B., Rotter, M., & Yanos, P. T. (2015). The influence of mental illness and criminality self-stigmas and racial self-concept on outcomes in a forensic psychiatric sample. *Psychiatric Rehabilitation Journal*, *38*(2), 150–157. https://doi.org/10.1037/prj0000133

Wolff, N., Morgan, R. D., Shi, J., Huening, J., & Fisher, W. H. (2011). Thinking styles and emotional states of male and female prison inmates by mental disorder status. *Psychiatric Services (Washington, D.C.)*, *62*(12), 1485–1493. https://doi.org/10.1176/appi.ps.000432011

7 Community Reintegration of Long-Term, Psychiatrically Hospitalized Forensic Patients

Heidi Camerlengo, Louis Martelli, and Nancy Fenning

Legally involved, psychiatric patients often spend a significant amount of time institutionalized due to the severity of their charges as well as the many obstacles to discharge that they encounter within the state psychiatric hospital and judicial systems. In the United States in 2020, there were approximately 40,000 patients utilizing an inpatient psychiatric bed, 60% of whom were classified as forensic (National Association of State Mental Health Program Directors Research Institute, 2020). While discharge planning technically begins from the day a patient enters the hospital system, forensic psychiatric patients, such as those who have been designated not guilty by reason of insanity (NGRI), incompetent to stand trial (IST), or who have committed sex offenses, typically spend significantly more time than the average civilly committed patient waiting for this to occur. In some cases, the wait for discharge planning can be decades. According to Finch (2014), in the United States, the average length of stay for patients adjudicated NGRI ranged from months to years, while civilly committed patients were typically hospitalized for one week to 10 days. Furthermore, in his same study, Finch (2014) found that patients in the United States adjudicated Guilty But Mentally Ill remained institutionalized anywhere from two months to 20 years based on data provided by four states.

As a result, it is challenging to reconnect this longer-term, institutionalized population with the larger community and to assist them with successfully transitioning into a more independent and self-satisfying lifestyle while remaining psychiatrically stable. Forensic psychiatric patients frequently have concerns about reentering the community after prolonged periods of institutionalization, in part because of rapidly changing societal norms and the ever-increasing difficulty of effectively performing essential life tasks in this evolving world. One way to address these concerns is through participation in community exposure programs that provide a supportive bridge for forensic patients to safely begin this frequently complex and anxiety-provoking process, a process that is often overlooked during discharge planning.

DOI: 10.4324/9781003360926-10

This chapter will discuss the creation and implementation of one such program, the *Community Reintegration Group*, a group designed and co-facilitated by the authors to focus on these critical needs. Grounded in extensive, personal, clinical experience, "*Community Group*" as it came to be known, offered legally involved psychiatric patients' opportunities to gain vital knowledge and skills to increase the likelihood of successful reintegration through involvement in structured community outings facilitated by treatment team members familiar with each participant.

The experiences and support provided in the *Community Group* were aimed at assisting this population with the development of appropriate independent living and socialization skills in conjunction with improved self-awareness and quality of life. The ultimate goals of this group were to help legally involved patients achieve discharge and reduce rates of rehospitalization and criminal recidivism. Over time, the *Community Group* evolved into a unit-wide program, involving clinical, nursing and direct-care staff and forensic patients at every level of functioning, motivating them to focus their energies on discharge rather than succumb to institutionalization. Patients' friends and family became involved with the *Community Group* as well, joining scheduled activities and attending annual functions in an effort to build and strengthen community connections and interpersonal relationships. In addition to the above dimensions of the group, this chapter will include a discussion of the unanticipated outcomes of the group and measures of its effectiveness, the systemic challenges that needed to be overcome, and the administrative and other supports necessary to ensure the success of a program such as *Community Group*, both in terms of stated outcomes and general safety. Finally, ideas for group sustainability will be presented for consideration.

There is a paucity of empirical research demonstrating the effectiveness of therapeutic groups that provide modeling and in vivo learning experiences to enable long-term, legally involved, psychiatric patients to practice critical independent living, socialization and leisure skills in order to promote a successful transition from the highly structured forensic hospital to the community setting. While much forensic inpatient treatment centers around participation in therapeutic groups, the majority of these groups are based within the confines of the hospital. This restriction severely limits patients' exposure to larger society and the many changes that occur outside the hospital over time, something individuals outside of this system may take for granted. As this segregation persists, successful community reintegration becomes increasingly more challenging since this population not only has the typical discharge issues to manage, such as adapting to a new community, they often have judicial obligations as well, which must be factored into the mix. The typical forensic inpatient spends many years confined to an institution. The amount of world change that can occur during this period, for example, COVID-19-related changes that began in 2020, is astounding.

At the same time that we were learning about obstacles to discharging people from our forensic unit and attempting to strategize remedies for these obstacles, our institution was actively implementing programmatic changes to address patient discharge in response to the U.S. Supreme Court's 1999 Olmstead decision (U.S. Department of Health & Human Services, 2018). According to Olmstead, unjustly segregating people with disabilities is a form of discrimination; therefore, states are responsible for providing community-based services to facilitate community reintegration of this population and avoid unnecessary institutionalization. Thus, the Olmstead decision was an additional impetus for us to create a community exposure experience for our long-term, forensic patients to promote positive attitudes and planful, graduated movement toward discharge.

Discharge planning for forensic psychiatric patients often involves a series of steps toward lower levels of supervision. On the hospital grounds, this may include transfers to less restrictive units and increasing unsupervised off-unit activities. This may also include supervised and, in some settings, unsupervised off-ground activities. Patients' success with increasing independence is required before more active forms of discharge planning are initiated (for example, locating housing and securing aftercare services). All of these measures are designed to address risk reduction and increase the likelihood of a safe community transition. While civilly committed patients often navigate through their hospitalization and are discharged to the community faster than forensic psychiatric patients, it can be argued that the average legally involved patient is better prepared for return to the community as a result of receiving significantly more active treatment due to their longer hospitalization. As forensic patients progress toward leaving the hospital, the programming focus shifts to providing them with more opportunities to develop and hone their independent living skills with the hope that discharge will one day come to fruition.

The *Community Group* was developed by seasoned clinicians working on a 40-bed, inpatient male forensic/psychiatric unit in the Northeast region of the United States. After nearly a decade of observing and working with these long-term, hospitalized patients, we witnessed them develop a fear of leaving the hospital due to the familiarity and comfort that it provided, lose hope for their future, and ultimately disengage from treatment, thus succumbing to their situation. Some of these patients became suicidal or unleashed their frustrations on peers and staff in the form of verbally aggressive and violent outbursts, thus causing even more isolation from their immediate environment and, in some cases, additional legal problems or time added to their involuntary commitment status.

Group members were initially selected by unit staff and treatment team consensus based on such factors as their current level of supervision, mental status, frequency and participation in programs, adherence to unit policies and procedures, including medication administration and activities of daily living, and general conduct among peers and staff on the unit. These standards remained the benchmark upon which future members were evaluated for inclusion in the *Community Group*, as safety was the paramount concern. Additionally, for those patients adjudicated IST and NGRI or who fell under Megan's Law due to a sex offense, the approval of the hospital's and division's forensic oversight committees was mandatory prior to participation in any community trips. NGRI patients also required Superior Court orders specifying not only the level(s) of supervision that they were permitted but also the activities within which they were allowed to engage (i.e., off-ground activities). Every team member involved with *Community Group* ensured that court authorization was in place and that approvals by the forensic oversight committees were obtained so that group members could engage in the planned group activities. Such attention to detail helped us to avoid placing ourselves or our institution in a position of contempt by violating participants' court-ordered privileges.

As success is typically the best way to increase the likelihood of continuance, we kept the *Community Group* small at first (three members), with 1:1 supervision provided by the authors. When considering facilitators for the group, it made sense to utilize those hospital staff who were integrally familiar with the patients and responsible for providing treatment and discharge planning. Thus, the team's psychologist (HC), treatment team leader (LM), and social worker (NF) were self-selected for these roles. At the time, this type of interdisciplinary collaboration was a unique feature of our group since the majority of available treatment modalities offered at the hospital were provided in a discipline-specific format. The *Community Group's* inaugural trip consisted of a three-hour visit to the local library, where each member was assisted with obtaining a library card and provided with a tour of the facility. Members were encouraged to identify a subject of interest and check-out media in their chosen area for which they were responsible to return at the next group outing. After several months of incident-free group excursions, we began to add a luncheon to the trip at a mutually agreed upon venue as an incentive to existing and potential group members. For many of these members, the ability to choose a restaurant and order their own food was a significant motivator, as a common complaint of hospitalized patients is poor food quality and a lack of dietary options.

To prepare for events where funding was necessary, patients were assisted with budgeting their monthly stipends and income that they earned by participating in the hospital's vocational rehabilitation program. As the group progressed, members were required to demonstrate the ability to independently manage monies needed for community trips. They were provided with individualized instruction if needed. Failure to appropriately maintain their budget resulted in additional training on money management strategies and, if necessary, temporary suspension from off-ground group activities unless there were extenuating circumstances, such as a Social Security check that had not cleared. In those rare cases, a petty cash fund was maintained and used to cover expenses.

Once the *Community Group* had been running successfully on a monthly basis for six months, we decided to expand the membership and offer three additional patients the opportunity to participate, as well as diversify the locations that we visited to include a balance of skill development and social/leisure activities. The group was being discussed on the unit, even by those patients who seemed unaware of their surroundings and others who were unmotivated to engage in any type of programming. As a result, we began to feel more assured about the positive effects of our hands-on approach. Our approach itself seemed to engender patient interest and cooperation since, at the time, it was unusual for psychiatrically hospitalized forensic patients to participate in activities with treatment team members outside of the secure forensic hospital setting. It was also rewarding to experience the increasingly relaxed atmosphere created among facilitators and patients during the *Community Group* outings that prompted members to remark that the group "Made us feel like normal people again." Research has shown that providing this population with such normalizing experiences helps to reduce the stigma associated with mental illness, develop resistance to prejudice and increase the likelihood of successful reintegration (Dubreucq et al., 2022; Zheng et al., 2022).

With confidence high, we began including existing members in a collaborative process of nominating and selecting new group participants. Group members also helped impart necessary information regarding group rules and norms consistent with concepts fundamental to evidence-based, peer support programs that utilize peer specialists with similar experiences to provide services (Addo et al., 2022; Baron, 2011; Barrenger et al., 2020). Such programs have been found useful in assisting psychiatric patients to adjust to their communities, promote recovery, and improve quality of life (Bellamy et al., 2017; Yokoyama et al., 2022). Our goal during this collaboration was to model a rational and unbiased decision-making process while emphasizing the qualities we felt were important for group membership. We hoped that our standards would be influential in reinforcing these positive qualities and behaviors for both existing and future *Community Group* members. Fortunately, our methods were successful.

Group members started to internalize these standards and display increasing self-assurance and diplomacy; subsequently, the culture of the unit began to change in positive ways. For example, more reclusive patients began to take an interest in the activities that the *Community Group* was planning for the month and started asking group members questions as well as bringing up the topic during daily unit meetings. Additionally, negative incidents, such as contraband possession, arguments, and assaults, decreased.

Suddenly, many patients on the unit who had previously seemed disengaged or uninterested in programming began asking how they, too, could become a part of this experience. Thus began the expansion of the group through monthly community excursions. Additional weekly groups were held on the unit to prepare for future groups as well as to begin initiating prospective members to the rules and expectations of the group. Current *Community Group* members were integrally involved in this process and, at times, served as co-facilitators, introducing new members to the group and sharing the rules and norms by which it operated, as well as assuming the role of mentors.

After a year of *Community Group* operation, we decided to further expand the experience to include more members (maximum of eight), make it a full-day event (seven hours), and include direct-care staff to further enhance unit-wide investment in the program. Members began to decide by way of a majority vote about preferred activities consistent with the group's goals for community reintegration. We required that activities include an educational component, such as visiting a museum or county agency to increase community connection and awareness of available resources; a shopping experience (usually Walmart or other types of discount stores) to practice myriad skills related to selecting and purchasing items within a budget; and leisure elements, such as bowling or going to a park, because hospitalized forensic patients often forget how to have genuine fun. Consistent with empirically derived models for the development of independent living skills (MacKain & Streveler, 1990; Sanchez et al., 2016; Wallace et al., 2000), knowledge and skills consequent to participation in the *Community*

Group included, but were not limited to:

- Budgeting and money management
- Comparison shopping and use of coupons
- Banking and ATM use
- Use of computers
- Introduction to community resources (Social Security, DMV, self-help centers)
- Use of public transportation and community navigation

- Food shopping and meal preparation
- Ordering from a menu and tipping
- Cultural and historical appreciation
- Time management and scheduling
- Socialization and leisure
- Planning and decision-making
- Impulse control and limit-setting
- Self-awareness and personal empowerment

Examples of the *Community Group* activities that afforded members opportunities to develop and practice the aforementioned skills included visits to:

- County self-help centers
- County vital records
- Social Security Administration
- United States Post Office
- Farmer's markets/thrift stores
- Shopping malls
- Grocery stores
- State planetarium
- Battleship New Jersey
- State aquarium
- Local, non-profit zoos
- State and local museums
- National wildlife refuges
- Historic Smithville Village
- Beach and boardwalk
- Minor league baseball game
- Bowling
- Movies

Upon the group's return from community outings, all members were required to submit their receipts and calculate the day's spending to determine if they remained within their budget. At one time, group members were permitted to purchase items for peers who were unable to leave the unit or were awaiting their turn in the group; however, due to concerns with the potential misuse of funds and contraband possession, this practice was stopped by hospital administration despite the multitude of benefits that it had on group members' self-esteem and unit morale, as well as reinforcing many of the skills consistent with group goals. Post-group discussions were also held to facilitate feedback from participants about the usefulness of reintegration activities and troubleshoot any difficulties encountered by the *Community Group* members. We also used this time to celebrate members' accomplishments toward treatment goals that they achieved through group participation, such as identifying a community in which to pursue discharge or learning how to use an ATM machine.

As *Community Group* became established, camaraderie among some of the senior members developed since, together, they had faced new, formerly daunting experiences related to hospital discharge and were successful in their endeavors. In response to these successes, members expressed feeling more confident in their ability to navigate life outside of the hospital and were significantly more motivated to pursue discharge. We, ourselves, experienced growing levels of trust with group members. This trust was implemented therapeutically, translating to increasingly independent community activities, allowing group members to utilize skills learned through the group within a culture of safety. For example, during some outings, the *Community Group* was broken down into smaller groups of two to three patients that were led by senior members with a staff member available on the periphery if guidance was needed. These subgroups were given a time frame within which to "independently" conduct their business, whether it was to shop for desired items, get a "real" haircut, or walk about the mall or beach.

The first time that we enacted this model, there was some trepidation as to how members would handle any dissent with the subgroup's agenda and how their decision-making process would meet each patient's individual needs. On a practical level, we also hoped not to lose anyone during these more independent activities! It was rewarding to observe members engage in egalitarian processes (voting), much like the processes that we modeled for them when making decisions concerning *Community Group* functioning. We also observed a host of prosocial behaviors among our members that research has shown are crucial aspects of recovery from mental illness (Bjorlykhaug et al., 2021; Kapse, 2016) and serve as protective factors for reducing criminal behavior (Swinkels et al., 2020). For example, group members began to socialize more with one another on the unit and develop deeper, increasingly personal relationships that, in some cases, have been maintained despite each person being discharged to their respective communities.

The *Community Group* alumni also remained connected with current members and were invited to join the group at monthly events. For example, several alumni met the group at a mall food court and shared a meal while discussing their very personal journeys since being discharged from the hospital. It was inspiring for current legally involved patients to see how their discharged peers successfully managed similar judicial issues while balancing the many demands of court-ordered aftercare services and monitoring. An event that stands out for the authors concerns one of our long-term, forensic patients who had been institutionalized for nearly 20 years before achieving discharge. He was one of the founding members of the *Community Group* and wanted to give back to his peers and the group because of how rewarding the experience had been for him. This generous man invited the entire group to his apartment, cooked us a full-course meal, and candidly shared the many challenges and successes that he had encountered since his discharge. It was a fun and educational time for all participants, as we were able to ask questions and experience directly what it was like for a former, long-term, forensic patient to survive and thrive in his new community environment...and the food was fantastic!

One of the most popular *Community Group* activities was the annual family picnic that was usually held during the month of June at a local park where there were picnic facilities, a river in which to fish (many of our members were avid fishermen), and ample open space where one could reconnect with nature. In order to make it a more family-like experience, the authors volunteered to prepare the dishes that were selected and voted on by group members. Every participant (including group facilitators and staff) contributed their share of money toward the final cost, and we also collectively decided how to cover the expense of additional guests such as the graduates of the *Community Group* and family members of current and former participants.

Each group member was given a responsibility for the picnic commensurate with their individual capabilities to facilitate their success in making a positive contribution to the event. For example, members were assigned to fill coolers with ice, ensure that we had all necessary supplies, load the van, or perform waste management. We found that the buddy system worked well in organizing larger groups of forensic patients so that there was a senior peer readily available to newer members for consultation and support if necessary. It also assisted us in keeping track of folks, especially as the size of the group and the number of its guests increased. During our tenure as facilitators, we are happy to report that we did not have any negative incidents while out in the community with our group, nor did we lose anyone! All participants, including alumni and family members, were encouraged to respect patient confidentiality consistent with group norms. To date, we are not aware of any breaches of such protected information by group participants or guests.

Similar to the findings of Birt and Klingenberg (2022), who developed a creative arts therapy group as a means to promote long-term psychiatric patients' interest in and preparedness for discharge, the *Community Group* alumni completed a written questionnaire and telephone interview

(NF) in 2022, revealing some of the more personally meaningful outcomes of the group:

- The feeling of freedom and relief experienced while away from the forensic hospital, where there is minimal choice for patients
- The development of a sense of dignity for being courageous and venturing into the "unknown" community
- Learning the ability to adapt to new and changing circumstances and feeling more comfortable reaching out for assistance when needed
- Reducing the feeling of prejudice against people with mental illness who have committed crimes
- Encouraging patients to keep a positive frame of mind while hospitalized and engendering hope
- Providing motivation to gain hospital oversight committee and court permission for increased privileges for movement toward discharge

Former members described *Community Group* as providing a very normalizing experience that allowed them to feel more comfortable and less paranoid outside of the forensic hospital and gave them multiple opportunities to see what resources were available in the various communities that they were considering for discharge. There was a consensus among group alumni that these experiences were instrumental in moving them toward discharge and helping them to avoid rehospitalization by teaching them how to stay connected with community providers and effectively communicate their needs. Of the 70 legally involved, psychiatric patients who participated in community trips during the group's eight-year tenure (2008–2016), 97% achieved discharge while only 16% were re-hospitalized as of the group's termination. Furthermore, of the 11 patients who returned to the state hospital, only two (3% of the total group) had incurred additional legal charges. This is well below national averages for similar legally involved, psychiatric populations (Finch, 2014).

We are proud to share that some of the *Community Group* alumni have purchased or leased their own homes and vehicles, have returned to school, have earned their real estate license, have resolved their legal situations and/or maxed out on their NGRI status, and have obtained and maintained part- and/or full-time employment. In one case, a group graduate worked his way off of state and federal subsidies and is now fully self-supporting. Additionally, some of our alumni have become integrally involved in their communities, for example, by becoming members of their local churches and self-help centers, including Alcoholics Anonymous and Narcotics Anonymous, volunteering at the Salvation Army, or providing transportation and meals to neighbors in need.

In addition to the many benefits of the *Community Group*, some unanticipated outcomes that we view as further demonstrations of the program's effectiveness are that during their hospitalization, members became viewed as unit leaders and, as such, took responsibility for reinforcing a positive milieu consistent with institutional policies and regulations. They were regularly called upon by staff and peers alike to offer their input on changes to unit functioning, selecting group activities, nominating future group members, and addressing patient concerns that arose both on the unit and within the group.

Moreover, group members became unit ambassadors, welcoming new patients and orienting them to the forensic hospital and the way in which to go about appropriately getting their individual needs met. Such hospitality and ongoing support provided by respected peers became an integral part of increasing patient unity and reducing violence. During the active phase of the *Community Group*, there was a reduction in the number of negative behavioral incidents, including restraint episodes, that occurred on the unit. For example, our unit was the only one in the entire hospital that went restraint-free for several consecutive months at essential times, largely due to the efforts of the patients, many of whom were in some stage of preparedness for group admittance. Informal discussions with unit residents revealed that nobody wanted to risk jeopardizing their eligibility for *Community Group* membership or discharge planning, nor did they desire to incur additional legal charges by getting involved in a fight or other reportable offense. Additionally, the negotiation skills learned by members, in part because of their group participation, helped to quell incidents before they became more difficult to manage.

In order to implement such a potentially risky program as the *Community Group*, it is critical to have the support of hospital administration. I (HC) sometimes humorously reflect on the reaction of those in charge of the forensic unit when I and my fellow team members (LM and NF) requested to take some of our violent offenders on a trip into the community in order to find new and creative ways to prepare and motivate them toward discharge. Luckily, at the time that we were designing the *Community Group*, not only was our institution actively responding to the Olmstead Decision, but our building was also managed by a fellow psychologist who understood the benefits of reintroducing this population to life outside of institutional walls and was not averse to the risks inherent in such a project. He was instrumental in giving us the endorsement to begin developing this experiential group and also in arranging for us to have regular, monthly access to a 15-passenger van for transportation as well as staff coverage on the unit when we took the group on our trips. After the group was established, our administrator authorized the release of patients' funds to cover their expenses for group activities, and he advocated for the *Community Group* to have official status within the therapeutic program scheduling system so that participants would get credit for their attendance.

Other supports that were essential to the *Community Group's* survival included an investment in the group by the direct-care staff members, who often felt empowered by the inclusive group process and were quick to report any concerns with a patient's ability to safely participate in group activities. Their involvement also helped to limit any animosity or jealousy experienced by non-group members through their reinforcement of the expectations for group inclusion. Equally important was the willingness of psychiatric and nursing staff to write off-ground group orders and change medication administration times for patients who were with us on community trips. Unfortunately, as within any large institution, administrative staff change, and so do executive priorities as well as tolerance for the risk associated with endeavors of this nature. When such changes occur, we have found it vital to involve hospital discipline heads sympathetic to our project who are also in positions of power to authorize its continuation and allocate the necessary resources for optimal functioning.

During one such administrative challenge to the group's existence, we enlisted the support of the Director of Psychology, who accompanied us on a community outing to see for himself how this program prepared its members for successful discharge. Our team psychiatrist, who was responsible for recommending and ordering patients' discharges, also supported the group for its usefulness in providing a means for clinicians to directly evaluate participants' discharge readiness and their individual strengths and challenges in this area for treatment planning and aftercare purposes.

Since the creation of the *Community Group*, the authors have moved on to other positions within the state and one of us has retired (NF). Unfortunately, the *Community Group* did not survive these changes despite its demonstrated effectiveness. One way to keep such programs running in anticipation of changes to staffing is to prepare new group facilitators by having them participate in unit-based groups and community trips to meet current members and experience first-hand how the group works. In this way, seasoned facilitators and participants can assist with the orientation process and avoid lapses in services. The authors also wish that we had developed a formal group curriculum and a detailed program manual to train new staff on the intricacies of group operation and to assist treatment team members with incorporating the *Community Group* goals and objectives into individualized treatment planning. Finally, we recognize the lost opportunity for comprehensive data collection in order to more accurately capture descriptive information concerning the participants, the nature and extent of their group participation, and their individual treatment outcomes, including length of time until discharged and rehospitalization/criminal recidivism rates.

Despite the dissolution of the *Community Group*, the authors remain a source of support and mentorship for seven group alumni who have remained successfully living in their respective communities anywhere from 3½ years up to 15 years and counting since they were originally discharged from the hospital. Several of these alumni are in regular contact with us, occasionally meeting for lunch as the unofficial *Alumni Group* and keeping us up to date with their progress as well as any challenges they may have encountered during the process of their community reintegration. This unique and underutilized component in forensic mental health care is crucially important for providing continuity, especially for newly discharged patients, many of whom have lost contact with family and friends after years of institutionalization and have a need for familiar and trusted people in their lives. Several group alumni have told us how important these mentorship relationships are to their continued progress and reduced anxiety in dealing with community-related and legal issues. In fact, 100% of the *Community Group* alumni agreed that the interpersonal relationships that they developed with the authors and their peers have helped to sustain their hope for continued success and have provided a positive support network within which to share their personal recovery stories and challenges and keep motivated to remain stable and avoid further legal problems. When engaging in such mentoring activities, it is vitally important to keep in mind one's ethical responsibilities so that everyone involved has a clear understanding of the clinicians' roles, professional responsibilities, and personal boundaries. Equally important when participating in these activities is maintaining an awareness of personal safety.

Research concerning outcomes of evidence-based programs for assisting mentally ill and legally involved patients with remaining stable in the community, such as Assertive Community Treatment (McKenna et al., 2015; Mohn, 2020), and its newer outgrowth, FACT; Forensic Assertive Community Treatment (Landess & Holoyda, 2017) stresses several important factors facilitating successful discharge and reducing episodes of psychiatric decompensation, hospitalization, and incarceration. An important factor is having a network of providers readily available to this population in order to troubleshoot issues and to provide support and encouragement when obstacles are encountered. Goulet et al. (2022) provided a systematic review and meta-analysis of the effectiveness of FACT programs among individuals with both mental illness and justice involvement. They found increased outpatient service utilization by participants as well as improved legal outcomes, such as less time spent incarcerated. Cusack et al. (2010)

also found that FACT participants had fewer days of hospitalization than clients receiving regular, non-forensic aftercare services, fewer bookings, and an increased likelihood of avoiding incarceration. Similar to Swinkels et al.'s (2020) concept of forensic network coaching, community exposure programs that incorporate this type of mentorship component can be an effective mechanism for enhancing the connection between discharged forensic patients and local FACT or similar aftercare programs, further supporting continuity in care.

Challenges to discharge for long-term, forensic psychiatric inpatients can be steadily conquered by incorporating experiential, community-based groups into the hospital's "programming as usual." While there are potential risks to any treatment modality of this type, it is hoped that administrators of institutions serving legally involved patients will recognize and value the many benefits derived by group participants. Such benefits include increased willingness to pursue discharge, improved self-confidence in community living, the ability to sustain social connections, adherence to post-discharge treatment, and a lack of criminal recidivism. These are some of the noteworthy outcomes of the *Community Group* that could be easily replicated in similar forensic psychiatric settings with proper administrative assistance. It is incumbent upon us as clinicians to advocate for initiatives of this type, not only to support patients' individual accomplishments in transitioning from forensic psychiatric hospitals to the community but also to prepare them to the greatest extent possible for the resumption of a more autonomous and fulfilling life outside of institutional care. The *Community Group* has proven to be one successful way to support this process.

References

Addo, R., Ginder, V., & Nedegaard, R. (2022). The role of peer support in recovery from psychiatric symptoms; A moderation analysis. *Community Mental Health Journal*, 58: 1141–1145. https://doi.org/10.1007/s10597-021-00923-5

Baron, R. (2011). *Forensic peer specialists: An emerging workforce.* New Brunswick, NJ: Center for Behavioral Health Services & Criminal Justice Research: Rutgers, State University of New Jersey. http://tucollaborative.org/wp-content/uploads/2017/03/Forensic-Peer-Specialists-An-Emerging-Workforce.pdf

Barrenger, S.L., Maurer, K., Moore, K.L., & Hong, I. (2020). Mental health recovery: Peer specialists with mental health and incarceration experiences. *American Journal of Orthopsychiatry*, 90(4): 479–488.

Bellamy, C., Schmutte, T., & Davidson, L. (2017). An update on the growing evidence for peer support. *Mental Health and Social Inclusion*, 21(3): 161–167.

Birt, D., & Klingenberg, J. (2022). Community reintegration of long-term psychiatric patients through a creative arts rehabilitation therapy group. *Journal of Applied Rehabilitation and Counseling*, 53(2): 150–158.

Bjorlykhaug, K.I., Karlsson, B., Hesook, S.K., & Kleppe, L.C., (2021). Social support and recovery from mental health problems: A scoping review. *Nordic Social Work Research*. https://doi.org/10.1080/2156857X.2020.1868553

Cusack, K.J., Morrissey, J.P., Cuddeback, G.S., Prins, A., Williams, D.M., (2010). Criminal justice involvement, behavioral health service use, and costs of forensic assertive community treatment: A randomized trial. *Journal of Community Mental Health*, 46: 356–363.

Dubreucq, J., Gabayet, F., Couhet, G., Demily, C., Guillard-Bouhet, N., Gouache, B., Legrand, G., Pommier, R., Quiles, C., Straub, D., Verdoux, H., Vignaga, F., & Franck, N., (2022). Stigma resistance is associated with advanced stages of personal recovery in serious mental illness: Patients enrolled in psychiatric rehabilitation. *Psychological Medicine*, 52(11): 2155–2165.

Finch, L.W., (2014). Assessment #3: Forensic mental health services in the United States: 2014. Alexandria, VA: National Association of State Mental Health Program Directors. https://www.nasmhpd.org/sites/default/files/Assessment%203%20-20Updated%20Forensic%20Mental%20Health%20Services.pdf

Goulet, M.H., Dellazizzo, L., Lesage, A., Crocker, A.G., & Dumais, A., (2022). Effectiveness of forensic assertive community treatment on forensic and health outcomes: A systemic review and meta-analysis. *Criminal Justice and Behavior*, 49(6): 838–852.

Kapse, P.P., (2016). Efficacy of social skills training among persons with schizophrenia. *International Journal of Psychosocial Rehabilitation*, 20(1): 45–50.

Landess, J., & Holoyda, B., (2017). Mental health courts and forensic assertive community treatment teams as correctional diversion programs. *Behavioral Sciences & the Law*, 35: 501–511. Retrieved from https://doi.org/10.10002/bsl.2307.

MacKain, S.J., & Streveler, A., (1990). Social and independent living skills for psychiatric patients in a prison setting, *Behavior Modification*, 14(4): 490–515.

McKenna, B., Skipworth, J. Tapsell, R., Madell, D., Pillai, K., Simpson, A., Cavney, J., & Rouse, P. (2015). A prison mental health in-reach model informed by assertive community treatment principles: Evaluation of its impact on planning during the pre-release period, community mental health service engagement and reoffending. *Criminal Behaviour and Mental Health*, 25: 429–439.

Mohn, E. (2020). Assertive community treatment (ACT). *Salem Press Encyclopedia of Health*.

National Association of State Mental Health Program Directors Research Institute. (2020). Use of State Psychiatric Hospitals, NRI's 2020–2021 State Profiles. www.nri-inc.org

Sanchez, J., Chan, F., Yaghmaian, R., Johnson, E.T., Pfaller, J.S., & Umucu, E., (2016). Assessing community functioning and independent living skills of individuals with severe mental illness. *Journal of Applied Rehabilitation Counseling*, 47(3): 6–14.

Swinkels, L.T.A., van der Pol, T.M., Popma, A., ter Harmsel, J.F., & Kekker, J.J., (2020). Improving mental wellbeing of forensic psychiatric outpatients through the addition of an informal social network intervention to treatment as usual: A randomized controlled trial. *BMC Psychiatry*, 20(418): 1–15. https://doiorg/10/1186/s12888-020-02819-2

U.S. Department of Health and Human Services, Office for Civil Rights (2018). *Serving people with disabilities in the most integrated setting: Community living and Olmstead.* https://www.hhs.gov/civil-rights/for-individuals/special-topics/community-living-and-olmstead/index.html

Wallace, C.J., Liberman, R.P., Tauber, R., & Wallace, J., (2000). The independent living skills survey: A comprehensive measure of the community functioning of severely and persistently mentally ill individuals. *Schizophrenia Bulletin*, 26(3): 631–658.

Yokoyama, K., Miyajima, R., Morimoto, R., Ichihara-Takeda, S., Yoshino, J., Matusyama, K., & Ikeda, N., (2022). Peer support formation and the promotion of recovery among people using psychiatric day care in Japan. *Community Mental Health Journal*, 58: 78–86. https://doi.org/10/1007/s10597-021-00793-x

Zheng, S.S., Zhang, H., Li, X., & Chang, K., (2022). Why I stay in community psychiatric rehabilitation: A semi-structured survey in person with schizophrenia. *BMC Psychology*, 10(1): 213. https://doi.org/10.1186/s40359-022-00919-0

8 Psychological Intervention with Adolescents with Sexual Behavior Problems

Ricardo Barroso, Eduarda Ramião, Daniel Mendonça, and Patrícia Figueiredo

Introduction

Sexual violence easily evokes a strong emotional response, given the severe impact and control actions exerted on the victims (Ryan et al., 2018). A study by Lieberman et al. (2003) on perceived moral wrongness found that child sexual abuse is perceived as a more severe crime than homicide. For this reason, several international institutions (e.g., the World Health Organization, the European Union) have been recognizing the impact of this problem, requiring not only an urgent and adjusted professional intervention or new on-site research but also requiring concrete and specialized policies to combat the problem. This includes both the standardization of psychological assessment procedures and the need to implement specialized interventions (Barroso et al., 2018, 2020, 2022).

From the point of view of clinical sexology, sexual behaviors can be defined as either normative or atypical, and the latter can have deviant and criminal characteristics (Bancroft et al., 2004; Worling, 2012). Normative and atypical/deviant sexual interests reflect two ends of a continuum along which individuals may engage in risky sexual behaviors and experience sexual difficulties. Regarding atypical sexual behaviors in adolescents, it is possible to find three distinct groups, namely individuals with coercive sexual interests or peer/adult offenders, child sexual offenders, and adolescents with pedophilic sexual interests (Barroso et al., 2016, 2018).

Adolescents who engage in sexually abusive behaviors are a diverse group of individuals (Barroso et al., 2019, 2022). Behavior, by itself, does not define the acts that comprise sexual aggression. The relationships, dynamics, and impact of these behaviors should also be considered. This polymorphism is reflected through the type of aggression or behavior (e.g., rape, child sexual abuse, and pedophilic interests, among others), as well as through the offenders' specificities, such as gender, age, the intentions that lead to the deviant behavior, and other individual characteristics (Aebi et al., 2013; Malin et al., 2014; Ramião et al., 2023).

DOI: 10.4324/9781003360926-11

Despite this typological differentiation of adolescents who have committed sexual offenses, it is important to note the existence of versatility at this level. In other words, some individuals may only commit a single offense throughout their lives. Others, known as specialized offenders, may commit several similar sexual crimes. Another group, called versatile/generalist offenders, may commit several different offenses, be they of a sexual nature, related to theft or robbery, or possibly related to substance trafficking (Harris et al., 2009). The varied characteristics of offenders and the range of factors related to their behavior must be taken into account in the psychological assessment and intervention process.

Conceptual and Theoretical Models of Sexual Violence

An intervention program should be empirically supported by theoretical models. These theoretical models allow for a better understanding of this phenomenon and, at the same time, support the interventions considered most effective.

Risk-Need-Responsivity Model

In Andrews and Bonta's (2010) original conception, the primary aim identified in the Risk-Need-Responsivity Model (RNR) is to ensure that interventions with at-risk populations are effective in reducing recidivism rates. As the name suggests, the principles of *Risk*, *Necessity,* and *Responsiveness* stand out in this theoretical model. The *Risk* principle assumes that the intensity of interventions is adjusted to the level of risk presented by sexual offenders. The intensity is defined by the length and frequency of clinical intervention and supervision. Thus, more intense levels of intervention should be applied to individuals who have a high risk of reoffending, while a low intensity of intervention should be applied to individuals with a lower recidivism risk.

Regarding the *Necessity* principle, interventions must be focused on appropriate factors related to criminal behavior, i.e., specific risk factors, for the purpose of decreasing the risk of recidivism (Andrews & Bonta, 2010). In contrast, non-criminal needs should not be targeted so that the focus of intervention is not diverted. Specifically, the criminal needs of SO include risk factors such as sexual deviance and an antisocial lifestyle. Finally, according to the *Responsiveness* principal, the intervention should be applied in ways consistent with the individual's specific characteristics (e.g., culture, personality, cognitive skills, and language; Andrews & Bonta, 2010). Therefore, the treatment should not be static and standardized. It is important that the treatment has a flexible character and is adapted to the individual's characteristics and skills to maximize the effectiveness.

Although the RNR model has strong empirical support, some authors (Ward & Stewart, 2003; Ward & Gannon, 2006; Ward et al., 2007b) suggest that certain additional factors should be considered. It is essential, for example, to associate the therapeutic alliance with this model, given its relevance in any interventional process, including interventions with adolescents who have committed sexual offenses (Marshall et al., 2003; Yates, 2003). Another important factor is that, even if not directly related to the risk factor for recidivism, it is important to address certain non-criminal dimensions, such as motivation and low self-esteem (Ward & Stewart, 2003).

Cognitive-Behavioral Model

Intervention programs with adolescents who have committed sexual offenses have been planned based mostly on the theoretical model of cognitive-behavioral therapy (CBT) (Hanson et al., 2002; Lösel & Schmucker, 2005). This therapeutic model was developed based on behavioral learning models (Skinner, 1953), the cognitive model (Beck, 1976), and, also, the social learning model (Bandura, 1986). CBT has a particular focus on cognitive (i.e., distortions in thought patterns and assumptions) and behavioral components to promote the development of suitable skills and behaviors.

Applied to adolescents who have committed sexual crimes, CBT focuses on changing patterns of behavior and cognitions related to sexual aggression, such as non-adaptive responses, with the purpose of replacing them with more adaptive schemas, behaviors, and prosocial responses. To achieve behavior change, CBT promotes the alteration of cognitive distortions and non-adaptive schemas and empowers individuals with problem-solving skills. This therapy is conceptualized as promoting the development of adaptive processes of thought, affect, and behavior that will have an impact on sexual, intimate, and social relationships and on the management of affective states, resulting in a decrease in deviant sexual arousal (Yates, 2003; Barbaree & Marshall, 2006; Barnett & Fitzlan, 2018).

Essentially, CBT works at the level of cognitive, emotional, and behavioral risk factors that may be linked to recidivism risk. In the dynamics of recidivism prevention, characteristics associated with denial and behavior minimization and distorted thoughts about sexual behaviors are addressed, with a focus on sexual arousal and sexual activation problems (Print et al., 2013).

Good Lives Model

Reviewing intervention models applied to adolescents who have committed sexual offenses, several clinical psychologists (Marshall et al., 2003; Barroso et al., 2018; Ryan et al., 2018) suggest that intervention models should consider the knowledge of prosocial pathways to meeting the needs possessed by sexual offenders. Along these lines, the *Good Lives Model* (GLM; Ward & Gannon, 2006; Ward et al., 2007a) proposes that this population be treated as goal-oriented and as seeking to acquire fundamental primary human values and principles, as actions, experiences, and activities that are beneficial to the individual's well-being and that are sought for one's own good (e.g., relationships/intimacy, action/autonomy, happiness/pleasure, and emotional balance). Thus, the GLM suggests that the consequences of sexual violence are not the result of desire but of the methods and strategies that individuals create to fulfill it. According to this model, the strategies used by individuals are developed in the context of their backgrounds, problematic developmental trajectories, and internal and external capacities to achieve their goals. Thus, as an intimacy-seeking sex offender, the focus is no longer on the intimacy the individual seeks, which is similar to that of all human beings, but on the problematic approaches the individual uses to achieve it (e.g., seeking out children).

The GLM applied to adolescents who have committed sexual offenses may contribute to risk reduction and increase motivation and engagement with the intervention through increased attention to responsiveness needs and the creation of a strong therapeutic alliance (Ward & Stewart, 2003; Yates, 2009). Recently, the self-regulation model has been incorporated into the GLM to provide the inclusion of risk factors (Yates & Ward, 2008), thus remaining consistent with the principles of clinical and forensic practice with sexual violence perpetrators.

Program for Psychological Assessment and Intervention with Adolescents Who Have Engaged in Sexually Abusive Behaviors (PBX)

Based on conceptual models that explain sexual aggression, the Program for Psychological Assessment and Intervention with Adolescents who have Engaged in Sexually Abusive Behaviors (PBX; Barroso et al., 2020) was developed. PBX aims to intervene with adolescents who have been involved in sexual aggression, using the period of measure/sentence to which they are subjected, to drive the intended behavioral change to sexual violence risk mitigation. Instead of a deficit-based approach, the perspective adopted in this intervention program is to "reinforce the skills" that the individual already has or will acquire, with the goal of facilitating safe future integration into society. For this integration, there is individual work focused on the future (anticipating problematic situations) and on the development and practice of new personal and social skills.

This intervention program is a 36-session manualized program that runs on a weekly basis. The program's structure follows a progressive strategy of change, which occurs in three sequential modules: (a) the initial phase; (b) general modules; (c) and specific modules. The main aim of the initial phase is to identify the main risk factors and dynamics of functioning, to determine the needs, the ability and motivation of the individual to accept responsibility for their actions, and to adopt strategies to promote change. The general modules, corresponding to six modules with 19 sessions for psychoeducational intervention, aim to develop skills and coping strategies. Through this process, participation in the program aims to prevent maladaptive behavior and promote safety and psychological health. Psychoeducational intervention is not only effective in inducing attitudinal changes, but research has shown that it has the potential to result in behavioral change (Colom et al., 2004). The four modules of the final component of the program, the "specific modules," consist of 17 sessions of psychotherapeutic intervention and training relating to life skills essential in society.

PBX Program Implementation

This chapter aims to describe the implementation of the PBX program (i.e., the initial phase, general modules, and specific modules) using a case presentation and analyze the behavior change through the analysis of a semi-structured interview. The initial phase describes the case report and assessment presentation. As mentioned above, PBX aims to intervene with adolescents who have committed sexual offenses. Psychological intervention takes place during the period of the sentence, whether the adolescent is in a juvenile detention center or in the community, with the aim of achieving the intended behavioral changes during this period.

Case Introduction

Arthur (name, data, and identifying information are fictitious) is a 13-year-old boy who is being housed in a juvenile detention center. According to the information obtained in the assessment, Artur spent a summer vacation at the home of a six-year-old cousin and his family, during which his cousin was sexually abused. During this vacation period, he and his cousin used to take naps together. During one of these naps, his cousin woke him up and showed him his buttocks, asking him if he "*wanted to*" (sic) and that he "*felt seduced*" (sic) and had the desire/willingness (and an erection). As a result, Artur had sexual intercourse with his cousin without, he says, actually penetrating him. In view of what happened, Artur says he feels bad about himself, not only because he knows that "*what he did was wrong*" (sic) but also because of the problems he is now having as a result of this situation. He also mentions that, during the sexual act, he took care to ask his cousin if he was enjoying it and says that he answered in the affirmative.

Personal History

Artur is part of a household made up of his 39-year-old mother and his 16-year-old sister. When he was just one year old, Artur and his mother emigrated to Portugal due to conflicts between his parents, especially because his father wouldn't accept his paternity. However, the process of adapting to this new country was described by his mother as being very difficult, as she was forced to entrust Artur's care to several caretakers, to sign up for the a job in order to earn money to meet family expenses.

When Artur was about 5/6 years old, he was allegedly sexually abused by a neighbor's son (3/4 years older) during his mother's working hours. Artur's mother says that this situation lasted for several years, until Artur was seven or eight years old, when the neighbor moved out and Artur stopped living with the alleged abuser. When the relationship with this alleged aggressor ceased, Artur began to show hypersexualized behavior, both through obscene gestures and showing his penis to girls at school and through what his mother calls "*outbreaks*" (sic) on his sister (over three years old). During these *outbreaks*, Artur would get into her bed, inviting her to have sex, a situation that was reported by her daughter (which was allegedly not consummated). When Artur was confronted by his mother about his sexual behavior, he confided that he had been repeatedly abused by the neighbor's son, saying "it was the neighbor who taught me how to have sex" (sic), without expressing any resentment or anger toward the aggressor for the alleged abuse he had suffered. On the contrary, Artur explained that he missed having sex, felt pleasure, and had difficulties controlling his impulses.

The information gathered at the school describes Artur as a diligent student who generally shows an interest in school activities. He is characterized as a student who follows the rules of the school and the classroom and who accepts the guidance and authority of teachers very well, responding politely. His relationship with his classmates seems easy, but he is also characterized as a very sensitive youngster who gets angry easily, showing low self-esteem. As far as other complementary activities are concerned, Artur has regularly taken part in sporting activities, maintains healthy lifestyle habits, and there is no evidence of risk indicators for alcohol and drug use.

Assessment

Measures

- Analysis of the procedural documents sent by the Court;
- Individual interviews with the juvenile's mother;
- Individual interviews with the juvenile;
- Articulation and collection of information from the currently and previously educational establishment attended by the juvenile;
- Articulation with CPCJ[1];
- Liaison with the Public Security Police (PSP) to assess the existing police reports;
- Application of a risk assessment tool/criminogenic needs – Youth Level of Service/Case Management Inventory (YLS/CMI, Hoge and Andrews, 2002);

Application of Psychological Assessment Instruments

- Raven's Progressive Matrices – PM38 – General Scale (Raven et al., 2001). It evaluates general intelligence, namely the subject's ability to deduce relations using non-verbal material.
- MACI – Millon's Clinical Inventory for Adolescents (Llagostera, 2004) is a self-report test to assess personality traits in adolescents.
- ow I Think" Questionnaire – HIT (Gibbs et al., 2001): A self-assessment instrument for cognitive distortions in youth with antisocial behavior.
- Protocols A, B, C, D, and E for the Assessment of Youth Sex Offenders. Translation and adaptation from Graham et al. (1997).
- Sexual Abuse Beliefs Scale (Machado et al., 2000).
- Juvenile Sex Offender Assessment Protocol (JSOAP – II; Prentky & Righthand, 2021; Barroso et al., 2019).

Case Conceptualization

Throughout the assessment process, Artur showed a collaborative attitude when analyzing his life circumstances, his personal functioning characteristics, and the facts of his criminal charges. His verbal self-censorship and non-verbal communication (crying) were consistent with his speech, revealing discomfort and internal suffering over what had happened. The data obtained through all the assessment methodologies seemed to converge on the hypothesis that Artur was an adolescent whose personality structure was strongly associated with a functioning of depressive traits, with difficulties in experiencing pleasure and enthusiasm in social interactions, tending toward self-depreciation and devaluation, adoption of a passive and submissive relational pattern, and internal experience of feelings of inadequacy, insecurity, and low self-esteem.

Their psychological and sexual development process was marked by victimization and early and repeated exposure to sexual practices. This seems to have conditioned their learning of what it is to experience and explore sexuality at an early stage of development, which explains the hypersexualized behaviors. Psychological assessment suggests cognitive distortions about sexual desire and fantasies with younger male children. Beliefs and thought patterns legitimize or minimize the unacceptability of the existence of sexual practices between adolescents and children, either due to a poor assessment of age indicators, a distorted perception of the existence of mutual pleasure associated with these practices, or the perception of the child as an active agent of sexual seduction. In this regard, Artur seems to be at significant risk of reoffending.

However, the assessment also indicated an awareness that these fantasies, desires, and behaviors are unacceptable from a social and legal point of view and deserve the strong disapproval of his surroundings, particularly his mother. This awareness, on the one hand, causes him embarrassment, shame, and internal suffering; but, on the other hand, it places him, at the time of this assessment, in an attitude of receptivity and possible adherence to a psychotherapeutic intervention and, expressed and verbalized, "*I just want to change my behavior*" (sic). Finally, it is important to note that during this assessment, no significant risk indicators were identified for antisocial behavior in general.

Course of Treatment and Assessment of Progress

It was considered that the main intervention should focus on the cognitive restructuring of dysfunctional beliefs and attitudes that lead to sexually abusive behavior and the acquisition of personal and social skills conducive to experiencing and expressing sexuality in a way that respects the rights and self-determination of others. In this sense, the PBX program was applied in such a way as to reinforce personal and social skills (namely with the application of the General Module) and at the level of cognitive restructuring and dysfunctional beliefs and attitudes toward sexual expression and behavior (through the General Model, but mainly through the Specific Module). Over the course of a year, all the PBX modules and sessions were applied in a standardized way. A semi-structured interview was then carried out, which made it possible to highlight Arthur's acquisition of personal and interpersonal skills, namely in terms of the perception of the notions of equality, intimacy, consent (i.e. in sexual behavior), behavioral change (e.g. avoiding risky situations), cognitive restructuring (i.e. automatic/alternative thoughts, satisfaction/masturbation, and self-confidence), and the identification of risky situations and projection into the future. The semi-structured interview made it possible to assess the various elementary themes that served as the basis for a thematic analysis. During the interview, the concepts of equality, intimacy, and consent appeared several times in association with each other. The definition of these concepts and what they covered were unclear to Arthur at an early stage of the intervention, but as the program developed, the meaning became more concrete and applicable. Arthur admits that because of the age discrepancy, there was no equal relationship, and, subsequently, as an older person, he had an obligation to know that the act performed was not an appropriate way for him to get sexual satisfaction.

PSYCHOLOGIST (P): "Is this way that you have satisfied your penis, with your cousin, the right way?"
ARTHUR (A): "No."
P: "Why in your opinion is it not the most suitable?"
A: "Because there was no equality...I was older than him and old enough to know the consequences, but he did not."

As sessions progressed, it became clear to Arthur that beyond an existence of equality in relationships, the intimacy between peers must also be developed, through approximation, friendship, communication, and fraternization.

P: *"Imagine you know someone with whom you would like to have sex. How, in the long run, could you get there?"*
A: "Become friends, get to know each other well, and if there is consent from that person."
P: "Ok. And when you are getting to know each other better, what are you creating?"
A: "Intimacy".

Along the same lines, Arthur also identified the consent domain as a third essential element when it comes to the practice of sexual relations. According to Arthur, if there is permission from both partners, through tone of voice as well as non-verbal expressions, there is consent.

P: "How do you see if a person is consenting, if he/she consents or not to a more intimate relationship, how can you observe that or be aware of that?"

A: "If the person says yes with that... that yes with a little fear you can tell."
P: "And what does that slightly fear lead you to think?"
A: "That the person doesn't want to."
P: "Ok, so you have to be sure that that yes is really a yes..."
A: "A strong yes."

It became clear during the interview that one of the focal points of the program, related to the themes, is sexual behavior and the development and reflection of the themes were modified in the course of the sessions.

P: "In your opinion, what was your biggest, motivating thing that led you to carry out this abuse with your cousin?"
A: "As I didn't know anything about it I thought it was a play/joke."
P: "Do you think you behave now the same way as you did a year ago? More or less?"
A: "Yes, I have the same behavior, but it is not the same sexual behavior."
P: "What has changed in terms of sexual behavior?"
A: "I already... for example, I already know how to avoid things."

Thus, Arthur recognizes the existence of risky situations that can compromise sexual behavior. However, throughout the sessions, there are clear strategies, acquired by Arthur, that allow him to get around this type of situation.

P: "I'm remembering a situation you told me about a girl at school, remember? From a girl at school...who was like that, she hung out with a lot of boys and was a little older (...). From what you told me, you realized that there was a risky situation there. Which you avoided. (...) What made you not move forward? Because you, if I remember correctly, you got excited and would have liked to have had sex with that girl, right?"
A: "Because she is much older than me, and I don't know her well."
P: "You realized that this could be a problem. So, what you did there was to avoid a difficult situation, thinking about what we have already talked about here, about equality, inequality, intimacy, right? And it was also, following an automatic thought was "I want to have sex with that girl" what came up? Was it a thought...?"
A: "Alternative."

The adolescent confirms that when faced with risky situations, automatic thoughts can arise that are uncontrollable and often compromise behavior.

However, Arthur learns to control himself and mentions that it is possible to avoid unwanted behavior by attending to alternative thoughts.

A: "Automatic thinking doesn't... we can't, for example, control it, but if we think differently, we can always correct something we've done."

P: "Ok. So, we can have automatic thoughts that can lead us to do something wrong, like that kind of behavior, is that it? And if these thoughts arise, how can you now deal with them?"

A: "With the alternative thoughts, for example, we cannot change automatic thoughts. And alternative thoughts are for us... for us to think twice about thinking a positive thing or doing a worse thing."

In sum, alternative thoughts can help us find more acceptable ways of behaving, such as through masturbation, in a respectful way, as well as without harming others.

P: "How can you satisfy your penis, right? Without harming anyone, without hurting anyone? Respecting other people."

A: "By masturbating."

P: "At that moment, if you feel like it, you can masturbate, right? Ok, that's a way to satisfy the penis, isn't it? And you can do this masturbation anywhere?"

A: "No. If it's in public it will be malicious intent...and people will find it disgusting."

Conclusion

The PBX program has been tested in the Portuguese treatment environment. It is currently being implemented in services belonging to the Ministry of Justice for adolescents who have committed sexual offenses. The program was structured in 36 sessions according to the latest international guidelines and following clinical research that supported the effective results of the intervention. The sessions feature periodic reinforcement and/or continued therapeutic support focused on atypical sexual interests and skill gain, seeking over time to anticipate problematic scenarios that the individual may meet upon return to the community. The semi-structured interview demonstrates cognitive change and describes behavioral changes seen in the adolescent participating in the program. However, additional and complementary methodologies to provide further support for the PBX program involve follow-up data and quantitative verification of recidivism in abusive sexual behavior.

A clinical intervention with adolescents must take into account their developmental characteristics (psychological and behavioral). Research on this topic (Barroso et al., 2019) has suggested that a psychotherapeutic intervention that does not take into account the 'offender's developmental stage, cultural and family context, personality, and other unique characteristics is ineffective and, in some cases, counterproductive (McGrath et al., 2013). The human and social impact of these interventions, as well as their high technical complexity, highlight the need for specialized training in forensic assessment procedures and clinical intervention practices, and it is important that professionals (e.g., psychologists or psychiatrists) working in this area have specific training and are equipped with up-to-date models and techniques for intervening with adolescents or young adults who have committed sexual crimes.

Note

1 CPCJ are official non-judicial institutions with functional autonomy that aim to promote the rights of children and young people and prevent or end situations that may affect their safety, health, training, education or integral development.

References

Aebi, M., Giger, J., Plattner, B., Metzke, C. W., & Steinhausen, H. C. (2013). Problem coping skills, psychosocial adversities and mental health problems in children and adolescents as predictors of criminal outcomes in young adulthood. *European Child & Adolescent Psychiatry, 23*(5), 283–293. https://doi.org/10.1007/s00787-013-0458-y

Andrews, D. A., & Bonta, J. (2010). *The psychology of criminal conduct* (5th ed.). Cincinnati, OH: Anderson.

Bandura, A. (1986). *Social foundations of thought and action: A social cognitive theory*. Englewood Cliffs, NJ: Prentice-Hall.

Bancroft, J., Janssen, E., Carnes, L., Goodrich, D., Strong, D., & Long, J. (2004). Sexual activity and risk taking in young heterosexual men: The relevance of sexual arousability, mood, and sensation seeking. *The Journal of Sex Research, 41*(2), 181–192. https://doi.org/10.1080/00224490409552226

Barbaree, H., & Marshall, W. (2006). *The juvenile sex offender*. New York: Guilford Publications.

Barnett, G., & Fitzalan, F. (2018). What doesn't work to reduce reoffending? A review of reviews of ineffective interventions for adults convicted of crimes. *European Psychologist, 23*(2), 111–129. https://doi.org/10.1027/1016-9040/a000323

Barroso, R., Borduin, C., & Munschy, R. (2016). Terapia multissistémica com adolescentes agressores sexuais (MST-PSB). In A. Sani, & S. Caridade (Eds.), *Práticas de Intervenção na Violência e no Crime* (pp. 127–145). Lisboa: Pactor.

Barroso, R., Pechorro, P., Figueiredo, P., Ramião, E., Manita, C., Gonçalves, R. A., & Nobre, P., (2020). Are juveniles who have committed sexual offenses the same everywhere? Psychometric properties of the juvenile sex offender assessment protocol–II in a Portuguese youth sample. *Sexual Abuse: A Journal of Research and Treatment, 32*(7), 606–825. https://doi.org/10.1177/1079063219858070

Barroso, R., Pham, T., Greco, A., & Thibaut, F. (2019). Challenges in the treatment of sex offenders. In B. Vollm & P. Braun (Eds.), *Long-term in forensic psychiatric care: Clinical, ethical and legal challenges* (pp. 169–180). New York: Springer Publishing Company. https://doi.org/10.1007/978-3-030-12594-3_12

Barroso, R., Ramião, E., & Figueiredo, P. (2020). *Programa de avaliação e intervenção psicológica com adolescentes que se envolveram em comportamentos sexualmente abusivos* (PBX). Direção Geral de Reinserção e Serviços Prisionais (DGRSP) e Universidade de Trás os Montes e Alto Douro (UTAD). ISBN: 978-989-33-0512-6

Barroso, R., Ramião, E., Figueiredo, P., & Pechorro, P. (2018). Processos neurobiológicos na etiologia dos interesses sexuais pedófilos. In M. Paulino & L. Alho (Edt.) *Comportamento Criminal e Avaliação Forense* (pp. 145–155). Pactor.

Barroso, R., Figueiredo, P., & Ramião, E. (2022). Comportamento sexual em adolescentes: do desenvolvimento sexual normativo à conduta sexual problemática. In A. Anciães & R. Agulhas (Coords.). *Grande livro da violência sexual: Compreensão, prevenção, avaliação e intervenção* (pp. 378–392). Sílabo.

Beck, A. T. (1976). *Cognitive therapy and the emotional disorders.* New York, NY: International Universities Press.

Colom, F., Vieta, E., Sánchez-Moreno, J., Martínez-Arán, A., Torrent, C., Reinares, M., Goikolea, J. M., Benabarre, A., & Comes, M. (2004). Psychoeducation in bipolar patients with comorbid personality disorders. *Bipolar Disorders, 6*(4), 294–298.

Graham, F., Richardson, G., & Bhate, S. (1997). Assessment. In M.S. Hoghughi, S.R. Bhate, F. Graham (Eds.) *Working with Sexually Abusive Adolescents* (pp. 74–91). Sage.

Llagostera, G. A. (2004). MACI. Inventario Clínico para Adolescentes de Millon [Millon Adolescent Clinical Inventory]. Pearson.

Lieberman, D., Tooby, J., & Cosmides, I. (2003). Does morality have a biological basis? An empirical test of the factors governing moral sentiments relating to incest. *Proceedings of the Royal Society: Biological Science, 270*, 819–826. https://doi.org/10.1098/rspb.2002.2290

Lösel, F., & Schmucker, M. (2005). The effectiveness of treatment for sexual offenders: A comprehensive meta-analysis. *Journal of Experimental Criminology, 1*(1), 117–146. https://doi.org/10.1007/s11292-004-6466-7

Gibbs, J, C., Barriga, A. Q., & Potter, G. B. (2001). *How I Think (HIT) questionnaire.* Champaign, IL: Research Press.

Hanson, R. K., Gordon, A., Harris, A. J. R., Marques, J. K., Murphy, W., Quinsey, V. L., & Seto, M. C. (2002). First report of the collaborative outcome data project on the effectiveness of psychological treatment for sex offenders. *Sexual Abuse: A Journal of Research and Treatment, 14*(2), 169–194. https://doi.org/10.1177/107906320201400207

Harris, D. A., Smallbone, S., Dennison, S., & Knight, R. A. (2009). Specialization and versatility in sexual offenders referred for civil commitment. *Journal of Criminal Justice, 37*(1), 37–44. https://doi.org/10.1016/j.jcrimjus.2008.12.002

Hoge, R. D., & Andrews, D. A. (2002). *The youth level of service/case management inventory manual and scoring key*. Multi-Health Systems.

Machado, C., Gonçalves, R., & Matos, M. (2000). *Escalas para avaliação do enquadramento cultural da violência contra mulheres e crianças*. Universidade do Minho.

Malin, H., Saleh, F., & Grudzinskas, A. (2014). Recent research related to juvenile sex offending: Findings and directions for further research. *Current Psychiatry Reports, 16*(4), 440. https://doi.org/10.1007/s11920-014-0440-5

Marshall, W., Fernandez, Y., Serran, G., Mulloy, R., Thornton, D., Mann, R., & Anderson, D. (2003). Process variables in the treatment of sexual offenders. *Aggression and Violent Behavior, 8*(2), 205–234. https://doi.org/10.1016/s1359-1789(01)00065-9

McGrath, R., Hoke, S., & Lasher, M. (2013). The Sex Offender Treatment Intervention and Progress Scale (SOTIPS): Psychometric properties and incremental predictive validity with Static-99R. *Sexual Abuse: A Journal of Research and Treatment, 24*(5), 431–458. https://doi.org/10.1177/1079063211432475

Prentky, R. A., & Righthand, S. (2021). The Juvenile Sex Offender Assessment Protocol-II (J-SOAP-II). In K. S. Douglas & R. K. Otto (Eds.), *Handbook of Violence Risk Assessment* (pp. 294–321). Routledge/Taylor & Francis Group. https://doi.org/10.4324/9781315518374-17

Print, B., Fisher, D., & Beech, A. (2013). The development of practice with adolescents who sexually harm. In B. Print (Eds.), *The Good Lives Model for adolescents who sexually harm* (pp. 19–34). Vermont: The Safer Society Press.

Ramião, E., Figueiredo, P., Azeredo, A., Moreira, D., Barroso, R., & Barbosa, F. (2023). Neurobiological characteristics of individuals who have committed sexual offenses: A systematic review. *Aggression and Violent Behavior, 72*, 101858. https://doi.org/10.1016/j.avb.2023.101858

Raven, J. C., Court, J. H., & Raven, J. (2001). *Raven matrices progresivas* (3ª edition). TEA Ediciones.

Ryan, M., McCauley, M., & Walsh, D. (2018). The virtuous circle: A grounded theory exploration of the good lives model. *Sexual Abuse, 31*(8), 908–929. https://doi.org/10.1177/1079063218780730

Skinner, B. F. (1953). *Science and human behavior*. New York: McMillan.

Ward, T., & Gannon, T. (2006). Rehabilitation, etiology, and self- regulation: The good lives model of sexual offender treatment. *Aggression and Violent Behavior, 11*(1), 77–94. https://doi.org/10.1016/j.avb.2005.06.001

Ward, T., Mann, R. E., & Gannon, T. A. (2007a). The good lives model of offender rehabilitation: Clinical implications. *Aggression and Violent Behavior, 12*(1), 87–107. https://doi.org/10.1016/j.avb.2006.03.004

Ward, T., Melser, J., & Yates, P. M. (2007b). Reconstructing the risk need responsivity model: A theoretical elaboration and evaluation. *Aggression and Violent Behavior, 12*(2), 208–228. https://doi.org/10.1016/j.avb.2006.07.001

Ward, T., & Stewart, C. (2003). Criminogenic needs and human needs: A theoretical model. *Psychology, Crime & Law, 9*(2), 125–143. https://doi.org/10.1080/10683160310001l6247

Worling, J. (2012). The assessment and treatment of deviant sexual arousal with adolescents who have offended sexually. *Journal of Sexual Aggression, 18*(1), 36–63. https://doi.org/10.1080/13552600.2011.630152

Yates, P. M. (2003). Treatment of adult sexual offenders: A therapeutic cognitive-behavioral model of intervention. *Journal of Child Sexual Abuse, 12*(3–4), 195–232. https://doi.org/10.1300/j070v12n03_08

Yates, P. M. (2009). Using the good lives model to motivate sexual offenders to participate in treatment. In D. S. Prescott (Ed.), *Building Motivation for Change in Sexual Offenders* (pp. 74–95). Safer Society Press.

Yates, P. M., & Ward, T. (2008). Good lives, self-regulation, and risk management: An integrated model of sexual offender assessment and treatment. *Sexual Abuse in Australia and New Zealand: An Interdisciplinary Journal, 1*, 3–20.

9 Implementing Group Cognitive-Behavioral Therapy for Psychosis (CBTp) in a Forensic Psychiatric Context

Peter Sheridan, Melissa Coelho, Kyrsten Grimes, Gary A. Chaimowitz, and Andrew T. Olagunju

Introduction

Cognitive behavioral therapy for psychosis (CBTp) is an evidence-based treatment approach for schizophrenia spectrum and other psychotic disorders (Health Quality Ontario, 2018; Wright et al., 2014). CBTp helps individuals normalize their experience of psychotic symptoms, improve insight and coping, and learn to reduce distress by recognizing and managing those symptoms. Evidence suggests CBTp is effective in reducing symptoms of psychosis and may be particularly helpful in managing breakthrough or residual symptoms.

In this chapter, we describe the implementation of group CBTp treatment in our forensic psychiatry program. The CBTp group is offered by trained clinicians to eligible individuals who have completed pre-treatment screening. This chapter details our experience delivering this intervention under the following subsections: overview of the literature on CBTp, adapting CBTp for forensic patients, implementation of the program, preliminary outcomes, and summary and recommendations.

Overview of CBTp

Psychotic disorders are mental illnesses characterized by positive (e.g., hallucinations and delusions), negative (e.g., flat affect and anhedonia), and cognitive (e.g., disorganized thinking and slow thinking) symptoms. They can include schizophrenia, schizoaffective disorder, bipolar disorder with psychotic features, major depressive disorder with psychotic features, and substance- or medication-induced psychotic disorders. Although antipsychotic medication is considered the first-line treatment for many of these disorders, only a proportion (about one-third in the case of schizophrenia) of individuals fully recover (Kane, 1999; Langlois, Samokhvalov & Rehm,

DOI: 10.4324/9781003360926-12

2012). As a result, a number of psychosocial interventions have been developed, with CBTp being one of the most well established (Chadwick, Birchwood & Trower, 1996; Fowler, Garety & Kuipers, 1999; Kingdon & Turkington, 1991, 1994, 2005; Wright et al., 2014). CBTp aims to teach individuals how to manage their symptoms and associated distress, as well as improve their insight, by challenging beliefs about their symptoms (i.e., their cognitive distortions) and by introducing strategies to address unhelpful thinking styles and unpleasant or distressing sensory experiences (mainly voices) and/or thoughts/beliefs.

Meta-analytic studies indicate CBTp has medium-to-large effects on positive symptoms and small effects on negative symptoms in general psychiatric settings, but little is known about its efficacy in forensic psychiatric settings (Jauhar et al., 2014; Mehl, Werner & Lincoln, 2015; Sarin, Wallin & Widerlöv, 2011; Slater & Townend, 2016; Wykes, Steel, Everitt & Tarrier, 2008).

Implementing CBTp in Forensic Psychiatry

Within the Canadian forensic psychiatric system, individuals found Unfit to Stand Trial (UST) or Not Criminally Responsible (NCR) on Account of Mental Disorder are detained under a provincial review board. Approximately 71% of these individuals have a psychotic disorder diagnosis, with a preponderance diagnosed with schizophrenia spectrum disorder (Canadian Institute of Health Information, 2016).

The Forensic Psychiatry Program at St. Joseph's Healthcare Hamilton, Ontario, provides a group CBTp intervention for individuals found UST or NCR in this province who have a diagnosis of schizophrenia spectrum disorder, other psychotic disorders, or major mood disorder with psychosis (Grimes & Sheridan, 2019). In our service, approximately 98% of individuals are diagnosed with one of these disorders. Our group CBTp intervention was piloted about five years ago by two of the chapter's authors, PS (the lead author and psychologist) and KG (then a psychology resident), for eligible individuals who experienced psychosis. It has since undergone many revisions and updates as other clinicians have shared their expertise.

Adapting CBTp in our forensic context combines elements of a manualized CBTp approach (Wright et al., 2014), Acceptance and Commitment Therapy (ACT; Hayes, Strosahl & Wilson, 1999), and mindfulness. Group members and clinicians work collaboratively and non-judgmentally to identify and manage the symptoms of psychosis. This is particularly important as psychotic symptomatology is nearly always associated with the offences that have resulted in detention in the forensic mental health system.

There is significant emphasis placed on the medical and psychopharmacological management of major mental illnesses in our service. The group CBTp program is presented as an adjunct to this treatment, offering individuals the possibility of learning and practicing cognitive and behavioral strategies that may prevent increases in medications that have serious side-effects and may help mitigate the potential negative impacts of treatment-resistant symptoms. CBTp, therefore, offers individuals the experience of being more in control of both their symptoms and their medications.

The group CBTp program also offers a "safe space" for individuals to discuss concerns about their diagnosis and treatment, their beliefs about mental illness, and their involvement in the forensic system, and to share their experience of their symptoms without fear of consequences such as the holding of privileges, negative reports to the provincial review board, or increases in pharmacological treatment. Indeed, group members are encouraged to use the CBTp group to express concerns and engage other group members and group facilitators in collaborative investigation and problem-solving. Examples include individuals who report being told they should not discuss their symptoms because it upsets others, who report justified changes in mood that have been mistaken for symptoms, or who believe their treatment teams are not open to hearing about the thoughts or voices that continue to distress them.

Every group member's experience is approached with a gentle, curious, and non-judgmental stance. We attempt to use language that is non- (or less) stigmatizing and demonstrates greater neutrality about the experience of psychosis. For example, as much as possible, we refer to symptoms as "experiences," auditory hallucinations as "voice hearing," and delusions as "thoughts and beliefs." When group members or facilitators inevitably refer to symptoms, hallucinations, or delusions, we engage group members in discussion about the importance of using language that reflects a neutral and curious stance with regard to the phenomena, reduces stigma, and allows for the normalization of their experiences along a continuum that respects historical, ethnocultural, and spiritual differences.

When referring to the difficulties group members have encountered as a result of their symptoms, we use terms such as unusual, unhelpful, unpleasant, or problematic experiences. As a group, we adopt the view that an individual's experiences must have been unhelpful or problematic in some way because they have resulted in their involvement in the forensic system, i.e., the behavior has resulted in significant legal sanction, including the restriction of their liberties. We adhere to the understanding that mental illness is differentiated from other experiences because the symptoms/experiences are intrusive, persistent, and cause distress to self or others. When group members question whether their own experiences meet those criteria, we engage the group in carefully reviewing them. For example, a woman who maintained she was the Queen of England claimed her behavior hadn't caused her or others any distress – until group members pointed out she had been arrested for shoplifting clothes she believed she shouldn't have to pay for because of her royal lineage.

Implementation

Screening and Introduction to the Group Program

The Forensic Psychiatry Program comprises a secure assessment unit, four rehabilitation units (two secure and two general), and an outpatient clinic. The program supports approximately 160 individuals found UST or NCR at any given time. Once the treatment team identifies a need for CBTp, screening is conducted to assess each individual's insight and treatment needs, introduce the program, and begin to identify treatment goals.

Our CBTp screening interview is semi-structured and utilizes open-ended questions in order to gather relevant information while developing therapeutic rapport. Questions are phrased in a neutral, non-judgmental manner. What brought you into the hospital? What is your understanding of why you are here and not in the correctional system (i.e., in hospital instead of prison)? Do you know what diagnosis you've been given? Do you agree with your diagnosis? What has your mental health been like in the past? What about now? Has anyone ever told you that you have experienced symptoms? What do you make of that? Do you experience anything like that now? Is there anything you can tell me that would help me appreciate what your experience is like?

The rationale for the CBTp group is shared, and the individual is invited to participate. If the individual agrees, the informed consent process and pre-treatment questionnaires are completed. An overview of the group program is provided below.

We have very few exclusionary criteria for our CBTp program. Individuals are eligible to be included if they are able to participate in some meaningful way and are able to tolerate two one-hour sessions per week for ten weeks. There is no expectation that the individual's symptoms will be managed or that they will take medication. In fact, we have found it quite helpful to include group members at various stages of treatment and at different points of progression through the forensic psychiatric system. This is because of the significant impact of learning through role-modelling, the credibility bestowed on peers (as opposed to professional facilitators), and the lived experience of major mental illness. We have therefore included individuals who are treated with medication and are asymptomatic, who experience residual or breakthrough symptoms, and those who are not treated or are suboptimally treated with medication and are considered "unwell" by our service. The only caveat to this is that, in accordance with Risk-Need-Responsivity principles (Andrews, Bonta & Hoge, 1990), we have modified content for individuals diagnosed with intellectual disability to meet their specific responsivity needs.

Early "Pre-Treatment" Group Sessions

Early "pre-treatment" sessions of CBTp in a forensic context focus on introduction to mindfulness and the CBT model, discussion of the symptoms and stigma associated with psychosis and the forensic system, individualized case formulation (for illness onset and/or the index offence), and enhancement of existing coping strategies.

In our group CBTp program, we ask members to brainstorm reasons for practicing mindfulness and accept that they recognize mindfulness primarily for bringing a calm, peaceful, restful, focused beginning to the group. We encourage them to conceptualize mindfulness very broadly as the practice of noticing what is happening "inside and outside." We stress the importance of observing ourselves, our environment, our feelings, and our thoughts as means of identifying and managing experiences. Every session begins with a mindfulness practice chosen to complement the strategies being taught.

We also adopt the stance that "thoughts are just thoughts." We encourage group members to consider their thoughts without judgment or attachment. They can be noticed with curiosity but not held onto, valued, or criticized. Thoughts can simply be "passing by," as though on a cloud in the sky or a leaf ona stream. This sets the stage for noticing but not holding onto the problematic thoughts associated with mental illness.

Group members are re-introduced to basic CBT concepts. In our service, nearly all therapeutic programs are framed from the CBT perspective, but it is nonetheless surprising how few individuals have learned some of the basic concepts. Early on, we re-introduce the "cognitive triangle," illustrating the interconnectedness between emotions, thoughts, and behaviors, using examples relevant to the group members' experiences (e.g., responses to review board decisions, denial of privilege requests, behavioral activation). We stress the importance of noticing, identifying, and changing thoughts to impact feelings and actions. We return to the cognitive triangle frequently to improve our understanding of CBT concepts and enhance the benefits of CBTp. Understanding how thoughts/beliefs influence feelings and behavior when considering how anger works, for example, is fundamental to understanding how distressing thoughts/beliefs, such as "My father wanted to kill me," influence feelings and behavior in the experience of psychosis.

In the early phase of group CBTp, we also provide psychoeducation regarding major mental illness, diagnoses, symptoms, and treatment from the psychiatric perspective. It has been eye-opening to discover how many of our group members have no or very limited understanding of these issues, even after many years in hospital. This speaks to the profound lack of insight experienced by many individuals living with a psychotic disorder. We use a combination of group discussion, short videos, and didactic teaching to provide group members with information about their diagnoses and the experience of psychosis in particular. We highlight the experience of positive, negative, and cognitive/disorganized symptoms from the psychiatric perspective.

This is a good opportunity for group members to share their experiences with each other. We have found that they are often excited to have a forum for openly discussing their experiences, and we are mindful of maintaining that neutral, non-judgmental stance. We are careful to point out when the language used is medical or psychiatric and that individuals may choose to describe or label their experiences in different ways.

At this point in the group cycle, the issue of stigma is also purposefully raised, and group members are invited to discuss their experiences in the mental health and forensic systems. We point out that individuals found UST or NCR experience multiple sources of stigma: stigma related to living with mental illness, stigma related to being involved in the legal/judicial system, as well as stigma related to intersecting minority statuses (e.g., on the basis of race or ethnocultural identity, sexual orientation, gender presentation, disability, etc.).

Finally, group members are provided with information about how mental illness develops. Because of our patient population, this is most often information about the cause, onset, and course of schizophrenia, although we also provide the same kind of information about schizoaffective disorder, major mood disorders with psychotic features, and substance-induced psychotic disorders. Group members are provided with a basic understanding of current theory and the limitations of that theory, framed in the stress-vulnerability model of illness development (Zubin & Spring, 1977).

Next, each group member is asked to consider how their own illness developed (or, if they don't believe they have an illness, how they came to be involved in the forensic mental health system) by reviewing predisposing, precipitating, perpetuating, and protective factors (Moritz, Woodward, Hauschildt & Metacognition Study Group, 2015). The resulting case conceptualizations, or "formulations," are referred to going forward as the group considers strategies for preventing a recurrence of these experiences.

An understanding of the course of one's illness is critical in managing the risk forrecurrence or relapse of symptoms as well as the risk forrecidivism, particularly violent recidivism, as mandated by the review boards. Effective cognitive and behavioral strategies are developed for each group member to address precipitating and perpetuating factors and enhance protective factors, balancing the principles of recovery and risk management.

Understanding and Normalizing Experiences

One of the cornerstones of our group CBTp program is helping group members view their experience of symptoms of psychosis as falling on a continuum of "normal" human experiences (Wright et al., 2014). For example, hallucinations are considered to be exaggerated or extreme versions of perceptual experiences or distortions many of us have, although such symptoms are experienced as intrusive, persistent, and distressing to oneself or others. Helping group members to see their experiences as an "extension" of common experiences, as well as see them as problematic or aversive at the extremes, reduces stigma and encourages the implementation of strategies to better manage them.

In our CBTp group, we first introduce the idea of a "mood continuum" in order to set the stage for later discussion of experiences associated with psychosis. Not only can group members relate to the idea of variations in mood being "normal," but discussing affective or mood states appears far less anxiety-provoking to begin with. On a large piece of paper or on a smart board, we draw a line (continuum) and ask group members to anchor it with as many examples of mood experiences as they can. Typically, group members will quickly identify depression and mania, and we ask them where along this line those two experiences should fall. We then add additional experiences the group identifies, such as sadness, loss, mourning, grief, contentment, satisfaction, elation, euphoria, etc. We may be given specific examples and include those as well (e.g., feeling like Superman, on top of the world, ecstatic, or having no energy/motivation, being unable to get out of bed, feeling suicidal, attempting suicide, etc.). As group members make suggestions, we encourage dialogue and debate about where along the continuum these various mood experiences should be placed.

Once there are several dozen points along the continuum, each of the group members is asked to mark off "normal human experience." This part of the exercise inevitably results in many group members choosing a very narrow range of emotional experiences. Group facilitators suggest a much wider range of experiences would be considered "normal" (particularly cross-culturally) and point out that only the very extremes of the continuum are likely to be truly problematic (i.e., when the experiences are intrusive, persistent, or distressing).

Over the course of the next few sessions, the group considers a continuum for sensory experiences and a continuum for thoughts and beliefs. The former generally elicits experiences ranging from optical illusions, seeing something in your peripheral vision, déjà vu, hearing your name called when no one is there, feeling the vibration of your phone when it's not with you, seeing or hearing a loved one who is not there, dreams/nightmares, seeing ghosts, commanding voices, etc. The latter often elicits examples such as childhood myths (Santa Claus, Easter Bunny, and Tooth Fairy), magic, spells, witchcraft, voodoo, religion, reincarnation, fear of being surveilled, followed, or targeted, paranoia, alien abduction, believing you have a special relationship with God or that you are God, etc. Again, facilitators encourage group members to view a wide range of experiences as "normal human experience."

"Treatment" Sessions: Strategies for Coping with Unpleasant Experiences

The remainder of our CBTp group program comprises multiple "treatment" sessions involving teaching and practicing strategies for coping with unpleasant or distressing experiences (mood, hallucinations, and delusions). These sessions are largely drawn from treating psychosis (Wright et al., 2014) but also incorporate strategies or skills taught generally in CBT (Beck, 2011) and DBT (Linehan, 2015). Below is an overview of the key concepts and strategies taught and rehearsed in these sessions.

For coping with unpleasant or distressing emotions, strategies taught include distraction, emotion surfing, behavioral activation, and various skills from DBT. One full session on forgiveness of self and others is also included in our group CBTp program. This is because, in early groups, members spoke often about their experience of guilt and shame, profound feelings of remorse, and anger at their mistreatment in legal, correctional, and forensic settings.

For coping with sensory phenomena, strategies such as questioning the experience, checking the facts (evidence for/against), visualization and grounding, and voice time are helpful. As an example, a group member described voice hearing, during which they felt criticized and derogated. Using strategies from CBTp, the distressing voice was visualized as a giant pair of ruby-red lips that was stuffed into a box; the box was then set on a raft floating on a deep blue ocean, and the group member visualized it drifting away onto the horizon, getting smaller and smaller, and the voice growing quieter and quieter until they could not hear it anymore.

With respect to coping with unpleasant or distressing thoughts/beliefs, strategies such as challenging, thought-stopping, adopting a helpful thought, checking the facts, and behavioral experiments are particularly beneficial. For example, one group member completed a Thought Record for the distressing ("hot") thought, "My father wanted to kill me." When reviewing the individual's Thought Record, group members pointed out that, in fact, the description of the situation indicated the father had said, "I hope you die alone in bed." The individual was then able to work through evidence supporting and not supporting this distressing thought to arrive at the alternative thought, "I was unwell and giving my father grief. He was angry and said he wanted me to die alone and unhappy."

Table 9.1 Overview of key concepts and strategies

Experience	*Key concepts*	*Key strategies*
Unpleasant Mood	Passenger on a bus Avoidance of emotions Cycle of avoidance Cognitive triangle (change thoughts or behavior to change emotions)	Mindfulness Avoid avoidance Distraction (short-term only) Emotion surfing Behavioral activation DBT distress tolerance and emotion regulation skills (e.g., TIP, ACCEPTS, IMPROVE, PLEASE) Forgiveness of self (for guilt and shame) Forgiveness of others (for anger)
Sensory Experiences (Hallucinations)	Selective attention Confirmation bias Cognitive triangle These are just visions/voices… Thought record Self-compassion	Mindfulness Improve self-awareness Question sensory experiences Voices: Check the facts (evidence for/against content or origin of voices) Alternative explanations Use of imagery/visualization Grounding Voice Diary and Voice Time Test the power of voices Coping affirmations
Distressing Thoughts/Beliefs	Cognitive triangle Unhelpful thinking styles Thoughts are just thoughts Thought Record Self-compassion	Mindfulness Cloud in the sky/leaf on a stream Question/challenge thought/belief Thought-stopping Adopt a helpful thought Check the facts (evidence for/against current distressing belief) Check the facts (evidence for/against distressing belief related to illness or index offence) Alternative explanations Behavioral experiments Coping affirmations

Finally, each group member is engaged in developing a wellness plan (relapse prevention plan) to maintain their health going forward. These plans are meant to identify individualized coping strategies for each unpleasant experience (symptom) as well as triggers and early warning signs for a possible relapse or recurrence of symptoms. Group members are asked to consider their personal strengths as well as resources or supports they find helpful in maintaining their well being.

One-to-one follow-up sessions are scheduled with group members to review their individualized case formulations, one completed Thought Record for sensory experiences or distressing thoughts/beliefs, and their wellness plans. These three exercises were chosen for review based on our belief that completed, practical, concrete exercises and strategies would be most useful in managing a recurrence of symptoms and the associated risk for recidivism in our forensic service.

Program Evaluation

The following measures are completed by group members pre- and post-intervention: Brief Psychiatric Rating Scale (BPRS; Overall & Gorham, 1962); Davos Assessment of Cognitive Biases Scale (DACOBS; van der Gaag et al., 2013); Expectations (about Change) Questionnaire (Smith et al., 2003); and Client Satisfaction Questionnaire (unpublished). Efforts are underway to review data from approximately 45 individuals who completed the CBTp group program prior to the onset of the COVID-19 pandemic. A preliminary review suggests modest changes on the BPRS and DACOBS, indicating a reduction in psychotic symptomatology and problematic cognitions. Group members spoke positively about the CBTp group, and the rate of attrition from this intervention (20%) was substantially lower than from other therapeutic interventions in our forensic program.

Conclusion and Recommendations

This chapter outlines our implementation of a manualized group CBTp intervention in a forensic psychiatric context. Our experience suggests that such an intervention can be tailored to meet the specific needs of individuals in this setting: in conjunction with other interventions, including pharmacotherapy, in the treatment of their psychotic disorders; to help them respond to unpleasant or distressing emotions, sensory experiences, and/or thoughts/beliefs with cognitive and behavioral strategies; and to help them manage their risk for recidivism, particularly violent recidivism, flowing from treatment-resistant symptoms of psychotic mental illness.

Our group CBTp program was delivered in two parts. "Pre-treatment" sessions consisted of general concepts including introduction to mindfulness and the CBT framework, basic education about illness and symptom management, stigma associated with involvement in the forensic system, and individualized case formulation. "Treatment" sessions then consisted of specific concepts and strategies to manage negative and positive symptoms, such as increasing behavioral activation and coping with unpleasant or distressing sensory experiences (mainly voices) and thoughts/beliefs.

In addition to this adaptation in the delivery of group CBTp, the concepts and strategies taught were also simplified as it became apparent that group members had difficulty understanding some of the vocabulary and abstract concepts presented. Delivering some of the content in more explicit, concrete terms was very helpful in improving comprehension of the material as well as willingness to engage in practice and rehearsal. It goes without saying that using examples from the forensic psychiatric experience helped group members appreciate the relevance to their own lives, both currently and at the time of their first involvement in the forensic system.

While our clinical experience delivering such groups suggests implementing group CBTp in a forensic psychiatric context is feasible and beneficial, further research is required to establish the efficacy of CBTp for individuals involved in this system. Some research questions include whether and to what degree CBTp results in a reduction in negative versus positive symptoms, how often CBTp strategies are utilized when an individual experiences residual or breakthrough symptoms, and how long gains observed at the end of treatment persist after it has concluded.

References

Andrews, D. A., Bonta, J., & Hoge, R. D. (1990). Classification for effective rehabilitation: Rediscovering psychology. *Criminal Justice and Behavior, 17*, 19–52.

Beck, J. S. (2011). *Cognitive behavior therapy: Basic and beyond* (2nd ed.). New York: Guilford.

Canadian Institute of Health Information. (2016). *The national trajectory project.*

Chadwick, P. D. J., Birchwood, M., & Trower, P. (1996). *Cognitive therapy for delusions, voices and paranoia.* New York: Wiley.

Fowler, D., Garety, P., & Kuipers, E. (1995). *Cognitive behavior therapy for psychosis: Theory and practice.* New York: Wiley.

Grimes, K. M., & Sheridan, P. (2019). The implementation of Cognitive Behavioural Therapy for psychosis (CBTp) in a forensic setting: Lessons learned and future directions. International Journal of Risk and Recovery, *2(1)*, 18–22. https://doi.org/10.15173/ijrr.v2i1.3703

Hayes, S. C., Strosahl, K., & Wilson, K. G. (1999). *Acceptance and commitment therapy: An experiential approach to behavior change.* New York: Guilford.

Health Quality Ontario. (2018). Cognitive behavioural therapy for psychosis: A health technology assessment. *Ontario Health Technology Assessment Series, 18(5)*, 1–141.

Jauhar, S., McKenna, P. J., Radu, J., Fung, E., Salvador, R., & Laws, K. R. (2014). Cognitive-behavioral therapy for the symptoms of schizophrenia: A systematic review and meta-analysis with examination of potential bias. *British Journal of Psychiatry, 204(1)*, 20–29.

Kane J. M. (1999). Management strategies for the treatment of schizophrenia. *The Journal of Clinical Psychiatry, 60(Suppl 12)*, 13–17.

Kingdon, D. G. & Turkington, D. (1991). Preliminary report: The use of cognitive behavior therapy and a normalizing rationale in schizophrenia. *Journal of Nervous and Mental Disease, 179*, 207–211.

Kingdon, D. G. & Turkington, D. (1994). *Cognitive-behavioral therapy of schizophrenia*. New York: Guilford.

Kingdon, D. G. & Turkington, D. (2005). *Cognitive therapy of schizophrenia: Guide to individualized evidence-based treatment*. New York: Guilford.

Langlois, K. A., Samokhvalov, A. V., & Rehm, J. (2012). *Health state descriptions for Canadians: Mental illnesses*. Ottawa, Ontario, Canada: Statistics Canada.

Linehan, M. M. (2015). *DBT skills training manual* (2nd ed.). New York: Guilford.

Mehl, S., Werner, D., & Lincoln, T. M. (2015). Does Cognitive Behavior Therapy for psychosis (CBTp) show a sustainable effect on delusions? A meta-analysis. *Frontiers in Psychology, 6*, 1450.

Moritz, S., Woodward, T. S., Hauschildt, M., & Metacognition Study Group. (2015). *Metacognitive training for psychosis (Version 6.2)*. Hamburg: VanHam Campus Press.

Overall, J. E. & Gorham, D. R. (1962). The brief psychiatric rating scale. *Psychological Reports, 10*, 799–812.

Sarin, F., Wallin, L., & Widerlöv, B. (2011). Cognitive behavior therapy for schizophrenia: A meta-analytical review of randomized controlled trials. *Nordic Journal of Psychiatry, 65*, 162–174.

Slater, J. & Townend, M. (2016). Cognitive behaviour therapy for psychosis in high secure services: An exploratory hermeneutic review of the international literature. *Behavioural and Cognitive Psychotherapy, 44*, 652–672.

Smith, L., Nathan, P., Juniper, U., Kingsep, P., & Lim, L. (2003). *Cognitive behavioural therapy for psychotic symptoms: A therapist's manual* (p. 135). Northbridge, WA: Centre for Clinical Interventions: Psychotherapy, Research & Training.

van der Gaag, M., Schütz, C., Ten Napel, A., Landa, Y., Delespaul, P., Bak, M., Tschacher, W., & de Hert, M. (2013). Development of the Davos assessment of cognitive biases scale (DACOBS). *Schizophr Res. 144*(1–3), 63–71. https://doi.org/10.1016/j.schres.2012.12.01

Wright, N. P., Turkington, D., Kelly, O. P., Davies, D., Jacobs, A. M., & Hopton, J. (2014). *Treating psychosis: A clinician's guide to integrating acceptance and commitment therapy, compassion-focused therapy, and mindfulness approaches within the cognitive behavioral therapy tradition*. Oakland, CA: New Harbinger Publications.

Wykes, T., Steel, C., Everitt, B., & Tarrier, N. (2008). Cognitive behavior therapy for schizophrenia: Effect sizes, clinical models, and methodological rigor. *Schizophrenia Bulletin, 34*, 523–537.

Zubin, J. & Spring, B. (1977). Vulnerability – A new view of schizophrenia. *Journal of Abnormal Psychology, 86(2)*, 103–126.

10 Not Just a Comic Relief

Medical Clowns in the Forensic Mental Health Setting[1]

Hilik Peri, Mickey Bash, and Etay R. Nachmias

The work of medical clowns at the 'Sha'ar Menashe' Mental Health Center (MHC) in Israel began in 2010. This work evolved from a collaboration between two partners: the MHC staff and management and the "Dream Doctors" association, founded by the 'Maggie and Philnor Foundations'. We are all used to seeing medical clowns in children's wards in general hospitals, and in the last few years, even in medical facilities serving adults and seniors. But in mental health settings, it is an unfamiliar sight, especially in forensic wards. In developing this program, we knew that we were expanding this intervention to a new population and would need to clarify our conceptualizations and adapt our implementation. Together, clinical psychologists and medical clowns struggled to give sense of and find an accurate adaptation for such encounters.

After more than 10 years of working together, it seems natural to see medical clowns working with patients in the various psychiatric wards. These days, they work in eight wards, in weekly sessions. Settings include acute, psycho-geriatric and forensic wards. In this chapter, we will describe the unique work that is done in the 'Sha'ar Menashe' forensic facility, which contains four forensic wards, also known as maximum security wards. This facility is a government national center where some of the most complex patients in Israel are committed. Therapeutic encounters are mostly carried out in group settings, although for the past five years we have also gained experience with one-to-one interactions, especially with patients for whom verbal communication is difficult or who need to be reached in different and creative ways.

We experience how the entrance of the clowns onto the wards changes the atmosphere; it becomes more vital and vibrant, full of magic, music and laughter. From the very beginning, the patients showed a lot of interest and curiosity in the new and exciting possibilities that the clowns brought with them, possibilities that can only be found in the unique way medical clowns perform and relate.

DOI: 10.4324/9781003360926-13

Let's Imagine. You are walking on a sidewalk and suddenly you catch in the corner of your eye some people gathering, laughing and enjoying music. It's a colorful scene; a clown is performing in an improvised arena. Some will rush to their business, telling themselves, "It's all nonsense, a waste of precious time", while others will come near and take part in something funny or exciting, something they didn't plan for or predict was coming. In a way, they take a risk because, with clowns and jokers, you can suddenly become the joke yourself. The experience of medical clowning in the forensic wards has some resemblance to the scene portrayed here, but it has many other characteristics that make it full of tension, extreme emotions and even danger.

Here, the sidewalk is a hall surrounded by clean walls and locked doors. Psychiatric nurses are watching through a big window with tempered glass. The participants are not free to move on to carry out their day-to-day matters elsewhere; these are people who suffer from extreme mental health states. Some of them experience confusion, anxiety and emotional instability. Others present deep sadness and despair; some have difficulties grasping reality and can be fearful and suspicious. They find themselves coping, apart from their own mental difficulties, with social alienation and stigma. The stigma has a way of being internalized, and one feels ill, weak, incompetent, violent and unpredictable (Corrigan & Watson, 2002). They are a group of patients that are considered to be unstable and, at times, even dangerous. The experience of danger is grounded in reality, as some of them committed serious crimes harming others, may it be an innocent bystander, a close relative or a medical staff member, and even in the most tragic circumstances, attacks that ended in murder.

With the entrance of the clown into the ward, we invite the patients to a 'potential space', where the clown gives an opportunity to experience 'play' in a safe environment. A place to be creative and imaginative that "facilitates growth and therefore health" (Winnicott, 1971, p. 40). Most of our patients have experienced traumatic events and environments early in their lives. Such experiences can damage one's sense of self, provoke pathological and defensive responses, and impact individuals' development and personality organization (Khan, 1963; Winnicott, 1953, 1965). From a clinical point of view, we meet patients whose fragile personality structure is defined by difficulties distinguishing between reality and imagination, whose boundaries between the self and others are blurred, and whose profound difficulties may be experienced in the ability to maintain emotional stability and control (Kernberg, 1995).

This invitation to step with our patients into this fragile 'potential 'space' is a complicated, not to say threatening, challenge for the medical clown, as he or she must be sensitive, attentive and alert, recognizing delicate clues that might indicate disturbances and dysregulations in our patients.

Though this is true for all of the wards that the medical clowns are working on, it is a far greater challenge on the forensic wards. Elsewhere, one of us (Peri, 2019) described the complex therapeutic work with patients that is being committed in the forensic ward. Patients who acted on their aggressive impulses in reality crossed the line between fantasy and reality, inflicting pain and damage on another person. Many of them suffer from comorbidity between severe mental disturbances and antisocial tendencies confronting the laws of society. This kind of background makes it emotionally loaded and frightening for the patient and therapist to be close and to relate (Minne, 2008).

Understanding the subjective experience of the patients, especially while in the acute phase (Eissler, 1951), was a very important step in letting the medical clowns step into the forensic wards. The next step was getting to know the MHC setting. In other words, after getting to know the "audience", it was important to get to know the "stage".

There is a growing understanding that it is better to help people in emotional distress in their own natural surroundings by encouraging self-help and help from family and friends (Cooke, 2017). Unfortunately, for many, community resources are not enough, limited, if not absent. And some need a more protective setting for their own safety and the safety of others (Fisher, Geller and Pandiani, 2009, Wyder, Bland and Crompton, 2016).

The hospital is not a familial and homey environment, especially when you are committed without consent. It's a medical institute that follows rules, restrictions, procedures and bureaucracy. There is a risk that patients will be assessed through a lens of biological deficits or pathology and through the use of labels that can miss the person with their unique personality (Turel, 2019). When patients experience the staff as emotionally reserved and distant, it may lead to expressions of anger and frustration. Sometimes the setting itself makes it hard for the patients to benefit from the compassion and care that is provided by professional health care staff. Working in such a complex environment carries with it the burden of holding harsh emotions and the danger of some defensive maneuvers from the side of the staff, such as creating a split between those who have control over their lives, "healthy, mature and normal", and the patients who are "sick, childish and unpredictable" (Hinshelwood, 1986). This split corresponds with the social stigma mental health patients experience outside the hospital. In the middle of this split, the medical clown has an important role.

In order to better understand the complexity of the unique encounter, it's important to review the nature of the clown as a figure that goes back in human history. There is rich and profound writing about the social and cultural role of the clown mentioned in myths, legends, philosophy and religion. "The Fool" is one example of what Jung called an "Archetype", a deep structure in the social and cultural collective unconsciousness, a role with a "Special spell", peculiar and fascinating (Jung, 1964, p. 79). The fool (or the clown) derives his or her strength and characteristics from the archetype of the trickster. The trickster is at the heart of a developmental journey, from a childish and impulsive position to a mature and integrative stance. The trickster is manifested in myths as displaying an amorphous identity and as often failing to adjust and be a part of society and the "good order". But when you look deeply into the journey he goes through, he touches on broad and complex human issues, reveals the truth and points out the distortions in the familiar social structure. (Henderson, 1964; Radin, 1948).

Van Blerkom (1995) points out that one can see the clown as a liminal figure, the figure of the shaman, mysterious and full of impression, evoking fear and curiosity. Anthropological research presents the shaman as a central figure in the ritual as a rite of passage. The shaman allows transitions, building a bridge between nature and culture, past and future, life and death (Turner, 1969). From this standpoint, you can imagine power and control, but on the other side of the coin, the clown stands as a scapegoat. Baroch (2017) notes that the archaic clown is a container for what society refuses to contain: physical deformity, illness, death and madness. This role puts the clown in danger of being condemned and even sacrificed as a way for society to expel unwanted drives and characteristics. It seems that the clown has a certain freedom to test boundaries and challenge society. He is called a *fool*, but in many ways he is *full* of wit, the one who sees the true, certain parts that society doesn't want to emotionally hold and process (Netzer, 2008). This is the beauty of the clown. It makes him an essential participant in the social structure. But it can also make it challenging for the scientific and medical establishments to contain and accept him.

In the early 80s of the last century, medical clowning appeared as a therapeutic field, first with the introduction of professional clowns to children's wards in general hospitals (Van Troostwijk, 2006). The encounter between the medical clown and the child's world, a world where fantasy and play are available, seems natural and intuitive. The main therapeutic goals of medical clowning were defined as easing the suffering of the patients and encouraging recovery with the help of humor, acting and imagination. Linge (2012) describes the connections that are built between the hospitalized child and the medical clown as 'magical attachments'. This short-term relationship helps the child to process feelings of anxiety, helplessness, confusion and vulnerability.

Raviv (2014) notes that the act of the show itself is a central aspect of the medical clown's healing power. "The healing performance" helps relieve difficult feelings and anxiety, sadness and despair and allows observing reality from a different, humorous and fresh angle. In exploring the "Family resemblance" between medical clowning and drama therapy, Pendzik and Raviv (2011) further elaborate on the medical clown and his therapeutic assets. They conclude that unlike the therapist, who exists for the patient as a containing and holding frame of the therapeutic process and is identified as coming from the world of reality, the clown acts as someone who appears in front of an audience and shares and sweeps the audience into the experience, when he himself is identified as coming from a space of imagination and fantasy.

The entry point of medical clowning into the general hospital was through the work with children, and the adults that enjoyed the benefits of this work were the companions of the hospitalized child or the adult staff member caring for the child. Medical clowns began to join various therapeutic procedures in hospitals, and a record of the healing benefits of their presence and intervention became apparent. Better compliance, better mood and better communication with the staff were found. An important effect was also found with the parent that accompanies the child. Examples where effects were found include blood test procedures (Meiri, Ankri, Hamad-Saied, Konopnicki, & Pillar, 2016), burn treatments (Yildirim, Koroglu, Yucel, Senay Kirlak, & Sen, 2019), and an experience with tests related to sexually abused children (Tener, Lang, Ofir, & Lev-Wiesel, 2010).

The next step that occurred was for the adult in a situation of hospitalization or treatment himself to be at the center of the medical clown intervention (Nuttman-Shwartza, Scheyer, & Tzioni, 2010). Here, research is limited, but there is important data showing benefits such as the reduction of patients' agitation and stress and changes in the atmosphere to be more playful and even amusing (Dionigi & Canestrati, 2016). It is important to note here that there is some research that points out that the clown should carefully watch for signs of adult patients who do not want to be involved in humorous interaction. With grownups, it is apparent that being open to amusement on a "bad day" isn't obvious and depends on personal traits that should be evaluated (Auerbach, 2017; Efrat-Triester, Altman, Friedmann, Margalit, & Teodorescu, 2021).

Introducing the clowns to the MHC's turned out to be a complicated task. Gelkopf (2011) reviews clinical and empirical studies about the use of humor and laughter as a therapeutic tool for those suffering from serious mental disorders. At the end of his review, he points out that there is a poor experience in this setting. He presents two main explanations for that: First, the socialization process of the medical staff, which emphasizes hierarchical relationships and social distancing, the second one is rooted in social stigma, with the perception that those who suffer from serious disorders are impaired in their ability to understand and enjoy humor.

Of the few studies in this field of experience, the following three studies are most relevant to the work described in this chapter. Higueras et al. (2006) found a positive effect of a "therapeutic clown" approach, using humor-centered activity to address disruptive behavior in psychiatric patients in a general hospital psychiatric ward. In addition to significant decreases in attempted escapes, self-injury and fighting, there were warm responses from patients and relatives. Gruber, Levin and Lichtenberg (2015) described a program held in a psychiatric ward using psychodramatic group therapy held by a medical clown. In this inspiring work, they presented the developmental gains patients can achieve when invited to a dramatic role play. They report the revealing of one's voice, gaining back self-confidence and building or exercising new ways to be with others. Although their case study, reporting on only an individual case, limits generalization, their observations of the effects of the intervention they described in this study were similar to the effects we observed and documented in our program. Sviridov and Grinshpoon (2019) conducted a survey in the forensic facility in 'Sha'ar Menashe' to assess the staff's perception of the impact of our own program on the patient population. The majority of the staff recognized the medical clown's positive effect on the patients and the atmosphere in the ward. Alongside that perception, some staff members experienced it as a disturbance to the daily routine and felt it even as creating pressure for the staff that take part in facilitating the activity. We ourselves experienced the staff's enthusiastic responses: "I never saw Mr. K. laughing", "I didn't know he is such a good dancer", "Did you hear the song he wrote?" And to other comments as well, especially when the days are busy and in the face of outbursts and violence: "Please turn the music down, you are too noisy", "Don't make such sharp movements, don't you see what's going on here". Those kinds of responses are natural and may reflect a worried and overloaded staff that tries to keep things quiet and under control.

The encounter between the psychiatric institution, the complex patients hospitalized there and the medical clown can create collisions and discomfort. The clown brings with him drama, challenge, ridiculous and ludicrous behaviors, and above all, stretches the boundaries between what is conventional and what is surprising, extraordinary and even provocative (Citron, 2014). We had a deep understanding that was accompanied by anxiety that we were offering our patients an important space for experiences, but we recognized that the experiences should be carefully guided and thought through.

The necessary guidance is provided in the form of supervision sessions, or consultation, with an experienced therapist who directs the medical clown, who may be a novice in mental health treatment. This has become a fruitful joint space for both the experienced supervisor and medical clown, the latter with limited prior experience in mental health settings. We introduced medical clowns to psychological thinking about the emotional world, psychoanalytical ideas and developmental theories, personality and psychopathology, and learned about the deep essence of clowning and performance. It felt like a parallel process that had to be delicate and playful, so we could respect and give place to intellectual understanding and knowledge and also respect the clown's intuition and inner freedom. What worked for us was encouraging emotional openness in a safe environment that is free of judgment, working hard to understand different languages and enjoying sharing and being together through this special journey.

In order to build between us a joint 'compass' to direct our work, we found it helpful to focus on three main goals: the first one was to enhance the patient's individuality, reassure their self-identity and their emotional experiences. The second one was to help them learn new ways to experience social interaction and positive cooperation. And the third one was finding new ways to sublimate harsh feelings, such as anger and frustration. The diagram below summarizes the model that we formulated:

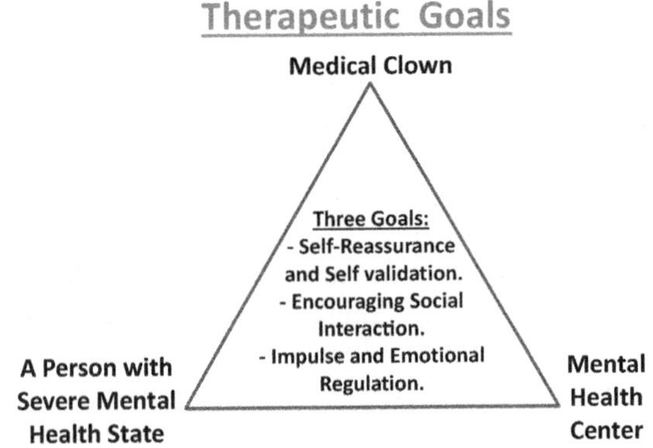

Figure 10.1 This diagram shows the three main goals of the Medical Clown intervention in working with people with severe mental health states: (1) Self-Reassurance and Self-Validation (2) Encouraging Social Interaction (3) Impulse and Emotional Regulation.

We will now explore four vignettes, glimpses into the medical clowns' work in the forensic wards. You will notice that the frame of the sessions is familiar, but the content of the session remains a bit vague, which allows the clown to bring something spontaneous, surprising and challenging:

VIGNETTE 1

Medical clown M. holds in his hand a bouquet of flowers that he has just collected on his way to the maximum security unit. This is a bouquet of Lantana flowers in purple, white, red and pink colors. In the maximum security ward, patients are preparing for the group session with him, sitting down in a familiar circle of chairs, as happens once a week. The session begins with an activity of music and movement, and patients can choose their favorite song. You find here diverse musical choices: hip-hop, trance, soul, and even songs with a religious tone. Each participant introduces his own special taste in music and the reason they chose a song. The group is required to adapt to and contain the different rhythms. While the music is being played, the clown calls on the participants to get into the circle. He himself proposes to diversify the dance movements and turn familiar movements into non-functional, impulsive and unusual movements. It looks odd and strange; the clown moves in inconceivable ways. A few patients join him after hesitation, others sitting with their eyes wide open in astonishment, and others laughing and calling toward the clown: "If someone from the outside sees you, he would think that you are the crazy one!" How hard it is for people whose actions are suspected of anomalies and oddities to join the invitation to play weird. The music stops, and the group moves on to practice breathing. M. fills his chest with air: "Today we will learn how to breathe, to breath is very important!" His statement is accompanied by pathos and a deep voice; the shaman within him appears. "Here it's the rib cage, we're all confined inside this cage. Today we will learn to produce movement in it and breathe". This short exercise works like magic; M. connects at this moment to an inner experience of the patients in the closed ward. Some of the patients indeed describe the wards as cages or prisons. And M. examines with them how this difficult and complex place can be brought into a dynamic space. All the while, the Lantana flowers are placed on the 'clown's chair, as if he holds a secret he brought from a distant, faraway place. Toward the end of the session, he begins to hand out the flowers using noble gestures and bends on his knee in a somewhat romantic gesture: "Oh, red flower for you". It seems both surreal and elegant and puts smiles on the faces of the participants. At the end of the group, M. puts a familiar song, and the participants dance in a circle, tapping each other on the back. With the last note of the song, they all look at each other and call out loud, "I know!" A way to say that what they experienced just now is in a place in space between imagination and reality.

In this vignette, it seems that M. expands the space between the walls of the ward hall. He creates a bridge between the outside world, where there is nature, color and freedom, and the secured and locked ward. The clown, who let himself be "crazy", enters a dramatic space without worrying that there is no way back. "Who is the crazy one?" the patients ask him. A description of this dramatic space while working with children in the general hospital can be found in Raviv's (2012) work. Hospital corridors are transformed into magical-imagined journeys, and staff members become captive to the children themselves. And here, M., in his noble gestures, gives our patients the feeling that they are special and deserve his "courting" efforts. The relationships between the hospitalized person and a member of the staff change dramatically, and the patient becomes the chosen one.

VIGNETTE 2

Medical clown E. enters the ward. Mr. A. is pleased to see him and they have a few moments together before the group session. Mr. A. starts by joking with the medical clown: "Does your wife knows that you took her panties?", and then: "Say Ra'anana" (a city in Israel), "The clown says: "Ra'anana", and the patient answers him "Banana!" with a victorious smile. After this known text, he is opening a discussion about music from the 80s, and in each conversation, he tries to challenge the clown and his knowledge on the music of this period, hoping to catch him with his "pants down". In a touching interaction, Mr. A. shares the death of his wife and his work as a musician that was interrupted because of his mental breakdown. Mr. A. is a sad "Joker", who finds a safe place to share with the clown.

The use of humor by this patient and many others gives us a lot of joy. For instance, in one of the first encounters of the medical clowns in the ward, one of the patients, very sensitive and full of wit, warned M., "People here are crazy. Be careful, if you ask them to behave as monkeys, don't be certain they will be able to get out of it", it was followed by a meaningful smile. The clown who comes from the outside is considered to be emotionally available and becomes a precious figure with whom our patients can relate. They can joke with him, be sincere and loose, and it can open new ways to share even in personal experiences of pain and loss. As one of the medical staff members expressed in his own words when he called to ask for medical clown intervention, "I believe that something formal won't work here".

VIGNETTE 3

Medical clown M. enters the ward; he meets a new patient who is in an acute psychotic/manic state. The patient is in his mid-twenties, tall and athletic, and moving around restlessly, like a lion in a cage. The session starts with a lot of tension. The patient stands in the middle of the arena, moves and dances in a way that nobody can get near. Patients are upset; some of them express frustration and anger, and others are frightened. The medical clown steps in and joins the ecstatic dance, jumping and throwing arms and legs everywhere. Next, he suggests to the patient that they hold hands, and they both start to spin together; their hands are firmly held together. The clown asks the patient to stop, and they turn back to back. They are leaning on each other, regaining their breath. They turn to each other, shaking hands, and the medical clown thanks the patient and asks him to sit down for the next activity. He initiates role play: "We will now play something that you might encounter outside the hospital. You are going to the bank to ask for a loan. One of you will act as the banker, and the other one will be the customer". It's easier for the patients to act as the banker; they portray him as a tough man who has no sympathy. The customers are usually more embarrassed and hesitant, M. helps them by encouraging them, and they all begin the interaction by saying a phrase M. is repeating continuously: "I exist, I matter, I can, and I will succeed!". In one of the acts, the patient we described earlier stands up and shouts: "Don't lend him the money, don't you see that he is crazy?!?". The moment of tense silence, the psychiatric nurses are getting closer, and M. tries to calm down and point out that it is a game. Help is coming from an unpredictable direction; the 'bank manager' comes to help: "You know, you look like a good guy, I will lend you the money". "A big applause to our bank manager!", says M. and the group has found new ways to get through another hard moment.

The medical clown 'can't work under these straining conditions without feeling safe. It is essential that, when entering wards, he ask for an update from the staff concerning the atmosphere on the ward, special events, and patients who are new to the ward or whose mental state has changed and who are not stable. There will always be a psychiatric nurse around and security guards; they are supposed to be alert and intervene when needed. In this vignette, we see how the inner experiences of a man who is in mental disarray are being acted on in his interpersonal interactions, so emotions and thoughts are being replaced by actions. He lost a fundamental aspect of mental health; the ability to "play" or pretend. Ogden (1985) discusses the dialectic qualities of the transitional space, a place that is between reality and imagination, between what is "me" and what is "not-me". On other occasions, we have witnessed this blending of imagination and reality, internal and external; one of our patients had the delusion that a medical clown had a plan to attack him, and another heard the voice of a medical clown commanding him to hurt another patient. The medical clowns are a part of the stimuli that the patients perceive, and they are "getting into their system", as one of our patients vividly described. Those instances are rare but need to be handled with professional guidance and collaboration with other staff members. Usually, it is a sign that a patient is very anxious and needs help in order to maintain his own safety and that of others around him.

VIGNETTE 4

Medical clown E. enters the ward. He is most welcome and, through the years, has built strong relationships with some of the patients there, but usually the motivation for participating and connecting is not high. Medical clown E. is used to hearing Mr. B. screaming at him: "Stop that noise, go away!". This patient is sitting in the corner of the hall with his back to the circle. The medical clown uses humorous gestures to catch the attention of his audience: "Let's start practice!" he says in a way you can imagine a gymnastic teacher. "But I don't want to!" he answers to himself in a childish manner while raising his shoulder like a child that is asked to follow an unwanted command. A big smile is spreading all around, and the participants start to follow his words, "I don't want to!" while starting to practice. Following the warmup, it's the turn of the "Fingers gym", and the hands and fingers are jumping from side to side on his knees. It's not very active training, but there is movement, and the room is filled with energy and laughter. At the end of the warmup, the medical clown reaches into his pocket and takes out a soap bubble toll. The participants then gather around the clown, who is blowing delicate and colorful bubbles. Most surprising is the way he creates small bubbles inside a big one with a very delicate blow of air. Not surprising is the fact that Mr. B. finds himself in the middle of the activity, attracted and involved. As with other patients in the ward, his cooperation won't guarantee his participation next week, and new, exciting and creative opportunities should always be offered by the medical clown.

This last illustration demonstrates in a very delicate and playful way how the medical clown has a way of overcoming resistance and rejection in a clownish way, amusing and at the same time human way. Creating motivation in patients, who may feel alone and distant from desired human contact, restricted and with limited resources, is a hard task but a very satisfying one.

Conclusion

We decided to 'close the curtain' on this chapter with a tribute to Stephen Sondhiem, the musical theater legend, who passed away two years ago (November 2021). The lyrics of his song "Send in the Clowns" accompanied us during the writing of the chapter ('A Little Night Music', 1973). This song became an inspiration for many performers and writers. Sondheim himself was surprised by the great attention this song has received and later explained that the clowns, or jokers, are the ones you send in when things don't go well on the stage (Horowitz, 2010; Sondheim, 2010). That's a good idea to use in times you feel confusion and disarray; it gives everybody, both the audience and actors, a form of relief in order to continue the show. Those of us working as traditional mental health professionals in inpatient settings can certainly relate to this need. Doing such work in such settings, you feel harsh feelings of fear and pain, sorrow and confusion, where notions such as hope and belief are under attack and failure and helplessness are familiar guests.

We learned during the years that inviting the clown doctors is not just a comic relief, but a new and surprising way to give our patients something that couldn't be found in the mental health institute. It can be considered another form of therapeutic intervention, one that gives the clown and his performance a central role in engaging and creating a playful environment that has many benefits for our patients. Following 'Sondheim's words, perhaps in saying, "We are out of words here", so, "Let's be creative"!

Note

1 We would like to thank Mr. Emanuel Amrami, clinical psychologist and psychoanalyst, who worked many years in the forensic facility in 'Sha'ar Menashe' Mental Health Center and initiated this program. Thank you for your courage, intuition and wisdom that made the entrance of the medical clowns possible.

References

Auerbach, S. (2017). Are clowns good for everyone? The influence of trait cheerfulness on emotional reactions to a hospital clown intervention. *Frontiers in Psychology*, 8, 1973.

Baroch, R. E. (2017). *The fool in European drama. Studies in European avant-garde drama: Jarry, wedekind, ghelderode, brechet, Beckett, weiss*. Safra Books.

Citron, A. (2014). Audacity and insane courage: Dream doctors' secret remedies. In *Performance studies in motion international perspectives and practices in the twenty-first century*. Eds: Citron, A., Aronson-Lehavi, S. and zerbib, D., Ch. 19, pp. 261–275. Bloomsbury/Methuen Drama

Cooke, A. (Eds.) (2017). *Understanding psychosis and schizophrenia. Revisited version*. Division of Clinical Psychology.

Corrigan, P. W. and Watson, A. C. (2002). The paradox of self stigma. *Clinical Psychology: Science and Practice*, 9(1), 35–53.

Dionigi, A. and Canestrari, C. (2016). Clowning in health care settings: The point of view of adults. *Europe's Journal of Psychology*, 12(3), 473–488.

Efrat-Triester, D., Altman, D., Friedmann, E., Margalit, D. L., and Teodorescu, K. (2021). Exploring the usefulness of medical clowns in elevating satisfaction and reducing aggressive tendencies in pediatric and adult hospital wards. *BMC Health Services Research*, 21(1), 15.

Eissler, K. R. (1951). Remarks on the psychoanalysis of schizophrenia. *The International Journal of Psychoanalysis*, 32, 139–156.

Fisher, W. H., Geller, J. L., and Pandiani, J. A. (2009). The changing role of the state psychiatric hospital. *Health Affairs*, 28(3), 676–684.

Gelkopf, M. (2011). The use of humor in serious mental illness: A review. *Evidence-Based Complementary and Alternative Medicine*, 2011, 8.

Gruber, A., Levin, R., and Lichtenberg, P. (2015). Medical clowning and psychosis: A case report and theoretical review. *The Israel Journal of Psychiatry and Related Sciences*, 52(3), 20–23.

Henderson, J. L. (1964). Ancient myths and modern man. In *Man and his symbols*. Eds: Gung, C. G. and Von Franz, M. L., pp. 104–157. Aldus Books Limited.

Higueras, A., Carretero-Dios, H., Munoz, J.P., Idini, E., Ortiz, A., Rincon, F., Prieto-Merino, D., and Aguila, M. D. (2006). Effects of a humor-centered activity on disruptive behavior in patients in a general hospital psychiatric ward. *International Journal of Clinical and Health Psychology*, 6, 53–64.

Hinshelwood, R. D. (1986). The psychotherapist's role in a large institution. *Psychoanlytic Psychotherapy*, 2(3), 207–215.

Horowitz, M. E. (2010). *Sondheim on music: Minor details and major decisions*. Scarecrow Press.

Jung. C.G. (1964). Approaching the unconscious, In *Man and his Symbols*. Eds: Jung, C. G. and Von Franz M. L., pp. 18–103. Aldus Books Limited.

Kernberg, O. F. (1995). *Object relations theory and clinical psychoanalysis*. Jason Aronson.

Khan, M. M. R. (1963). The concept of cumulative trauma. *The Psychoanalytic Study of the Child*, 18(1), 286–306.

Linge, L. (2012). Magical attachment: Children in magical relations with hospital clowns. *International Journal of Qualitative Studies on Health and Well-being*, 7(1), 11862.

Meiri, N., Ankri, A., Hamad-Saied, M. Konopnicki, M., and Pillar, G. (2016). The effect of medical clowning on reducing pain, crying, and anxiety in children aged

2–10 years old undergoing venous blood drawing—a randomized controlled study. *Euroopean Journal of Pediatrics*, 175, 373–379.

Minne, C. (2008). The dreaded and dreading patient and therapist. In *Psychic assault and frightened clinicians*. Eds: Gordon, J. and Kirtchuk, G., pp. 27–40. London: Karnac Books.

Netzer, R. (2008). *The magician, the fool and the empress*. Modan Publishing House.

Nuttman-Shwartza, O., Scheyer, R., and Tzioni, H. (2010). Medical clowning: Even adults deserve a dream. *Social Work in Health Care*, 49(6), 581–598.

Ogden, T. H. (1985). On potential space. *International Journal of Psycho-Analysis*, 66, 129–141.

Pendzik, S. and Raviv, A. (2011). Therapeutic clowning and drama therapy: A family resemblance. *The Arts in Psychotherapy*, 38, 267–275.

Peri, H. (2019). The Clinical Psychologist's Work in a Forensic Psychiatry Ward. In *Clinical Psychology in the Mental Health Inpatient Setting*, Eds: Turel, M., Siglag, M., Grinshpoon, A., Routledge. pp. 267–283.

Radin, P. (1948). *Winnebago hero cycles: A study in aboriginal literature* (No. 1–5). Waverly Press.

Raviv, A. (2012). Still the best medicine, even in a war zone. My work as a medical clown. *The Drama Review*, 56(2), 169–177.

Raviv, A. (2014). The healing performance: The medical clown as compared to African Kung and Azande ritual healers. *Dramatherapy*, 36(1), 18–26.

Sondheim, S. (1973). *A little night music*.Broadway, The Shubert Theatre.

Sondheim, S. (2010). *Finishing the Hat: Collected Lyrics (1954–1981) with Attendant Comments, Principles, Heresies, Grudges, Whines and Anecdotes*. Alfred A. Knop. pp. 277–278.

Sviridov, K. and Grinshpoon, A. (2019). Medical clowning in a amaximum secure forensic unit in a a mental health center: Impressions of the caregiving staff (Brief report). *Isreal Journal of Psychiatry*, 55(2), 54–55.

Tener, D., Lang. N., Ofir, S., and Lev-Wiesel, R. (2010). Laughing through this pain: Medical clowning during examination of sexually abused children: An innovative approach. *Journal of Child Sexsual Abuse*, 19(2), 128–140.

Turel, M. (2019). Weaving with a relarional thread: The clinical psychologist use of empathy in the mental health inpatient setting. In *Clinical psychology in the mental health patient setting*. Eds: Turel, M., Siglag, M. and Grinshpoon, A., Routledge. pp. 423–435.

Turner, V. (1969). *The ritual process: Structure and anti-structure*. Aldin.

Van Blerkom, L. M. (1995). Clown doctors: Shaman healers of western medicine. *Medical Anthropology Quarterly, New Series*, 9(4), (Dec., 1995), 462–475.

Van Troostwijk, T. D. (2006). The hospital clown: A cross boundary character. In *Making sense of stress, humour and healing*. Ed: Litvack, A., Inter-disciplinary Press Publishing Creative Research.

Winnicott, D. W. (1953). Psychoses and child care. *The British Journal of Medical Psychology*, 26(1), 68–74.

Winnicott, D. W. (1965). Providing for the child in health and in crisis. *International Journal of Psychoanalysis*, 64, 64–72.

Winnicott, D. W. (1971). Playing: A theoretical statement, ch. 3. pp. 38–52 in *Playing and Reality*. London: Tavistock Publications.

Wyder, M., Bland, R., & Crompton, D. (2016). The importance of safety, agency and control during involuntary mental health admissions. *Journal of mental health (Abingdon, England)*, *25*(4), 338–342. https://doi.org/10.3109/09638237.2015.1124388

Yildirim, M., Koroglu, E., Yucel, C., Senay Kirlak, S., and Sen, S. (2019). The effect of hospital clown nurse on children's compliance to burn dressing change. *Burns*, 45, 190–198.

11 Development of a Legal Competency Restoration Program within a Forensic Psychiatric Hospital

Susie Chung, Ashley Strathern, and Jeffrey Palmer

Introduction to Competency to Stand Trial

Competency to stand trial (CST) or competence to proceed, which involves a defendant's rational and factual understanding of the legal proceedings in court as well as the defendant's ability to assist the defense attorney, is the most frequently adjudicated psycho-legal issue in the American criminal justice system. While the exact number of competency assessments conducted annually is unclear (Morris et al., 2021), the assessment of CST and restoration efforts plays a major role in the practice of forensic psychology. Although the concept of CST as it relates to one's participation in the criminal judicial process can be traced back over 200 years (Melton et al., 2017), the focus of scientific pursuits from a forensic mental health perspective has been largely devoted to the assessment of an individual's competence to proceed rather than the restoration of competency.

In *Dusky v. United States* (1960), the U.S. Supreme Court defined the concept of CST as a defendant having the ability to rationally consult with counsel as well as possessing a rational and factual understanding of their criminal proceedings. This *Dusky* decision has become the minimum standard in federal court as well as in all state jurisdictions. *Drope v. Missouri* (1975) and *Godinez v. Moran* (1993) further elaborated or clarified that competent defendants must also have the capacity to assist their attorney in preparing their defense as well as possess certain decision-making abilities. When defendants are found incompetent to stand trial (IST), they have historically been sent to a psychiatric hospital – sometimes indefinitely – for inpatient psychiatric treatment to determine whether they can become competent. However, in *Jackson v. Indiana* (1972), the U.S. Supreme Court ruled that a defendant who is found IST cannot be held for more than the reasonable length of time necessary to determine whether there is a substantial probability that they will attain competency in the foreseeable future. Thus, research focusing on treatments specifically targeted toward competency restoration has been increasing over time.

DOI: 10.4324/9781003360926-14

Rationale for Developing a Legal Competency Restoration Program at a State Psychiatric Hospital

Defendants who are found IST typically remain in the criminal justice system until they are restored to competence or their charges are dismissed; some IST defendants require lengthy hospitalizations in state forensic psychiatric hospitals. Historically, standard hospital treatment for those defendants consisted of milieu therapy, participation in rehabilitation programs targeting psychiatric stabilization, and psychopharmacological treatment. In some cases, basic education of legal terms/concepts was also provided during hospitalization. In a state forensic hospital in New Jersey, about 2,000 defendants have been committed for competency evaluations between 2000 and 2023.

Despite the methods used to estimate these numbers varying in reliability, the number of competency evaluation orders has likely increased over the last five decades. Some studies suggest that between 1% and 8% of defendants in the United States may be referred for CST evaluations (Morris et al., 2021). Considering that 80–90% of defendants are restored to competency within six months (Zapf, 2013; National Judicial Task Force, 2021) and the limited number of beds in forensic or state psychiatric hospitals, it is even more essential that the most effective treatment is provided in efforts to restore defendants to competency. In New Jersey, defendants who are found IST are sent to one of three state psychiatric hospitals, depending on the severity of their charges and the county where the charges originate.

Individuals Requiring Competency Restoration

Most defendants referred to New Jersey's state forensic hospital experience symptoms of serious mental illness with a significant risk of either self-harm, self-neglect, or assault, conditions that preclude consideration of less restrictive settings for competency restoration. However, competency restoration in less-restrictive settings (e.g., outpatient) is not available in many states, including New Jersey.

Factors associated with a low likelihood of restorability of defendants found in several studies include older age, diagnoses of intellectual disability, a severe psychotic illness, a longer cumulative length of stay, and being on multiple medications; in contrast, defendants with predominantly mood disorders tended to have a favorable chance of restoration (Pirelli et al., 2011; Warren et al., 2013). A review of the defendants that have been hospitalized under an IST commitment court order and treated with the Legal Competency Restoration Program (LCRP) found that the average defendant was around the age of 40, male, and diagnosed with a psychotic illness, such as schizophrenia or schizoaffective disorder.

Background/History of CompKit and the Legal Competency Restoration Program

Florida State Hospital assembled the CompKit: Competency to Proceed Training Resources from a combination of locally developed materials as well as those developed across the nation. The CompKit package takes a multi-modal approach to enhance learning. It includes the printed documents, one compact disk containing the instructional materials, and one digital video disk containing videos (consisting of one mock court hearing, one mock trial, and competency restoration training presented as a television game show). It also includes brochures that summarize important materials for the defendants, which were translated into Spanish and Haitian Creole. In the manual's suggestions for teaching the materials, learning styles, cultural considerations, and educational achievement levels are all taken into consideration (Florida State Hospital, 2009). Exercises employ vignettes in which defendants role-play various court situations in order to apply acquired knowledge to assist in their defense. In addition, teaching approaches are discussed for different types of learners, labeled as IST typologies (Florida State Hospital, 2009). Each typology is a category defined by the psycho-legal deficits or symptoms of mental illness that impair an individual's competence.

CompKit was first introduced outside Florida State Hospital in 2007 at a national meeting (Florida State Hospital, 2009). A comprehensive program to address the unique treatment needs of the IST defendant population was long overdue in the state of New Jersey, not only for those who were not responding to standard hospital care but also in response to the courts' requests for such an intervention. As a result, the LCRP, based on the CompKit and adapted to New Jersey statutes in 2010, was created by Susie Chung, Ph.D., with the assistance of a legal expert, the late Melanie Griffin, Esq. The LCRP was implemented in 2011 with the assistance of Ashley Strathern, Psy.D., at a forensic psychiatric hospital. Prior to 2011, rehabilitation staff ran a group in which basic legal terms were taught to IST defendants. The LCRP extends beyond teaching basic legal terms by encompassing the standard for assessing competency that was defined by *Dusky* and elaborated by *Drope* and *Godinez*. Moreover, important components of the LCRP that were previously absent in other restoration efforts are psychological interventions such as individual social and verbal reinforcement, cognitive-behavioral techniques (e.g., to address defendants' delusional beliefs by generating alternate explanations or to develop adaptive responses), and in-group behavior plans with social and tangible reinforcements.

Description of the Legal Competency Restoration Program

The goal of the LCRP is to provide treatment to defendants who are psychiatrically hospitalized after being adjudicated incompetent to proceed. Treatment includes: (1) providing accurate and relevant information about the criminal justice system specific to the State of New Jersey; (2) setting social and behavioral expectations for participation in their legal case; (3) monitoring progress in the defendant's ability to factually and rationally understand the criminal justice system as well as to assist counsel; and (4) assisting the treatment team in identifying psychiatric symptoms that interfere with the defendant's competence. The group sessions are central aspects of the LCRP, but there are other important components of the program. In addition to the group sessions, the LCRP encompasses a screening assessment component, a targeted individual treatment component based on IST typology that involves individual sessions, clinical case management with the treatment team, and clinical documentation in the form of weekly and end-of-program summary progress notes (specifically designed to provide data needed by the evaluator who assesses the defendant's competence). The LCRP follows a structured curriculum and culminates with mock trials: one that is fully scripted and one that allows the defendants to come up with their own case and legal strategy. These mock trials prepare the defendants for court by providing them with an in vivo opportunity to build on and apply learned skills that are associated with participation in the legal process.

Two of the most important goals of the LCRP are: (1) monitoring the defendant's psychiatric symptoms; and (2) teaching skills to cope with those symptoms that may interfere with becoming competent. At the outset of each group, defendants are clinically screened to identify the IST typology that best fits their competency-related deficits. Defendants are separated into the following typologies based on the etiology of their incompetence: Delusional/Irrational, Psychotic/Confused, Low Functioning, Disruptive, and Advanced/Maintenance. Defendants who exhibit symptoms of delusional and/or irrational beliefs are classified within the Delusional/Irrational typology. Defendants who exhibit other symptoms of psychosis impairing their CST besides delusional beliefs would be classified in the Psychotic/Confused typology. Defendants who exhibit intellectual or neurocognitive deficits that would impair learning or cognition are classified within the Low-Functioning typology. Defendants who exhibit impulsive, belligerent, or attention-seeking behaviors that are interfering with their competency would be classified within the Disruptive typology. Finally, defendants whose competency-related knowledge is intact and whose behavior is stable but who may require continued interventions to maintain their competence would be classified within the Advanced/Maintenance typology. Those who are believed to be feigning symptoms or incompetence are also placed in this category. Often times, defendants may qualify for classification into two categories. In such cases, treatment interventions would be implemented for both categories. However, for purposes of data collection and program management, the most salient symptoms interfering with competency and their related typology would be used.

These typologies help guide interventions; for example, if a defendant's symptoms resulted in behavioral disruption within the group that could potentially prevent them from behaving appropriately in court, then part of the treatment would involve redirection, reinforcement, and/or other individual behavioral techniques during group sessions. In addition to two group sessions per week, individual competency psycho-education and/or psychotherapy sessions are conducted, as needed, to foster increased legal comprehension and active participation as well as to target the IST typology-specific deficits. Individual sessions also allow the defendant to discuss personal case concerns in a confidential learning environment. This approach is in line with the recommendations of the National Judicial Task Force (2021), which stated, "There is an evolving recognition that there is value in all three approaches – medication, individualized treatment, and legal education, to varying degrees depending on the individual defendant's overall needs."

One function of the LCRP is to closely observe defendants and to help differentiate diagnoses, such as determining the occurrence of malingering or ruling-in subtle intellectual impairments that interfere with competence. The information documented in weekly progress notes and a final summary can be incorporated into a defendant's competency evaluation, helping to improve its validity, especially in treatment-resistant cases, by providing examples to illustrate the defendant's skills/deficits related to the factual and rational aspects of *Dusky*. Such data and observations can be – and have been helpful – in suspected malingering cases as well as when making a final determination of non-restorability. When a defendant has completed the LCRP, clinical observations of the defendant during group and individual sessions, accounts of their interactions with other group members and staff, and the defendant's behaviors and understanding of their role during mock trial sessions provide valuable information that can be used to support or inform an evaluator's opinion in the report to the court.

Issues and Obstacles during Program Development and Beyond

In implementing the LCRP, there were a number of obstacles that had to be solved. First was the availability of a one-hour time slot in the rehabilitation wing where the group sessions could be held. Such slots were in high demand. Once a room was identified within the daily schedule of treatment programming, it was determined that it could be utilized only two times per week and could only fit about six to eight defendants, while taking into account the one required security officer and the two group leaders who needed to be present as well as table space for each defendant's binder containing the group materials. The LCRP was also in demand for additional defendants, and we recommended that if a larger space was available, more defendants could participate in a group at a time. When the LCRP was accommodated in a larger room, the group size was increased to a maximum of ten defendants, in addition to the mandatory security officer and two group leaders. More recently, during the COVID-19 pandemic, the groups were hosted the defendant's housing units, allowing for more participants per group.

Another obstacle was related to the method of obtaining referrals for the LCRP and the potential wait times to participate in a group cycle. Each potential participant was screened by a group leader with specific exclusion and inclusion criteria. Group participants had to be committed for 90 days rather than 30 days (to allow for enough time in the hospital to participate in the LCRP) and had to be sufficiently stable psychiatrically so that they were able to either leave their housing unit and attend rehabilitation programming or be able to participate safely in the group on the unit. The group was developed as a closed group, with the same start and end dates for all participants. This enabled defendants to learn competency-related factual terms and concepts before using them to build upon their rational understanding. To ensure adequate group size, the group would not start until at least five referrals had been screened and deemed appropriate for participation. An average of 25 sessions, or 3 months, was necessary for each group to complete the LCRP when groups were only able to be held two times per week (Chung et al., 2013). Each participant also received a minimum of two individual sessions. The LCRP accepted referrals at any time and created a waitlist consisting of defendants who had already been screened and deemed eligible so that as soon as one group finished, another could begin soon after. There were times, particularly in the early years of the LCRP, when obtaining referrals was a longer process. Referral packets containing important information on each defendant's case were often incomplete. Following up with staff members who were responsible for obtaining all the necessary documents took time. Referral packets included the completion of the referral form, a copy of the defendant's competency commitment court order, and the defendant's discovery, including the Grand Jury indictment; these items were used within the LCRP during group and individual sessions. Such documents were used to help teach defendants to read about and understand their charges, including their rational understanding of their legal case. Group facilitators needed to have the information contained in these documents to be educated about the defendant's case so that they could reasonably engage in discussion with defendants throughout the course of the program.

One of the biggest obstacles was finding psychologists within the forensic hospital who were willing to work as group leaders, as they often juggled several job duties already. We restricted group leaders to doctoral-level psychologists with appropriate training in group therapy because they were considered most likely to be familiar with running therapy groups as well as with IST-related skills and concepts. Later, the use of social workers was implemented, mostly due to the need for bilingual Spanish-speaking group leaders. Group leaders were trained through a rigorous process that involved becoming familiar with the LCRP materials, observing several groups led by experienced co-leaders, and then co-leading the group at least twice with an experienced group leader, with increasing involvement by the trainee. On at least one occasion, the training process demonstrated that a staff member was not a good fit for the program. Not only did the LCRP lose a potential group leader, but it was also difficult to explain to those not familiar with competency assessment or restoration treatment that a group leader needed to demonstrate enough understanding about competency to be able to teach it to others or to understand the specific clinical interventions.

Quality Assurance and Data Collection

Data were collected from individuals who participated in the LCRP, including demographic, clinical (e.g., diagnoses), and legal (e.g., type of charges) histories. Participants were also administered the CompKit Competency Screening Test (CCST) and the Competence Assessment for Standing Trial for Defendants with Mental Retardation (CAST*MR) prior to beginning treatment. Both measures were again administered after they completed the program. The CAST*MR was chosen because its content corresponds more closely to the areas of competency set by *Dusky* than other available instruments and could be used with defendants encompassing a wide range of intellectual functioning, even though most participants were not diagnosed with an intellectual disability. Scoring guidelines in Section 3 of the CAST*MR were modified to increase reliability in scoring and to capture specific data about an individual's rational understanding of their case. Moreover, each defendant's primary IST typology was collected.

In 2013, these data points were analyzed to determine if the program was effective at restoring defendants to competency faster than individuals who were receiving standard hospital treatment (Chung et al., 2013). It was hypothesized that by participating in the LCRP, more IST defendants court-ordered for inpatient commitment would be restored to competence (i.e., based on the outcome of an inpatient IST evaluation, which is typically conducted by a psychiatrist at the hospital). It was also hypothesized that LCRP participants would be restored more quickly (i.e., shorter length of hospitalization) than those defendants who were receiving psychopharmacological and standard hospital treatments alone. Using archival data to simulate two comparison groups (Comparison Group 1: $n = 11$ and Comparison Group 2: $n = 20$) because of logistical issues related to the delivery of treatment (e.g., a wait-list control group was not feasible), these comparison groups were created using the same inclusion and exclusion criteria as for the treatment group. Defendants in the treatment group ($n = 24$) and comparison groups were also admitted to the hospital during the same time period. Analyses of the data showed that participants in the LCRP improved significantly in their CCST [$n = 27$, $t(26) = -2.805$, $p = 0.009$] and CAST*MR scores [$n = 15$, $t(14) = -2.695$, $p = 0.017$] by the end of the program, but they did not differ significantly from those in the comparison groups in whether they were found competent by the evaluator [Treatment Group and Comparison Group 1: $X^2(2, N = 35) = 1.580$, $p = 0.454$; Treatment Group and Comparison Group 2: $X^2(2, N = 44) = 2.92$, $p = 0.318$]. Additionally, in contrast to what was hypothesized, the treatment group had a significantly longer average length of stay compared with those who did not participate in the LCRP [$n = 11$, $t(19) = 3.083$, $p =0.006$]. However, the small sample sizes and other variables (e.g., factors unrelated to competency that determined how long someone remained hospitalized) may have accounted for these results. It is hypothesized that one of these variables was related to how treatment teams selected defendants for referral to the program. Rather than concluding that hospitalizations were extended by participating in the LCRP, it was suspected that defendants who were referred to the program had a longer length of hospitalization because they had not responded to standard hospital treatment as quickly as other defendants.

In 2014, cumulative demographic as well as pre-/post-CCST and CAST*MR data were again analyzed (Strathern et al., 2014). Of those who had completed the program ($N = 75$), the average age of LCRP participants was 33.5 years; 86.6% of participants were male, whereas 13.3% were female. The results indicated that LCRP participants showed significant improvement in CCST (pre-test mean = 24.5 vs. post-test mean = 27.0; $p =0.009$) and CAST*MR (pre-test mean = 32.1 vs. post-test mean = 36.7; $p =0.017$) scores, suggesting gains in competency-related skills. These two studies showed that measurable improvements demonstrated by individuals who participated in the LCRP were promising and showed some effectiveness related to the program. Nonetheless, changes or refinements have been made, with the intention of improving the differential effectiveness of the LCRP as well as to make it more user-friendly and accessible to a more diverse population.

Changes to the Original Program

Since LCRP's initial implementation, modifications have been made to address new challenges as they have arisen and to improve the materials based on experience from running multiple groups. For example, two major revisions were made to the manual in order to streamline the lessons and make printed materials more user-friendly for both group leaders and participants. In addition, a Spanish version of the LCRP was created by Ashley Strathern, Psy.D., and bilingual social worker Amalia Adame, B.S., between 2018 and 2019. The development and implementation of a Spanish version posed its own obstacles, related to both human error and administrative oversight. After professional translation, the exact Spanish dialect was reviewed and adjusted to ensure that the legal terminology used throughout all materials was consistent and would target the most individuals in the geographical region. This determination was based on the history of Spanish-speaking defendants admitted to the hospital for competency evaluations. For example, the term "prosecutor" can be translated into Spanish as either "el fiscal," "el acusador," or "demandante." Amalia Adame, B.S., who assisted in the translation of the materials, recommended that "el fiscal" be utilized, as it was a more common term in the dialects of the Spanish-speaking population admitted to the hospital. The groups for Spanish-speaking defendants have since been led by this bilingual social worker.

Among the challenges addressed in providing the competency restoration groups has been the pressure to treat more defendants in less time. Since the LCRP began in 2011, the group size has ranged from 4 to 13 defendants. These groups historically included defendants from all housing units, each of which contained 25 defendants, including men and women with various diagnoses and cognitive abilities. Given that there were consistently more defendants at the hospital who needed restoration services than the psychology department was capable of providing at any one time, defendants were prioritized for any given group with the following criteria in mind: defendants who were at the hospital under a judge's order for competency assessment, were sufficiently stable in that they were not acutely dangerous, were deemed capable of benefitting from restoration treatment, and were in need of court-ordered competence restoration.

The COVID-19 pandemic caused major changes in how all clinical services were provided across the hospital, including the LCRP. In March of 2020, the LCRP that began in January 2020 stopped after 19 sessions due to the need to implement social distancing and isolation protocols. After the initial COVID-19 wave, when therapeutic groups were able to run again, the hospital ordered that all defendants only attend treatment programs with others from the same housing unit. This was done in an effort to reduce the potential spread of infection between units. Given that mixing defendants from different units was not possible, it was decided to adapt a unit-based model for the delivery of restoration services. Each restoration group would only contain participants from a single housing unit.

To facilitate this change, the hospital's total population of defendants needing restoration services, roughly 50% of the hospital's 200 beds, were divided into three sub-groups to better deliver treatment. The first sub-group consisted of women who required English-language restoration services (approximately 11% of the hospital's IST population), the second consisted of men who required Spanish-language restoration services (approximately 14% of the hospital's IST population), and the third consisted of men who required English-language restoration services (approximately 75% of the hospital's IST population). Since there is only one women's unit, which for much of the pandemic was split into a regular unit with 15 beds and a COVID quarantine unit with 10 beds, competency restoration programming was offered to the women who were appropriate for restoration services in a physical space on the unit.

A group of 25 male defendants, mixing English and Spanish language peers who required restoration services, were targeted for transfer to a single housing unit to facilitate two linguistically-separate restoration groups. The criteria to prioritize transfer to the male restoration unit were the same as those who were prioritized for referral to the LCRP pre-pandemic, with the added criteria of having not completed prior groups, in an effort to make sure that newer defendants had an opportunity to benefit from treatment.

Since March 2021, unit-based restoration service treatment has been offered, although this has not been without challenges. For example, the transfer of numerous non-IST defendants off the restoration unit required facilitating large numbers of transfers in a short amount of time, which put a heavy burden on both the transferring and receiving treatment teams. In addition, for various reasons, efforts to establish a unit that solely houses restoration defendants have not succeeded. Additionally, many defendants either benefit from repeating the restoration group or have been courtordered to repeat, meaning that there are cases in which a defendant who has already attended a LCRP group must participate in the next available group, which, in turn, prevents new defendants from gaining entry. Finally, due to personnel and space limitations, the psychology and social work departments were only capable of running three groups at a time: one women's group, one Spanish-language men's group, and one English-language men's group.

Once the LCRP transitioned to unit-based programming, there was an increase in the number of defendants who were able to receive services. For example, prior to March of 2020, a total of 171 defendants received restoration services, for an average of 6.8 defendants per group across

25 groups. Once programming was able to be restarted, from March 2021 to July 2022, a total of 87 defendants participated in the program, with an average of 12.4 defendants per group across 7 groups. The increase in the number of defendants who have participated is likely related to improved staffing, more groups being offered simultaneously, and the groups moving from a closed format to an open-group format that could accept defendants as soon as they were transferred to the units where the group was being offered. The change from closed to open groups arose from new defendants being moved to the various IST units while restoration groups were in progress. In these cases, the group leaders would assess the readiness of the defendant (i.e., psychiatric stability, risk/safety factors, willingness, intellectual ability, familiarity with the legal system, IST typology, etc.) and balance it against the current group's progress in the LCRP manual. If the defendant was deemed appropriate, they would join the group in progress; if not, they would be waitlisted until the balance of the above factors changed or the next group began. At times, it was deemed beneficial for a defendant who was willing to join a group in progress to do so, even if the leaders believed that it would be necessary for them to complete a full rotation of the group later, to increase their exposure to the materials.

Notwithstanding these improvements in the number of groups offered, there were still more defendants in need of restoration services. For example, recent numbers indicated that 58% of all eligible defendants in the hospital could still benefit from participating in the LCRP. Efforts to address these limitations included the additional training of staff to be able to run the program, such that more English or Spanish language groups could be offered simultaneously. Other efforts included training unit psychologists to provide individual competency education to defendants waitlisted for transfer to the restoration unit and consideration of establishing an additional restoration unit.

Ideas for Future Research and Program Development

As the LCRP continues to develop, we foresee improving on the current approach by adding more staff, including additional bilingual mental health professionals and a clinical case manager who can oversee the program while collaborating with treatment teams. This case manager would be able to complete a more comprehensive screening process to place defendants into their identified restoration category (e.g., IST typology), to develop more individualized treatment plans, and to provide consistent oversight related to a defendant's continued needs for competency restoration in preparation for discharge while assisting to reduce the length of hospitalization. Additionally, we foresee the ever-more important need for an outpatient or community-based legal competency restoration program that would be available to individuals who need the same treatment but whose symptoms of mental illness are not severe enough to warrant inpatient psychiatric treatment.

Future research should continue to focus on demonstrating the effectiveness of a comprehensive treatment program such as the LCRP in comparison with standard psychiatric hospital treatment or by IST typology as well as to examine how changes or revisions made to the program over time may have impacted its effectiveness. There are many obstacles to conducting such research in a state or even private psychiatric hospital, including staffing shortages, insufficient resources, and the fact that incarcerated individuals are considered a special population when conducting research. Further research could be better accomplished with sufficient resources and support.

References

Chung, S., Strathern, A., & Terranova, R. (2013, March). Effectiveness of the Legal Competency Restoration Program as an adjunct to psychopharmacological and standard hospital treatments. Poster Session presented at the meeting of the American Psychological-Law Society, Portland, Oregon.

Drope v. Missouri, 420 U.S. 162 (1975).

Dusky v. United States, 362 U.S. 402 (1960).

Florida State Hospital (2009). CompKit: Competency to Stand Trial Training Resources. Chattahoochee, Florida: Florida State Hospital.

Godinez v. Moran, 509 U.S. 389 (1993).

Jackson v. Indiana, 406 U.S. 715 (1972).

National Judicial Task Force to Examine State Courts' Response to Mental Illness (2021, August). Leading Reform: Competence to Stand Trial Systems (v2).

Melton, G. B., Petrila, J., Poythress, N. G., Slobogin, C., Otto, R. K., Mossman, D., & Condie, L. O. (2017). Psychological Evaluations for the Courts: A Handbook for Mental Health Professionals and Lawyers. 4th ed. Guilford Press.

Morris, N. P., McNiel, D. E., & Binder, R. L. (2021). Estimating Annual Numbers of Competency to Stand Trial Evaluations across the United States. *Journal of the American Academy of Psychiatry and the Law*, 49(4) online. DOI: 10.29158/JAAPL.200129-20.

Pirelli, G., Gottdiener, W., & Zapf, P. (2011). A Meta-analytic Review of Competency to Stand Trial Research. *Psychology, Public Policy & Law*, 17(1): 1–53.

Strathern, A, Chung, S., & Gurmu, S. (2014, October). Competency Restoration: A Psychology-Psychiatry Collaboration. Poster session presented at the Annual Meeting of the American Academy of Psychiatry and the Law, Chicago, Illinois.

Warren, J., Chauhan, P., Kois, L., Dibble, A., & Knighton, J. (2013). Factors Influencing 2,260 Opinions of Defendants' Restorability to Adjudicative Competency. *Psychology, Public Policy & Law*, 19(4), 498–508.

Zapf, P. (2013). Standardized Protocols for Treatment to Restore Competency to Stand Trial: Interventions and Clinically Appropriate Time Periods (Document No. 13-01-1901). Olympia: Washington State Institute for Public Policy.

12 Animal-Assisted Intervention

The "Paws for Wellness Program"

Andrew T. Olagunju, Angela Li, Ashley Palmer, John M.W. Bradford, and Gary A. Chaimowitz

Introduction

In forensic-correctional settings, treatment approaches are developed to promote remission of mental disorders, recovery, and risk management to mitigate recidivism and eventually reintegrate patients into the community. One of the prevailing approaches to recovery, risk management, and mitigation of recidivism in the forensic-correctional mental health system is the Risk-Needs-Recovery (RNR) model. The RNR model manages recidivism risk through a cognitive-behavioral-social learning framework (Crocker et al., 2017). However, some limitations identified with the RNR model include that it may not address the individual goals and preferences of service users. As such, emerging models (such as the Good Lives Model and the Recovery Model) of rehabilitation and the development of innovative programs are gaining traction to promote holistic and humanistic care. (Lutz et al., 2022). Furthermore, there has been movement in recent years toward improving patients' engagement and patient-centerd care through the provision of meaningful involvement in a range of activities in forensic-correctional mental health service delivery and improving the social milieu and comfort of the inpatient wards to support the safety of patients and staff (Crocker et al., 2017). These developments pave the way for non-traditional innovative interventions (including animal-assisted intervention [AAI]) among the forensic-correctional populations to aid learning prosocial behaviors, improve safe social interactions, develop a sense of purpose, and enhance community reintegration.

In this chapter, we discuss the *"Paws for Wellness"* program, an AAI implemented and utilized as an adjunctive intervention among forensic-correctional populations in a Canadian setting. The history and evidence base for AAI are highlighted to provide an appropriate background. We describe the implementation process and conclude with recommendations to promote adaptation in comparable settings and populations.

DOI: 10.4324/9781003360926-15

Overview of Literature on Animal-assisted Intervention

The earliest recorded use of animals as therapeutic agents appears to have existed since the 17th century, identifying a purported positive impact of animal interaction on mental and physical health (Serpell, 2000). Scientific interest in AAI grew in the 20th century as emerging evidence identified an association between animal visits or companion animals and a variety of positive health outcomes related to cardiovascular health, stress, anxiety, and depression (Davis, 1988; Francis et al., 1985; Friedmann et al., 1980).

AAI and Psychological Wellbeing

In individuals diagnosed with schizophrenia and receiving long-term inpatient care, canine-assisted therapy was shown to improve the severity of positive and negative symptoms of schizophrenic illness (Chu et al., 2009; Villalta-Gil et al., 2009). Notably, a significant proportion of people in forensic-correctional settings who present with psychiatric problems are diagnosed with schizophrenia and more likely to receive long-term inpatient care (Al Marzooqi et al., 2022; Chaimowitz et al., 2022). A systematic review of 20 studies by Villafaina-Domínguez et al. on the effects of dog-based AAI in the prison population, with mental illnesses and those in "psychiatric prisons" and "mental health prison units" with therapy sessions lasting 60–120mins occurring 1–3x/week demonstrated statistically significant improvement in multiple outcomes, including anxiety, depression, emotional control, empathy, and academic skills. However, the review was limited by the few number of included studies and the large heterogeneity with respect to study participants and outcomes (Villafaina-Domínguez et al., 2020).

Impact of AAI on the Risk of Violence

A randomized control trial (RCT) conducted by Nurenberg et al. assessed the effectiveness of equine-assisted psychotherapy (EAP) on chronic psychiatric inpatients with violent behaviors. Ninety participants were randomized to EAP, canine-assisted psychotherapy (CAP), environmentally enhanced social skills group psychotherapy (active control), or regular hospital care (standard control). Seventy-six percent of the participants had a diagnosis of schizophrenia or schizoaffective disorder, and 56% had been committed involuntarily for civil or forensic reasons. The primary outcome measured was the frequency of aggressive behavior identified by hospital incident reports. Other outcomes evaluated included the frequency of use of seclusion, restraint, one-to-one monitoring, and verbal and physical aggression on the Overt Aggression Scale. The study findings reported a statistically significant decrease in violent incidents in the EAP group, sustained for several months after the therapy. CAP did not demonstrate a statistically significant improvement in violent behaviors; however, there was a decrease in one-to-one observation in the CAP and EAP groups. The researchers noted that the CAP group had a relatively low incidence of pre-intervention violent incidents compared to other groups, which may have made it difficult to detect the effect of the intervention (Nurenberg et al., 2015).

Impact on Other Parameters of Wellbeing and Recovery

Improvements in social roles and interpersonal relationships were noted in two RCTs assessing the effectiveness of canine-assisted therapy in the correctional population (Jasperson, 2013; Seivert et al., 2018). Improved social contact and quality of life related to social relationships were also demonstrated in a study utilizing canine-assisted therapy in "chronic" inpatients with schizophrenia (Villalta-Gil et al., 2009). A meta-analysis of 11 studies evaluating the effect of prison-based dog programs found a significant reduction in the primary outcome, criminal recidivism (Duindam et al., 2020).

Epidemiological data studying the association between pet ownership and cardiovascular disease risk factors found beneficial effects of pet ownership on systolic blood pressure, cholesterol, and triglyceride levels (Anderson et al., 1992; Beetz et al., 2012). There are various hypotheses that may explain the benefits of AAI in reducing anxiety, depression, blood pressure, and cortisol. These include the biophilia hypothesis, whereby there is a genetic propensity for humans to seek connection with other living organisms (Besthorn & Saleebey, 2003), or an increase in oxytocin resulting in antidepressant and calming effects (Beetz et al., 2012). Other studies have demonstrated an increase in beta-endorphins and dopamine production (Odendaal & Meintjes, 2003). Nevertheless, there are methodological limitations to the studies, and only a small body of literature on AAI in the forensic-correctional population exists at the present time. There is a need for further research in this area.

Forensic-correctional Mental Health Services in Canada

Individuals fall within the forensic system if they are found unfit to stand trial (UST) or not criminally responsible (NCR). A finding of UST is rendered if the accused is unable, on account of a mental disorder, to understand the nature or object of trial proceedings, the possible consequences of the proceedings, or communicate with counsel. NCR is rendered if the Court determines that the individual was suffering from a mental disorder at the time of the offense or omission that rendered them incapable of appreciating the nature and quality of the act or omission or knowing that it was wrong ("Criminal Code," 1985). Those with a UST or NCR finding fall under the purview of their provincial Criminal Code Review Board. Review boards are independent, quasi-judicial administrative tribunals, holding meetings at least annually for individuals under their jurisdiction to render and review dispositions. Possible dispositions include a detention order (the accused can be detained at a facility), a conditional discharge order (the accused is to live in the community while subject to certain conditions), and an absolute discharge order (the accused is no longer subject to the oversight of the review board; Chaimowitz et al., 2022, Olagunju et al., 2022). Privileges are also outlined within a disposition. These may start with escorted visits off the unit but within the hospital and can progress to unaccompanied overnight leaves in the community. This is determined by the individual's mental status, behaviors, and treatment response. In Canada, the goal of forensic mental health services is the rehabilitation and reintegration of people into the community. On the other hand, correctional psychiatry deals with the treatment and rehabilitation of offenders with mental health conditions in correctional settings, including lock-ups, jails, detention centers, and juvenile correctional centers (Al Marzooqi et al., 2022, Bioku et al., 2021, Olagunju et al., 2018)

The Forensic Psychiatry Program (FPP) at St. Joseph's Healthcare Hamilton (SJHH) was started in 1972 and now consists of two general secure units, two higher security units, one assessment unit, and an outpatient unit linked with community-based resources and services for community living. Recently, the program created an acute stabilization unit to provide extended mental health services for offenders with severe and active psychosis in local detention centers (correctional psychiatry).

Background on Paws for Wellness

For many years, small-scale, brief AAIs, typically in the form of pet visits, were facilitated at SJHH by community-based programs and were well received by patients and staff alike. In 2019, formal AAI programs began within the FPP. The first program was weekly pet visits on alternating days, with the support of three volunteers and their dogs. An on-site petting zoo was also introduced, as was the launch of the *Pawsitive Strides* program, an animal intervention that helped patients build on their coping skills and work on strengthening family supports and bonding time while also enhancing their confidence through the use of animal obedience classes. Unfortunately, these programs were halted when the COVID-19 pandemic started. The *Pawsitive Strides* program was facilitated three times for a duration of eight weeks (Kahl et al., 2020).

As the pandemic continued, there were calls for pet therapy programs to resume. As community-based programs unfortunately closed permanently during the pandemic, the idea to develop a FPP Resident Dog was conceived. It was deemed most favorable for a dog to be raised as a pup, supported by the hospital, and fostered by a staff member. The other proposed scenario was for an adolescent dog that would be trained and supported by staff within the program and either live with the staff or within the building. In consultation with community groups, we were advised of the requirements for the resident dog, including personality traits and training requirements. Furthermore, a program proposal was developed and executed that included cost analyses and formal vetting of the handler by the FPP. Full details of the requirements and cost breakdown are provided under the subsection on the implementation of the AAI program.

Regarding the breed of dog, Leonbergers were deemed to be an appropriate breed for this role. Noble and powerful, a good Leonberger is calm and steady, yet bolder and more athletic than most giant breeds. The Leonberger enjoys swimming, tracking, agility, therapy work, pulling a cart or sled, and weight pulling – these are all productive outlets for their energy. They are a loyal and gentle giant, often referred to as "lean-on-berger," as they will lean in when enjoying a good friendly rub. Through connecting with a local breeder to discuss the nature of our program, the needs, and the requirements, the most suitable pup was identified.

While waiting for the suitable pup, we concurrently obtained formal approval for our program from the leadership of the FPP, followed by the leadership group for mental health and addictions at our hospital, and finally, the senior leadership of SJHH approved the program. When the pup was born, the breeder provided frequent updates on the pup's progress and information on how to raise the pup, including grooming instructions, training suggestions, securing a personal veterinarian, and arranging immunizations specific to this breed. Follow-up questions were raised along the way and easily addressed. Adequate consultation with clinical team members was conducted to make consensus decisions as needed. For example, a contest was completed throughout the service to identify a suitable name for the pup, and "Scout" was the winning name. See Table 12.1 for the program development timeline.

Table 12.1 Program development timeline

May 2021	*Sept 2021*	*Nov 2021*	*Dec 2021*	*April 2022*	*Sept 2022*
Initial proposal for the Paws for Wellness program structure	Final approval for the program granted Scout is born	Scout arrived at the program Weekly training begins	Scout's initial introduction to program staff and patients	Scout attended the risk and recovery conference	Patient engagement begins

Scout was presented to the FPP on November 5, 2021, and began formalized AAI training through the *Scholars in Collars* program immediately, per the recommendation of the breeder. He took up residence with the handler and their family, who would raise him. In December 2021, Scout met patients and staff on the hospital grounds, outside the building per SJHH policy at the time, as he was not yet fully trained or vaccinated. These policies were subsequently revised for the Scout's training purposes. Scout's formal patient engagement began in September 2022.

The *Paws for Wellness Program*: Purpose, Structure, Implementation, and Evaluation

Purpose

The purpose and goals of the *Paws for Wellness* program are:

1. To support and provide opportunities for patients to improve their social interaction skills
2. To provide an opportunity for safe touch and connection while mitigating risk
3. To provide opportunities to improve patients' confidence
4. To provide an alternative outlet for managing negative emotions and build on coping skills
5. To support patients with stress-related issues and foster recreational relaxation
6. To pioneer a research project, with the first "Resident Dog," that further puts us on the map, enabling us to help other hospitals change policies and offer the same intervention.

Program Evaluation

The effectiveness of the *Paws for Wellness* program is being evaluated through two research studies that received ethics approval in November 2022. Outcome measures being monitored include:

1. Patient attendance – documented in the patient's chart as therapeutic intervention and captured with MIS statistics.
2. Aggressive Incidents Scale and Electronic Hamilton Anatomy of Risk Management (eHARM) (Chaimowitz et al., 2020a & b; Mullally et al., 2018).
3. As needed, medication usage.
4. "Perception of dogs" – 5-question mini-survey generated by our program.

5 Quality of life – Quality of Life Inventory (Frisch et al., 1992)
6 Anxiety – Beck Anxiety Inventory (Steer & Beck, 1997).
7 Happiness – Oxford Happiness Questionnaire (Hills & Argyle, 2002).
8 Heart rate.
9 Staff burnout scale (unpublished).

Implementation of the *Paws for Wellness* Program

Animal Requirements

Through consultation with community AAI programs, we determined the following requirements for a suitable dog for the program:

1 A larger breed to be able to withstand the emotional demands that working with our population might make on a dog.
2 A dog breed with a good quality of endurance and patience.
3 Adolescent dogs would be ideal, but generally, this is tough to find.

With these recommendations and through past successful use within our hospital, we concluded Leonbergers would be a suitable breed and liaised with a community breeder who was consulted on our project and willing to donate a dog to our program that had the appropriate temperament.

Housing

Expert consultation concluded that the ideal living conditions for an AAI dog would be a steady family environment outside the hospital. This is due to the high expectations and demands placed on the dog, given the requirements to take in the emotions, sights, scents, and supports of its workplace. This would allow him to learn to maintain a calm demeanor and allow opportunities for play and affection. Scout also lives with a canine companion at home.

Training

Once Scout entered our program, he immediately began the *Scholars in Collars* weekly training program. This started with desensitization training and basic skills to help Scout adjust to various sounds, learning to be content on its own when not engaged by the handler, and bladder training. Training and orientation around the hospital building were graduated. He completed training and orientation to the three levels in the hospital (levels 1–3) and subsequently began orientation to specialty training at six months of age. This involved entering the hospital facility to work through fears around the floors and heights, calmly roam the hallways with the handler to remain focused on working, and not bark or approach those that do not wish to pet him. He also learned to lay on the floor to allow patients to come and pet him while being aware he could stand and remove himself safely with the handlers support at any time. He has also adjusted to learning commands and how to be supported by a second handler, who was also vetted through the program to ensure a good fit. Handlers must be committed and able to follow and respect the training guidelines.

Staffing Requirements

It was determined that the handler must be an employee of the SJHH FPP. The dog would be fostered by the handler and their family to enable opportunities for "downtime" and support the animal's wellness. This also enables the dog to be onsite with a trusted staff member while supporting our patients and staff.

Facility Protocols

Previous SJHH policy stated that an animal was only allowed to visit for up to one hour, could not be owned by a staff member, and had to be at least one year of age to enter the building. This was subsequently revised for our program to permit Scout to enter the building at six months old as part of his training to familiarize himself with the facility. Scout has been formally evaluated at the one-year mark, and a follow-up assessment was conducted in November after he started to officially visit with patients. These evaluations to ensure fidelity to the protocol and findings are provided to the director of the forensic psychiatric service periodically to ensure we are following and meeting proper expectations and safety standards for all.

Currently, the protocol for Scout's hospital visits involves:

1. Informing the manager when Scout is on site.
2. Calling the units ahead of time, should there be a staff that is afraid or has an allergy to be aware of his visit. The handler and the dog are both very aware of staff who are uncomfortable and keep a safe distance.
3. It is part of our policy and procedure that infection protection and control guidelines are followed, including washing hands pre- and post-visit with the dog.
4. Any messes he makes are to be cleaned up by the handler.
5. Scout has his own office to allow for downtime for him and his handler.
6. Scout must always be with a handler and on the lead.

Funding Considerations

Start-up costs, which may vary based on jurisdiction

1 Cost of animals
2 Veterinarian fees (neutering and microchipping)
3 Training
4 Miscellaneous costs (bed, collar, and slip lead)

Ongoing costs

- Annual
  1 Veterinarian fees
    1 Regular check-ups and medications
    2 Vaccinations
  2 Dog license with the city
  3 Bags for animal waste
- Monthly costs
  1 Pet insurance
  2 Dog food
  3 Dog treats

Visit Structure

The program consists of a dog that is owned by the hospital and housed by a handler who is an employee of the hospital. The dog has been trained to provide therapy to patients in the form of group visits, group walks, and individual programming for those needing intensive support. The AAI dog is available up to five days a week. The visits shall only take place in the agreed-upon location area between the designated pet handler and the unit managers. The visits can consist of referral-based/closed programming, courtyard visits, group walks, or a trial of independent visits for higher-risk individuals/those in need of greater support. These visits are conducted in the inpatient forensic visitor lounges, common areas within the unit, and courtyards. The visits last a maximum of two hours to allow the dog to have a break.

The size of the group depends on the nature of the visit – as the patient-to-staff ratio will differ. Initially, Scout is present Monday to Friday for half days, and then working full days within a year.

Early Observations from the Paws for Wellness Program

1 Patients who normally isolate to their rooms have come out to participate in visits with Scout. They often ask questions to enhance their knowledge of the program and awareness of dogs by asking about their care and interests while petting them.
2 Patients prioritize attending Scout's visits over independent time off units, which supports time management awareness.
3 Patients enjoy playing toss the ball or toy in courtyards. They treat Scout like their own pet while providing treats and training him for new tricks.
4 Patients have de-escalated during visits. In one patient interaction, the patient went from fists on the table for attention to calm hands petting Scout, stating "hands feel better this way" while brushing Scout's back.
5 Patients and staff were noted to have a brighter effect during and following interactions with Scout on the unit. It appears that Scout's visits boost the morale of the clinical environment.
6 Comments recorded by patients regarding Scout's visit include the following:

   a "He takes away the stress of the environment….its so calming to pet and love on him."
   b "He is the bestest boy."
   c "I look forward to his visits."
   d "[Scout] brings a feeling of home and helps to normalize the environment."
   e "It's so nice to pet and hug an animal that will not judge you."

7 As noted by one of the research assistants working on the AAI program: from my own personal observation, MANY patients and staff state they love Scout and love having him on the unit. One patient did say to another co-patient "Do you like my friend?" (referencing Scout). On a forensic inpatient unit, they call it a "code woof". I personally, from doing this research and observing, have seen many individuals positively benefit from interacting with Scout. Their mood increases and feelings of worry and anxiety reduce – it is evident through their behaviors.

Considerations and Recommendations of the AAI Program

The handler's main roles include dog walking, training, feeding, supporting, and grooming. These roles are intensive, often requiring regular and continuous activities. Consequently, it is important to arrange coverage for the handler roles with alternate staff to maintain the care of the dog and continue the program in special cases if the need arises (e.g., vacation or leave). The handler must balance and manage other roles and tasks with patient care, as well as supporting the dog.

The developmental-growth phases of the dog might present unique challenges that must be addressed. For example, the dog might show new fears or behaviors (e.g., becoming more playful or jumpy). These changes must be addressed and managed to ensure that the dog can engage the client safely and freely with no risk of harm. Training the dog is a lengthy process that is ongoing and continues on a regular basis to address novel situations encountered during engagement with patients.

It is important to be sensitive to an individual patient's attributes and cultural differences with respect to their perception of dogs, fears, allergies, or individual preferences. Furthermore, within the forensic-correctional population, adequate consideration must be given to individuals' index offenses that may involve animals, specifically dogs. This information is collected during pre-intervention screening surveys or assessments of patients for participation in dog visits. Furthermore, some forensic-correctional patients may not be used to animal touch, and as such, teaching the appropriate use of touch with a dog is needed and conducted.

Education, advocacy, and stakeholder engagement are needed to enhance uptake, sustain the program, and accommodate the lengthy process of training an AAI dog to work with patients and support them in a safe manner. Data collection and research to generate evidence to inform policy and program implementation are indicated.

Future Directions of the Program

Currently, the collection of empirical data for research on our program is in the early stages. Scout's attendance on units started with drop-in visits before progressing to half-day visits and then full-day visits. Since ethics approval was recently obtained in late November 2022, the early stages of data collection have begun. So far, initial feedback from inpatients and staff has been very positive, with patients requesting future visits and reporting improvements in anxiety after interacting with the dog. Evaluation of the program will be completed by patients and staff members, including an assessment of attendance and the collection of qualitative data based on direct feedback provided by patients. The *Paws for Wellness* program is also in the process of expanding to a second dog who will be a different breed and smaller in size to aid in supporting those individuals who fear larger dogs.

Conclusion

Overall, the *Paws for Wellness* program is a novel, canine-assisted intervention developed for the forensic-correctional population to support clients' wellbeing through social interaction and provide an outlet for developing new leisure skills. Optimally, the program can model proxy prosocial behaviors and emotional resources for safe engagement and interactions with patients. In addition to providing increased therapeutic support for forensic-correctional patients, this program extends the clinical application of AAI in forensic-correctional settings. We hope this chapter provides relevant knowledge to support the implementation of similar interventions in comparable populations.

Acknowledgments

We wish to express our sincere gratitude to Donna Jenkins (Zachary's Paws for Healing), Cindy Hunt (Concorde Ridge Leonbergers), and Kelly Bulley (SJHH) for their support and contributions to the implementation of the program.

References

Al Marzooqi, S., El Sheikh, A., Al Shehhi, N., Al Mesmari, A., Al Zaabi, M., Haweel, A., Wang, J., Prat, S. S., Chaimowitz, G. A., Olagunju, A. T. (2022). Forensic-correctional psychiatric services in Abu Dhabi: Lessons from a descriptive analyis of the attributes of a sample of service users. *Psychiatr Danub*, Winter; *34*(4):635–643. https://doi.org/10.24869/psyd.2022.635

Anderson, W. P., Reid, C. M., & Jennings, G. L. (1992). Pet ownership and risk factors for cardiovascular disease. *Med J Aust*, *157*(5), 298–301. https://doi.org/10.5694/j.1326-5377.1992.tb137178.x

Beetz, A., Uvnäs-Moberg, K., Julius, H., & Kotrschal, K. (2012). Psychosocial and psychophysiological effects of human-animal interactions: The possible role of oxytocin. *Front Psychol*, *3*, 234. https://doi.org/10.3389/fpsyg.2012.00234

Besthorn, F., & Saleebey, D. (2003). Nature, genetics and the biophilia connection: Exploring linkages with social work values and practice. *Adv Soc Work*, *4*, 1–18.

Bioku, A. A., Alatishe, Y. A., Adeniran, J. O., Olagunju, T. O., Singhal, N., Mela, M., Bradford, J. M., Chaimowitz, G. A., Olagunju, A. T. (2021). Psychiatric morbidity among incarcerated individuals in an underserved region of Nigeria: Revisiting the unmet mental health needs in correction services. *J Health Care Poor Underserved*. *32*(1):321–337. https://doi.org/10.1353/hpu.2021.0026

Chaimowitz, G., Moulden, H., Upfold, C., Mullally, K., & Mamak, M. (2022). The ontario forensic mental health system: A population-based review. *Can J Psychiatry*, *67*(6), 481–489. https://doi.org/10.1177/07067437211023103

Chaimowitz, G. A., Mamak, M., Moulden, H. M., Furimsky, I., & Olagunju, A. T. (2020a). Implementation of risk assessment tools in psychiatric services. *J Healthc Risk Manag*, *40*(1), 33–43. https://doi.org/10.1002/jhrm.21405

Chaimowitz, G.A., Mamak, M., & Olagunju, A.T. (2020b). Aggressive Incidents Scale (AIS) – A Measure of Aggression That Manages Violence Risk. Rossiiskii psikhiatricheskii zhurnal. *Russ J Psychiatry*, 6: 36–44. https://doi.org/10.24411/1560-957X-2020-10605.

Chu, C. I., Liu, C. Y., Sun, C. T., & Lin, J. (2009). The effect of animal-assisted activity on inpatients with schizophrenia. *J Psychosoc Nurs Ment Health Serv*, *47*(12), 42–48. https://doi.org/10.3928/02793695-20091103-96

Criminal Code, (1985). Criminal Code, RSC 1985, c C-46. Accessed on 20/08/2023 from: https://laws-lois.justice.gc.ca/eng/acts/c-46/

Crocker, A. G., Livingston, J. D., & Leclair, M. C. (2017). Forensic mental health systems internationally. In *Handbook of forensic mental health services*. (pp. 3–76). Routledge/Taylor & Francis Group. https://doi.org/10.4324/9781315627823-2

Davis, H. D. (1988). Animal-facilitated therapy in stress mediation. *Holist Nurs Pract*, *2*(3), 75–83. https://doi.org/10.1097/00004650-198802030-00013

Duindam, H. M., Asscher, J. J., Hoeve, M., Stams, G. J. J. M., & Creemers, H. E. (2020). Are we barking up the right tree? A meta-analysis on the effectiveness of prison-based dog programs. *Crim Justice Behav*, *47*(6), 749–767. https://doi.org/10.1177/0093854820909875

Francis, G., Turner, J. T., & Johnson, S. B. (1985). Domestic animal visitation as therapy with adult home residents. *Int J Nurs Stud*, *22*(3), 201–206. https://doi.org/10.1016/0020-7489(85)90003-3

Friedmann, E., Katcher, A. H., Lynch, J. J., & Thomas, S. A. (1980). Animal companions and one-year survival of patients after discharge from a coronary care unit. *Public Health Rep*, *95*(4), 307–312.

Frisch, M. B., Cornell, J., Villanueva, M., & Retzlaff, P. J. (1992). Clinical validation of the quality of life inventory. A measure of life satisfaction for use in treatment planning and outcome assessment. *Psychol Assess*, *4*, 92–101. https://doi.org/10.1037/1040-3590.4.1.92

Hills, P., & Argyle, M. (2002). The oxford happiness questionnaire: A compact scale for the measurement of psychological well-being. *Pers Individ Differ*, *33*(7), 1073–1082. https://doi.org/10.1016/S0191-8869(01)00213-6

Jasperson, R. A. (2013). An animal-assisted therapy intervention with female inmates. *Anthrozoös*, *26*(1), 135–145. https://doi.org/10.2752/175303713X13534238631678

Kahl, N., Palmer, A., & Hurlock, K. (2020). Pawsitive strides: Changing the face of animal-assisted interventions. *J Ther Recreat Ontario*, *14*, 54–64.

Lutz, M., Zani, D., Fritz, M., Dudeck, M., & Franke, I. (2022). A review and comparative analysis of the risk-needs-responsivity, good lives, and recovery models in forensic psychiatric treatment [Review]. *Front Psychiatry*, *13*. https://doi.org/10.3389/fpsyt.2022.988905

Mullally, K., Mamak, M., & Chaimowitz, G. A. (2018). The next generation of risk assessment and management: Introducing the eHARM. *Int J Risk Recov*, *1*(1), 21–26. https://doi.org/10.15173/ijrr.v1i1.3365

Nurenberg, J. R., Schleifer, S. J., Shaffer, T. M., Yellin, M., Desai, P. J., Amin, R.,… Montalvo, C. (2015). Animal-assisted therapy with chronic psychiatric inpatients: equine-assisted psychotherapy and aggressive behavior. *Psychiatr Serv*, *66*(1), 80–86. https://doi.org/10.1176/appi.ps.201300524

Odendaal, J. S., & Meintjes, R. A. (2003). Neurophysiological correlates of affiliative behaviour between humans and dogs. *Vet J*, *165*(3), 296–301. https://doi.org/10.1016/s1090-0233(02)00237-x

Olagunju, A. T., Bouskill, S. L., Olagunju, T. O., Prat, S. S., Mamak, M., & Chaimowitz, G. A. (2022). Absconsion in forensic psychiatric services: a systematic review of literature. *CNS Spectrums*, 27(1), 46–57. https://doi.org/10.1017/S1092852920001881

Olagunju, A. T., Oluwaniyi, S. O., Fadipe, B., Ogunnubi, O. P., Oni, O. D., Aina, O. F., Chaimowitz, G. A. (2018). Mental health services in Nigerian prisons: Lessons from a four-year review and the literature. *Int J Law Psychiatry*. May-Jun; *58*, 79–86. https://doi.org/10.1016/j.ijlp.2018.03.004

Seivert, N. P., Cano, A., Casey, R. J., May, D. K., & Johnson, A. (2018). Animal assisted therapy for incarcerated youth: A randomized controlled trial. *Appl Dev Sci*, 22(2), 139–153. https://doi.org/10.1080/10888691.2016.1234935

Serpell, J. A. (2000). Animal companions and human well-being: An historical exploration of the value of human—animal relationships.

Steer, R. A., & Beck, A. T. (1997). Beck Anxiety Inventory. In C. P. Zalaquett & R. J. Wood (Eds.), *Evaluating Stress: A Book of Resources* (pp. 23–40). Scarecrow Education.

Villafaina-Domínguez, B., Collado-Mateo, D., Merellano-Navarro, E., & Villafaina, S. (2020). Effects of dog-based animal-assisted interventions in prison population: A systematic review. *Animals (Basel)*, *10*(11). https://doi.org/10.3390/ani10112129

Villalta-Gil, V., Roca, M., Gonzalez, N., Domènec, E., Cuca, Escanilla, A.,... Haro, J. M. (2009). Dog-assisted therapy in the treatment of chronic schizophrenia inpatients. *Anthrozoös*, 22(2), 149–159. https://doi.org/10.2752/175303709X434176

13 Dialectical Behavior Therapy

A Full Fidelity Model in a Forensic Hospital

Sarah M. McKay

In a forensic inpatient setting, committed patients present with a variety of issues in addition to their legal adjudication. In addition to their qualifying mental health disorder, many of the patients also present with personality disorders and dysfunctional personality characteristics, which complicate the risk. Many times, these issues become a primary focus of treatment due to the significant risk such personality-fueled behaviors may pose, not only to themselves but to peers, staff, and the community at large. To address this, the Oregon State Hospital began implementing interventions specifically meant to target these behaviors and their related symptoms with a unit-based approach.

A gender-diverse unit, largely for patients adjudicated Guilty Except for Insanity (GEI), was identified as a unit for individuals who presented with underlying personality disorders or personality disorder characteristics that were determined to be primary drivers of risk. Specifically, behaviors including chronic suicidality, non-suicidal self-injury (NSSI), reactive and/or instrumental interpersonal violence, and/or highly conflictual and tumultuous relationships with staff that were impacting treatment efficacy were identified as key targets for intervention. Patients with these presenting issues were screened to rule out anyone high in Factor I psychopathy. If they met criteria for these behaviors and/or had a confirmed diagnosis of borderline personality disorder, they were recommended for placement on this specialized unit.

Dialectical Behavior Therapy

The intention was to develop a unit-wide curriculum utilizing dialectical behavior therapy (DBT) to address the target behaviors and provide patients with a therapeutic environment in which the entire staff was trained in basic theory and DBT interventions. DBT was originally developed by Marsha Linehan, PhD, and very early on was demonstrated to vastly improve the quality of life and reduce NSSI and chronic suicidality in women

DOI: 10.4324/9781003360926-16

with borderline personality disorder (Linehan et al., 1991). As more research was completed, it was found that DBT also demonstrated efficacy in substance use treatment (Axelrod et al., 2011; Linehan et al., 1999; Rizvi et al., 2011), reducing hospitalizations in adults (Comtois et al., 2007; McFetridge & Coakes, 2010; Sambrook et al., 2007; Turner, 2000; Williams et al., 2010), improved quality of life (Carter et al., 2010), eating disorder treatment (Chen et al., 2008; Courbasson et al., 2012; Kröger et al., 2010; Telch et al., 2001), reducing suicidality and NSSI in individuals with Post-traumatic Stress Disorder (PTSD; Feigenbaum et al., 2012; Harned et al., 2014), depression treatment (Axelrod et al., 2011; Perroud et al., 2010; Pistorello et al., 2012; Steil et al., 2011; Williams et al., 2010), reducing depression, hopelessness, and improving social connection in domestic abuse survivors (Iverson et al., 2009), PTSD treatment (Bohus et al., 2013; Steil et al., 2011), trichotillomania treatment (Keuthen et al., 2010), reducing anxiety (Steil et al., 2011; Williams et al., 2010), reducing depression, paranoia, hostile mood, violence, and psychotic behaviors in inpatient men with borderline personality disorder or antisocial personality disorder (McCann & Ball, 1996; McCann et al., 2000), reducing impulsivity and behavioral issues in adult correctional facilities (Shelton et al., 2009), reducing risk behaviors of adults with intellectual disabilities in forensic settings (Sakdalan et al., 2010), and reducing staff burnout on inpatient units (McCann & Ball, 1996; McCann et al., 2000), to name a few.

There are four primary components to DBT—individual therapy, skills groups, phone coaching, and provider consultation teams. A program must have these four components to offer "full-fidelity" DBT. In individual therapy, the therapist and patient identify goals for treatment and target behaviors. Individual therapy is a place for the patient to work through many of the struggles they are experiencing. It also provides opportunities for further exploration and practice of the skills they learn in the skills groups. Target behaviors and other key symptoms are tracked weekly with diary cards, and when target behaviors occur, comprehensive behavior analyses are completed to identify the triggers and antecedents and alternative responses for the future.

The skills groups are a place for individuals in the program to learn new skills and practice them with their peers. There are four primary skill modules: mindfulness, distress tolerance, emotion regulation, and interpersonal effectiveness. Each of these modules has various skill sets designed to help the individual manage different situations and learn new coping strategies to ensure that they will find skills that will work for them.

Phone coaching provides opportunities for patients to reach out to their coach or individual therapist during a crisis when they have reached skill failure and are on the verge of engaging in target behaviors. These coaching sessions are usually brief, and parameters are agreed upon beforehand as to what a patient must do before engaging in phone coaching (e.g., try X number of skills, connect with supportive others, etc.). These provide an opportunity for the patient to get extra help when they find themselves in a situation where their skills aren't working or they do not yet have a deep bench of skills to work from. This helps to reduce the likelihood of engaging in target behaviors as well as the likelihood of other behaviors leading to crisis services or emergency room visits.

Finally, provider consultation is an opportunity for providers to consult with one another about difficulties they are experiencing and to find support from their peers, as providing work to patients constantly in crisis can quickly lead to burnout or possible ethical violations if the provider is unsupported. Weekly consultation also helps ensure that providers are maintaining fidelity to the program and the treatment model. This also helps to reduce patient dropout rates and improve outcomes.

Program Development

In the development of the DBT unit's full-fidelity program, the leadership, or interdisciplinary team (IDT), which consisted of two psychologists, two psychiatrists/PMHNPs, a behavioral health specialist (a master's-level mental health clinician), a social worker, a nurse manager, and a treatment care plan specialist, were all extensively trained in DBT. All IDT members went to at least 24 hours (three days) of DBT training in a Linehan-boarded training program, with most of them attending an additional two-week training. At least two members of this team were even more extensively trained. While I was on the unit, the behavioral health specialist was a certified DBT provider, and I was working on certification and had completed a six-month training program with supervision in addition to the 24-hour training. Also, the IDT (and other providers throughout the hospital who provided DBT therapy) had weekly consultation groups that lasted 90–120 minutes. Many of the rest of the unit staff also attended the 24-hour training as well as being required to attend a hospital-led training offered twice a year that was 16 hours long. They were also invited to attend the weekly consultation groups.

Full-fidelity treatment for the patients was developed to as closely mirror Dr. Linehan's full-fidelity model as possible. DBT skills groups were developed and planned to be held four days per week to ensure several options for patient attendance; the groups were first made available to patients throughout the unit, then to other patients in the hospital as space was available, i.e., not just to those who were in the full program. The plan allowed for individual therapists to have a caseload of individual patients who joined the full program. These patients would also have access to phone coaching. For patients on the unit who decided not to join the full program, they would still have unit staff who would engage with them, utilizing the underlying philosophy of DBT.

Patients who were determined to be most likely to benefit from the environment and were considered appropriate to be placed on a gender-diverse unit were transferred to the unit as openings were made available. They were introduced to the team, the goals of the unit, and why it was believed they would benefit—ultimately intending to reduce the target behavior/s, improve their quality of life, and mitigate the risks that contributed to their GEI adjudication. They were also offered the opportunity to join the full DBT program. They met with a DBT provider, often several times, who gave them details about the program, the benefits, what it entailed, and the expectations that they would be held to in joining the program. Expectations included signing a six-month commitment to participate in the treatment; that contract was also a commitment to not engage in any egregious or "target behaviors[1]." If they did so, they would be required to complete a behavior chain analysis (a common DBT intervention), present it to a repair committee of three-to-five people comprised of DBT-trained staff and other DBT full program patients, and then complete the assigned repairs. Patients who engaged in target behaviors were also not able to meet with their therapist for 24 hours after engaging in a target behavior in order to reduce any inadvertent reinforcement of those behaviors through the attention of the therapist.

The unit itself was also set up to include several coping strategies based on interventions learned in the skill groups. There were ice packs and buckets that were available for those who utilized the TIPP skill, as well as access to various music selections, aromatherapy, and other items in a sensory room (IMPROVE skill). There were also posters and reminders around the unit about other skills that were often utilized by the patients. The unit also set up a token economy of DBT Bucks[2] that patients in the full program could earn when they were observed by staff utilizing their skills appropriately and/or attempting to use their skills rather than their target behaviors. These could be traded in to purchase money for the hospital cafe or store, extra video games or TV time on the unit, or other rewards as identified by the treatment team.

Outcome Measures and Data

Progress was tracked via administration of two measurement tools to program participants: Difficulties in Emotion Regulation Scale (DERS) and the DBT Ways of Coping Checklist (DBT-WCCL). Those in the full program were given measures at the onset of their first commitment signing and upon every re-signing thereafter (every six months). Patients who were only in the groups were tracked at each new group cycle (approximately every 9–12 weeks), filling out the same measures each time. The scores were tracked via Excel spreadsheets to monitor patient progress. Additionally, data was de-identified and aggregated to monitor treatment effects across modalities and pooled to remove bias that might be present regarding particular patients. We also tracked information regarding instances of egregious behaviors for each patient and monitored for trends and improvements (or regressions). Regarding egregious behaviors, we found that on the DBT unit, instances of assaults were reduced by 50% in two years. On another unit considered "maximum security" with much higher instances of assaults, on which DBT interventions were being heavily utilized but not to full fidelity, assaults were reduced by 21% in that same time frame. Instances of seclusion and restraints were reduced by 31% on the DBT unit and 27% on the maximum security unit. The outcomes on the DERS and DBT-WCCL were less definitive. As these were self-report measures, this outcome could be due to limited insight into improvements or changes that the patients may have been experiencing. That being said, there were some positive trends on the DBT-WCCL among patients in the full-fidelity program.

Certification

Once data had been collected for approximately three-to-four years, the unit applied to the Linehan credentialing board; the application required that there was at least one fully credentialed DBT therapist heading the program. We also had to send in our program plan, demographics of patients, and outcome data. Once the unit made it through the first round in the application process, a site visit was required, in which several advisors on the board came to the hospital, met with several of the DBT providers and unit staff, and interviewed several of the group and individual DBT patients. They also toured the unit and reviewed several of our individual therapy patient formulations, chart notes, and video and audio recordings. At the end of the site visit, which took two to three days, they gave the team preliminary feedback on things we were doing well and areas of improvement that would likely need to be addressed before we could be credentialed. Several weeks later, we received a tentative "yes" to becoming the first forensic inpatient DBT unit, with the understanding that certain portions of the program were addressed. These included better guidelines regarding the phone coaching protocols, testing out strategies for patients who have been through the full group program twice, and more training and consultation opportunities for the unit floor staff.

Challenges

One of the largest systemic challenges was the general reactive nature that healthcare systems have toward suicide and NSSI. Typically, these behaviors are met with swift intervention, serious provider support, and caretaking. However, in the case of individuals with borderline personality disorder, such reactions by hospital systems often reinforce these behaviors (Paris, 2002). Such unintentional reinforcement is why much of the research regarding borderline personality disorder indicates that hospitalization is contraindicated much of the time. The forensic hospital where our DBT unit is located was no different in that, ethically, it had an obligation to address NSSI and suicide attempts, and it had to do so in certain ways as outlined by the Joint Commission and Centers for Medicaid and Medicare Services (CMS) standards. Therefore, the DBT unit was often at odds with the standards that applied to such behaviors. Finding the balance between meeting the ethical and legal requirements and doing what is therapeutically indicated was often difficult and required the providers in our program to become advocates as much as therapists. Generally speaking, this balance continues to be a struggle as certification and credentialing boards continue to demand certain actions in the face of these behaviors, even when contraindicated by the empirical evidence for certain populations.

Another significant issue that the unit had to contend with was the delicate nature of the obvious power structure at the hospital. The participating patients were, by and large, GEI patients ordered by the various court systems of the state to serve their time at the hospital while receiving treatment. While engagement in treatment was voluntary, there were also underlying difficulties for patients who did not engage in treatment, namely, that it took longer for them to gain privileges and reach conditional release readiness status. Finding the balance between allowing the patient to invoke their autonomy while still attempting to do our due diligence regarding treatment and risk mitigation was not always a successful endeavor. However, this author believes that one of the largest safety nets for these struggles was the skillfulness of the providers in managing these difficult power dynamics and in their commitment to maintain as much transparency and partnership with the patients as possible. This allowed for a great deal of rapport to develop, which allowed for some grace on the side of the patients when the providers had to make unpopular decisions (or when they had to enforce unpopular decisions made by management or executive levels of the hospital's upper echelon).

Another obstacle that the unit often faced was one presented by the patients themselves. These patients were not in treatment simply because of their personality disorders or behaviors. They were GEI patients, which means that they also had a primary mental health disorder, often a bipolar or schizophrenia spectrum disorder, and sometimes a co-occurring trauma disorder, which complicated their presentation. The providers were not only having to help the patients learn to manage traits and behaviors associated with the disordered personality characteristics but were also sometimes contending with mania, severe depression, PTSD, or acute psychosis, which brought their own distinct behaviors and symptoms that also needed to be treated. Some of these symptoms are also successfully treated with DBT (PSTD and depression, namely), but medication is a frontline treatment for mania and psychosis. Often, medication can be a difficult intervention to get started when working with individuals experiencing severe paranoia, disorganization, and dysregulation. Often, the team was making split-second decisions to determine how best to help a patient in crisis. They would have to quickly determine if this was a crisis of emotion or thought disorder and how best to address it, while often the patient would be on the brink of NSSI or violence. The staff, due to their own skill set, their training, and their dedication to their patients and the philosophy of the unit, would walk into these often dangerous and volatile situations with a calm demeanor and caring attitude and, while being mindful of their safety, would focus on the patient's needs and encourage the patient to use skills, help them use their skills, and work with them to slowly return to baseline.

The other obstacle that often comes with working with such populations is provider burnout. Burnout, vicarious trauma, and compassion fatigue are all very real phenomena within the field, particularly when working with severe and persistent mental illness and/or borderline personality disorder in an outpatient setting. In an inpatient setting, the provider sees the patients (between 20 and 30 on the unit, depending on the census) every day rather than every week. There are fewer opportunities to take breaks and fewer opportunities to move away from a patient who is activating a countertransferential reaction in the provider. Unit staff members are inundated. Therefore, the IDT (who was also susceptible to all these consequences of working with the population but had more opportunities to leave the unit and take breaks than the unit staff did) knew early on that addressing these issues was going to be imperative. The consultation groups were one way to address this, as were the ongoing trainings. However, the IDT also knew that appreciation and recognition could go a long way in reducing compassion fatigue and burnout as well. Therefore, there were frequent social get togethers with all the staff, and the break rooms on the unit were almost always filled with various snacks and goodies (some healthy, some guilty pleasures). Additionally, the IDT pushed for the unit staff to receive differential pay for working on a DBT unit due to the highly specialized nature of the unit, and ultimately, the nursing staff (all the floor/unit staff) were able to get a 5% differential as long as they were able to pass a test demonstrating basic knowledge of the DBT fundamentals. That differential would apply any time they worked a shift on the DBT unit once they passed that fundamentals test.

A final challenge that was often difficult to navigate was the tendency to infantilize psychiatric patients and the overall restriction of their ability to explore their own sexuality. While the hospital had policies regarding "dating behaviors" due to the need to protect vulnerable patients from possibly predatory behaviors engaged in by some of our more antisocial patients, patients were also sometimes discouraged from exploring their sexuality in their own rooms. On one such occasion, a female patient was taken to seclusion due to masturbatory practices that one unit staff member deemed to be "self-harm" simply because the staff member believed it was inappropriate for the patient to be "rough" with herself, despite the patient explaining that she found this practice pleasurable and was not actually harming herself. The patient had been in her room at the time. Other patients often have their self-stimulation aids taken away as they are deemed "unsafe" or unsanitary, rather than teaching them safe practices on how to care for the aid. While these dimensions of the sexual needs and behaviors of patients are potentially outside the context of DBT in general, one of the principles of DBT is to encourage autonomy for the patient and to encourage the patient to act as their own advocate and believe that they are capable. Some of the responses and restrictions placed on sexual behavior in inpatient forensic settings are directly contrary to that principle.

The Current View and Looking to the Future

Prior to the COVID-19 pandemic, the program was well on its way to maintaining its upward trend. Obstacles frequently arose along the way, largely systemic, that highlighted areas of future growth for the unit. Often, these were made apparent either by changes in management and repeatedly changing decisions about patient treatment strategies or by the high staff turnover that the hospital was beginning to experience. Additionally, the hospital encountered some legal difficulties due to the large increase in competency restoration demand that resulted in court orders, changes in admission laws and time frames, and influenced the ways in which patient populations were distributed across the hospital. Among the challenges to the program was an administrative decision that, despite the overall success of the DBT unit, that success was not enough to insulate it from having to integrate patients on the unit who were hospitalized for competency restoration and were not necessarily appropriate for the DBT unit as it had been functioning. This significantly changed the way treatment was able to be offered on the unit.

As a result of changes that were initiated due to the pandemic and to accommodate the influx of competency restoration patients, the unit had to be altered significantly. The competency restoration patients were not psychiatrically stable enough to engage in DBT in the same way as their

GEI counterparts. The unit staff continued to follow the principles of DBT, and groups and individual therapy were still occurring. However, patients from different units could no longer commingle in groups that were held on the unit during the pandemic. The environment of the unit had to be heavily modified to meet the needs of a more acute population. This means that the posters were removed, and some of the sensory and other coping methods had to be either heavily modified or removed entirely. Then, a few months after some of these adaptations took place, a CMS review led to a host of new rules that prompted the further removal of many other patient coping tools.

Despite these changes, there have been some ongoing successes. Several patients have continued to engage in the full-fidelity program. Several patients were able to graduate from the program and demonstrate mastery of the skills taught in the groups. One long-term DBT patient who, upon arrival at the hospital, was not able to tolerate any type of frustration without significant outbursts and suicidal ideation and would often self-sabotage any type of personal success, went on to complete his bachelor's degree. Another patient who was in the program for several years prior to the pandemic has been violence-free now for several years. So while the program has undergone significant changes because of the significant shift in the demands of the community and the judicial system and because of hospital administration's decisions, there are still successes to point to and patients that have been able to make a life-changing recovery because of this unit and the program.

Once the pressures created by the pandemic pass and there is "a new normal," it may be possible to allow for competency restoration patients to be treated elsewhere in the hospital and for the unit to return to serving as a DBT unit with the GEI patient population. Should that not occur and if the hospital continues to see increasingly high numbers of competency restoration patients, it would be imperative that the hospital find a way to incorporate what it has learned about running a DBT unit and apply it to the restoration population, which would include alterations in the DBT program to be suited for higher acuity, cognitive and neuropsychiatric disorders, developmental delays, and other presentations that often impact competency.

Notes

1 e.g., violence, threats of violence, non-suicidal self-injury, suicide attempts, substance or medication abuse, or patient-specific factors such as possession of pornography for patients with SO charge adjudications.

2 The Bucks were a reinforcement only, and the patients could not lose Bucks for egregious behaviors or other rule-breaking behavior.

References

Axelrod, S. R., Perepletchikova, F., Holtzman, K., & Sinha, R. (2011). Emotion regulation and substance use frequency in women with substance dependence and Borderline Personality Disorder receiving Dialectical Behavior Therapy. *The American Journal of Drug and Alcohol Abuse*, *37*(1), 37–42. https://doi.org/10.3109/00952990.2010.535582.

Bohus, M., Dyer, A. S., Priebe, K., Krüger, A., Kleindienst, N., Schmahl, C., Niedtfeld, I., & Steil, R. (2013). Dialectical Behaviour Therapy for Post-Traumatic Stress Disorder after childhood sexual abuse in patients with and without Borderline Personality Disorder: A randomised controlled trial. *Psychotherapy and Psychosomatics*, *82*(4), 221–233.

Carter, G. L., Willcox, C. H., Lewin, T. J., Conrad, A. M., & Bendit, N. (2010). Hunter DBT project: Randomized controlled trial of Dialectical Behaviour Therapy in women with Borderline Personality Disorder. *Australian & New Zealand Journal of Psychiatry*, *44*(2), 162–173.

Chen, E. Y., Matthews, L., Allen, C., Kuo, J. R., & Linehan, M. M. (2008). Dialectical Behavior Therapy for clients with Binge-Eating Disorder or Bulimia Nervosa and Borderline Personality Disorder. *The International Journal of Eating Disorders*, *41*(6), 505–512. https://doi.org/10.1002/eat.20522.

Comtois, K. A., Elwood, L., Holdcraft, L. C., Smith, W. R., & Simpson, T. L. (2007). Effectiveness of Dialectical Behavior Therapy in a community mental health center. *Cognitive and Behavioral Practice, 14*(4), 406–414. https://doi.org/10.1016/j.cbpra.2006.04.023.

Courbasson, C., Nishikawa, Y., & Dixon, L. (2012). Outcome of Dialectical Behaviour Therapy for concurrent eating and substance use disorders. *Clinical Psychology & Psychotherapy*, *19*(5), 434–449. https://doi.org/10.1002/cpp.748.

Feigenbaum, J. D., Fonagy, P., Pilling, S., Jones, A., Wildgoose, A., & Bebbington, P. E. (2012). A real-world study of the effectiveness of DBT in the UK National Health Service. *British Journal of Clinical Psychology*, *51*(2), 121–141.

Harned, M. S., Korslund, K. E., & Linehan, M. M. (2014). A pilot randomized controlled trial of Dialectical Behavior Therapy with and without the Dialectical Behavior Therapy Prolonged Exposure protocol for suicidal and self-injuring women with Borderline Personality Disorder and PTSD. *Behaviour Research and Therapy*, *55*, 7–17.

Iverson, K., Shenk, C., & Fruzzetti, A. (2009). Dialectical Behavior Therapy for women victims of domestic abuse: A pilot study. *Professional Psychology: Research and Practice, 40*, 242–248. https://doi.org/10.1037/a0013476.

Keuthen, N. J., Rothbaum, B. O., Welch, S. S., Taylor, C., Falkenstein, M., Heekin, M., Jordan, C. A., Timpano, K., Meunier, S., Fama, J., & Jenike, M. A. (2010). Pilot trial of Dialectical Behavior Therapy-enhanced habit reversal for trichotillomania. *Depression and Anxiety*, *27*(10), 953–959. https://doi.org/10.1002/da.20732.

Kröger, C., Schweiger, U., Sipos, V., Kliem, S., Arnold, R., Schunert, T., & Reinecker, H. (2010). Dialectical Behaviour Therapy and an added cognitive behavioural treatment module for eating disorders in women with Borderline Personality Disorder and Anorexia Nervosa or Bulimia Nervosa who failed to respond to previous treatments. An open trial with a 15-month follow-up. *Journal of Behavior Therapy and Experimental Psychiatry*, *41*(4), 381–388. https://doi.org/10.1016/j.jbtep.2010.04.001.

Linehan, M. M., Armstrong, H. E., Suarez, A., Allmon, D., & Heard, H. L. (1991). Cognitive-behavioral treatment of chronically parasuicidal borderline patients. *Archives of General Psychiatry*, *48*(12), 1060–1064. https://doi.org/10.1001/archpsyc.1991.01810360024003.

Linehan, M. M., Schmidt, H., Dimeff, L. A., Craft, J. C., Kanter, J., & Comtois, K. A. (1999). Dialectical Behavior Therapy for patients with Borderline Personality Disorder and drug-dependence. *American Journal on Addictions*, *8*(4), 279–292.

McCann, R. A. & Ball, E. M. (1996). DBT with an inpatient forensic population: The CMHIP forensic model. *Cognitive and Behavioral Practice*, *7*(4). 447–456. https://doi.org/10.1016/S1077-7229(00)80056-5.

McCann, R. A., Ball, E. M., & Ivanoff, A. (2000). DBT with an inpatient forensic population: The CMHIP forensic model. *Cognitive and Behavioral Practice*, *7*(4), 447–456. https://doi.org/10.1016/S1077-7229(00)80056-5.

McFetridge, M. A. & Coakes, J. (2010). The longer-term clinical outcomes of a DBT-informed residential therapeutic community; An evaluation and reunion. *Therapeutic Communities*, *31*(4), 406–416.

Paris, J. (2002). Chronic suicidality among patients with Borderline Personality Disorder. *Psychiatric Services*, *53*(6), 738–742. https://doi.org/10.1176/appi.ps.53.6.738.

Perroud, N., Uher, R., Dieben, K., Nicastro, R., & Huguelet, P. (2010). Predictors of response and drop-out during intensive Dialectical Behavior Therapy. *Journal of Personality Disorders*, *24*(5), 634–650. https://doi.org/10.1521/pedi.2010.24.5.634.

Pistorello, J., Fruzzetti, A. E., MacLane, C., Gallop, R., & Iverson, K. M. (2012). Dialectical Behavior Therapy (DBT) applied to college students: A randomized clinical trial. *Journal of Consulting and Clinical Psychology*, *80*(6), 982.

Rizvi, S. L., Dimeff, L. A., Skutch, J., Carroll, D., & Linehan, M. M. (2011). A pilot study of the DBT coach: An interactive mobile phone application for individuals with Borderline Personality Disorder and substance use disorder. *Behavior Therapy*, *42*(4), 589–600. https://doi.org/10.1016/j.beth.2011.01.003.

Sakdalan, J. A., Shaw, J., & Collier, V. (2010). Staying in the here-and-now: A pilot study on the use of Dialectical Behaviour Therapy group skills training for forensic clients with intellectual disability. *Journal of Intellectual Disability Research*, *54*(6), 568–572. https://doi.org/10.1111/j.1365-2788.2010.01274.x.

Sambrook, S., Abba, N., & Chadwick, P. (2007). Evaluation of DBT emotional coping skills groups for people with parasuicidal behaviours. *Behavioural and Cognitive Psychotherapy*, *35*, 241–244. https://doi.org/10.1017/S1352465806003298.

Shelton, D., Sampl, S., Kesten, K. L., Zhang, W., & Trestman, R. L. (2009). Treatment of impulsive aggression in correctional settings. *Behavioral Sciences & the Law*, *27*(5), 787–800. https://doi.org/10.1002/bsl.889.

Steil, R., Dyer, A., Priebe, K., Kleindienst, N., & Bohus, M. (2011). Dialectical Behavior Therapy for Posttraumatic Stress Disorder related to childhood sexual abuse: A pilot study of an intensive residential treatment program. *Journal of Traumatic Stress*, *24*(1), 102–106. https://doi.org/10.1002/jts.20617.

Telch, C. F., Agras, W. S., & Linehan, M. M. (2001). Dialectical Behavior Therapy for Binge Eating Disorder. *Journal of Consulting and Clinical Psychology*, *69*(6), 1061–1065. https://doi.org/10.1037/0022-006X.69.6.1061.

Turner, R. M. (2000). Naturalistic evaluation of Dialectical Behavior Therapy-oriented treatment for Borderline Personality Disorder. *Cognitive and Behavioral Practice*, 7(4), 413–419.

Williams, S. E., Hartstone, M. D., & Denson, L. A. (2010). Dialectical Behavioural Therapy and Borderline Personality Disorder: Effects on service utilisation and self-reported symptoms. *Behaviour Change*, *27*(4), 251–264. https://doi.org/10.1375/bech.27.4.251.

Part III

System Wide Intervention and Transformation

14 Recovery-Oriented Cognitive Therapy (CT-R)

Empowering Individuals with Serious Mental Health and Justice-Related Challenges

Ellen Inverso and Shelby Arnold

Recovery-oriented treatment principles have been a mandate of mental health care since the release of the President's New Freedom Commission on Mental Health (2003) report. Forensic mental health settings often encounter difficulty incorporating these principles due to factors inherent to the justice system (e.g., length of stay, hierarchical decision-making), but also because legal constructs such as recidivism serve as markers of success rather than whole-person definitions of recovery (e.g., living one's desired life; Dorkins & Adshead, 2011; Mann et al., 2014). Recovery-oriented cognitive therapy (CT-R) is an approach that can improve forensic mental health care by operationalizing recovery principles and can be implemented in the most restrictive settings. Guided by Aaron Beck's cognitive model (1963; 2019), CT-R is an evidence-based practice that provides concrete, actionable steps to promote recovery and resiliency (Beck et al., 2021), thereby empowering individuals to take action toward a meaningful and desired life.

Importantly, CT-R also provides an efficient means to promote risk mitigation through the reduction of evidence-based criminogenic risk factors (e.g., antisocial cognitions, lack of educational/vocational activities) and bolstering protective factors linked to recidivism reduction (e.g., increased connection, meaningful ways to spend time). CT-R includes methods that lead to lasting belief change – helping individuals[1] view themselves as capable, other people as worth connecting to, and the future as more hopeful.

CT-R has been implemented in at least nine US states at many levels of care – from community teams to residences to highly secure forensic hospital units – by providers of all levels of education, holding myriad roles in care, including psychiatrists, psychologists, social workers, peer specialists, recreation and rehabilitation professionals, nurses, officers, and direct care staff, among others (Grant, 2019). CT-R can also be adapted to empower individuals facing hurdles that occur along the justice involvement continuum, such as competency restoration, agreeability to legal

DOI: 10.4324/9781003360926-18

processes, experiencing purpose rather than stagnation during long periods of confinement, and preparing for community reentry – a precarious process often filled with collateral consequences that can lead to a return to justice involvement, especially for individuals with serious mental health challenges (Baillargeon et al., 2010).

In high-security forensic implementation projects, programs have used CT-R skills despite limited access to resources and technology, as it allows for creativity and flexibility. CT-R was designed to be adaptable to any setting, regardless of its limitations, systemic challenges or inequities, and to embrace the diversity of individuals served. It can also be applied in any type of interaction (e.g., individual or group therapy, on the milieu, in a brief interaction; Morales et al., 2022). Further, CT-R is broadly applicable; techniques can be adapted for use with any individual, regardless of their level of insight or cognitive abilities.

Recovery-Oriented Cognitive Therapy

Background

CT-R meets two needs: one, the continued need for effective psychosocial treatment for individuals experiencing challenges associated with serious mental health condition diagnoses, such as schizophrenia, and two, the sociocultural shift toward a recovery model of mental health treatment. Building upon input from people with lived experience and their loved ones, providers, previous research, and original research utilizing clinical trials, CT-R was originally developed to improve outcomes for individuals who experience negative symptoms of withdrawal, isolation, limited access to energy and motivation, and reduced verbal expressivity (Grant, 2019; Beck et al., 2021). Negative and self-stigmatizing beliefs that contributed to individuals' disengagement included: "I can't do the things I like anymore," "I'm broken," "this is as good as it gets for me," and "I have to forget about having a life now." Individuals' beliefs concerning their interpersonal value and their sense of belonging or relatedness were also uncovered: "I'm better off staying to myself and away from others," "I'm not like everyone else," or "I'm not good with people." These beliefs have now been linked to negative symptoms, poorer psychosocial functioning, and limited social activity around the globe (Grant & Beck, 2009; Grant & Beck, 2010; Campellone et al., 2016; Thomas et al., 2017; Reddy et al., 2018; Raugh et al., 2019). Further, it was discovered that while these individuals did not see themselves as capable of doing much or connecting with others, the desire was still present. Most described wanting relationships, families, jobs, and life in the community. CT-R is a psychosocial method to address this paradox, providing a way for providers to partner with often cautious or mistrustful individuals to help them feel less defeated and more connected.

The personal and future-focused approach of CT-R matches the characteristics of the Recovery Movement that have become an important influence in the direction of mental health care and treatment. Originating in the 1960s as a political effort to bring about social justice (Davidson et al., 2011), the Recovery Movement involved individuals with lived experience and mental health advocates making demands for community-based care as opposed to chronic institutionalization. Two of the ways recovery-oriented treatment defines the process and outcome of care (Davidson et al., 2008) are: individuals should have an active role in treatment; goals should focus on their desired life. In CT-R, the concept of recovery is about people living the meaningful lives of their choosing and building empowerment and resilience related to challenges impeding the pursuit of that life.

Theory

CT-R's flexibility and broad applicability arise from three elements: the theory of modes (Beck, 1996), the cognitive model (Beck, 1963), and attentional narrowing (Gable et al., 2015; Hicks et al., 2015; Grant & Inverso, 2023).

Theory of Modes

Beck's theory of modes posits that people move between different modes of being when faced with different circumstances. Originally applied to personality disorders (Beck, 1996), the theory is now transdiagnostic (Beck & Haigh, 2014; Beck, Finkel, & Beck, 2021), describing how people experience and interact in their environment. In CT-R, the focus is on two specific modes: the *adaptive* mode and the *disconnected* mode (Beck et al., 2021; Grant & Beck, in preparation). The *adaptive* mode represents a person feeling at their best or more like themselves. Challenges or symptoms are less central; the person has greater access to energy, motivation, and seeing themselves more positively; and they are more likely to engage with others and the world. In contrast, the *disconnected* mode is when a person has less access to energy, motivation, hope, or possibility. In this mode, challenges or symptoms are dominant, and the person is less likely to engage or participate. People often either retreat (e.g., negative symptoms) or respond with reactive behavior (e.g., aggression, substance use).

The Cognitive Model

The second feature of CT-R theory is the cognitive model (Beck, 1963), which describes behavior and emotion in terms of underlying beliefs – how the person views themselves, other people, the world, and their future. These beliefs are active when the person is in either a disconnected or adaptive mode. The disconnected mode is driven by negative beliefs. Over six decades of research support Beck's cognitive model for understanding challenges commonly seen in forensic mental health settings: depression, anxiety, anger, personality disorders, substance use, positive symptoms (i.e., hallucinations, delusions), negative symptoms, and criminality (Beck, 1999; 2019). CT-R extends the cognitive model to understanding people's perceptions when they are thriving – or at least when the problems are less dominant. Positive beliefs become more accessible when people are in an adaptive mode (Beck et al., 2021). In CT-R, the aim is to support the strengthening of positive beliefs, as this has been shown to correspond with increased community participation and reduced symptomatology (Grant & Best, 2019).

Attentional Narrowing

The third feature of CT-R theory involves attention, which can vary in scope from broad to narrow. Narrow attentional fixation can, at times, be useful, such as focusing to complete a task (Gable et al., 2015; Hicks et al., 2015). However, CT-R theory (Grant & Beck, in preparation) posits that the challenges a person experiences (i.e., aggression, self-injury) become entrenched through a similar mechanism. For example, a person prone to aggressive behavior can experience attentional narrowing to the extent that alternative perspectives about a situation (and alternative actions they can take) are screened out. Strategies and interventions that shift a person into the adaptive mode broaden attentional scope.

Overview of CT-R in Forensic Settings

A principal aim of CT-R is to increase the amount of time individuals are spending in the adaptive mode; the five core elements are: accessing, energizing, developing, actualizing, and strengthening the adaptive mode. *Accessing* includes discovering what specifically gets a person into their adaptive mode (e.g., cooking, music, video games, cultural knowledge). *Energizing* involves increasing the frequency with which people participate in these interests, skills, and activities. Taken together, *accessing* and *energizing* provide practical procedures for building wellness factors of connection and trust between individuals and providers. *Developing* involves discovering and vividly exploring an individual's aspirations for the future, which can include specific targets but emphasizes the values, meanings, and positive beliefs they desire, enlivening the recovery principle of hope. The focus on more conceptual meanings allows forensically involved individuals to experience hope with fewer limitations. The focus on values also makes CT-R culturally conscious, which can help meet the needs of individuals from minority backgrounds who disproportionately find themselves in the forensic system (US Census Bureau, American Community Survey 2019; Arya et al., 2021). *Actualizing* turns aspirations into action by breaking them into achievable steps as well as locating activities to experience the meanings of aspirations regularly – actions that are a source of the recovery factor of purpose. *Strengthening* the adaptive mode is the fifth part of CT-R but is incorporated throughout the approach. This involves the use of targeted questions to support individuals in drawing meaningful conclusions about themselves, others, and possibilities for the future based on positive experiences and successes, including building beliefs about the person's resilience as they use strategies for handling challenges.

Challenges are then understood in the context of aspirations: what is interfering with progress toward, or achievement of, aspirations? This could include behaviors, legal factors, and beliefs. A CT-R formulation aids forensic providers and teams in understanding all aspects of the individuals they are serving and in selecting interventions that have a good likelihood of success for each person. Common beliefs in forensic populations include feeling demoralized, alone, isolated, mistrustful of providers or systems (e.g., mental health, judicial), hopeless, broken, and incapable. Individuals may also be impacted by trauma or institutionalization. Reluctance to engage in treatment is typical. Based on this understanding, interventions are selected that function to increase access to the adaptive mode, provide opportunities to strengthen positive beliefs, or provide tools for the individual to feel more in control of challenges, such as interfering symptoms.

The CT-R Recovery Map (Beck Institute, 2020) captures the formulation. All members of interdisciplinary teams are encouraged to come together to create recovery maps, as they each have unique interactions with the justice-involved and can bring important information. Interventions can be developed to fit team members' unique roles and resources. Recovery maps can also be a way to communicate a whole-person picture to legal teams and future providers.

Implementation

CT-R is best implemented following the theory-driven, evidence-based protocol (Stirman et al., 2010; Grant, 2019) that includes a comprehensive needs assessment, training, consultation, and sustainability plan. This approach to implementation ensures a high likelihood of training success by enhancing the skills of existing staff and allowing each to bring their unique experiences within their respective roles to bear.

Needs Assessment

Early sessions with administrative stakeholders help orient the organization to what is required of in CT-R training and to plan logistics. Subsequent quarterly meetings are typical, with special attention to feedback, effectiveness outcomes, and sustaining the training long-term. Staff to be trained participate in focus groups, which allow them to learn about the approach and provide insight into program strengths and typical challenges (e.g., reluctance to discharge, not engaging with legal teams, aggression). Focus groups can be an interesting phase, as participants often come in with little background on the endeavor and can be curious – or outright mistrustful – of the intentions of both administration and trainers. People ask if they're being monitored or reported; some ask if things will change systemically, such as policy or hiring changes. The dynamic is generally different depending on the presence or absence of administrators due to concerns about retaliation for expressing an unfavorable opinion. The best focus groups have been ones that prioritize trainers learning about trainees' best days at work and that acknowledge the experiences and expertise of direct care staff. One site shared that they feel most proud when people engage in holiday celebrations because everyone participates, but indicated they would benefit from strategies for managing the isolation and aggression that come after these events. They were assured that this could be addressed as part of the implementation. Meeting staff where they are is as important as meeting individuals receiving treatment where they are.

Workshop

Workshops provide the theoretical foundation, strategies, and practical interventions for each stage of CT-R, including emphasis on mental health and justice-involvement challenges and familiarizing teams with the Recovery Map. Sessions can be held in real time (in-person or virtual) or can be accessed through on-demand, web-based trainings, which expand access to a broader range of staff and programs (Grant, 2019). The length of a CT-R workshop can vary based on program needs. For example, in one locked residence, what worked best was one-and-a-half-hour abbreviated workshop sessions spread over several weeks, while in one forensic hospital, two seven-hour training days spread over two weeks were preferred. In both cases, staff had the opportunity to test-drive the strategies discussed and return with their own examples and feedback. Two to three days held consecutively is sometimes preferred, such as in the case of an outpatient case management program that saw clients weekly and did not want to cancel or reschedule them three weeks in a row. Because forensic treatment settings are not one-size-fits-all, the workshop structure can't be either.

Consultation

Research shows that workshops alone are not sufficient to bring skills into practice (Stirman et al., 2010). It requires technical assistance in the form of ongoing consultation – an opportunity to put learning on its feet through targeted discussions of individuals on the service, milieu programs, group therapy applications, and creating recovery maps. Consultation sessions are best done in a group format, either with a team or a number of individual providers, and are most effective when participants represent different departments and roles in justice-involved individuals' care. Six months of weekly consultation is the standard length for consultation, though different durations can be effective. Over time, consultation can shift from external CT-R expert-led sessions to internal CT-R champion-led sessions while receiving feedback.

Consultation can provide a venue for creative problem-solving. For example, in one state system, there was an opportunity to partner with providers in a large maximum security forensic facility. Here, many of the individuals had lengthy, if not life-long, sentences, and virtually all had been given serious mental health condition diagnoses. Aggression and high-risk interactions (e.g., gambling) were among the most reported challenges and were typically addressed with increased restrictions and limits. A pivotal point in the setting's implementation of CT-R happened during consultation, when the team agreed to use available and permitted resources as opportunities for the individuals to have a role in teaching staff or facilitating group activities. The energy and attention that had been put into conflict were shifted to opportunities to contribute to others, including officers and nurses, which opened opportunities for connection and more positive, meaningful experiences. One particular individual, who had double-digit numbers of assaults every month, began teaching staff how to work the equipment in a computer lab. Having hoped to go to school for technology in the past, this provided both an opportunity to demonstrate skills and strengths while also meeting the values of his aspiration. Incidents dropped to zero, as he could anticipate when he would be able to engage in this activity, and staff were intentional about helping him notice what he was doing for them and the whole ward, and most importantly, what it said about him as a person – that he was skilled, capable, and had something of value to offer others.

From the staff perspective, this led to team unification and more cohesive treatment, as they each had a role in learning about and from the individual and gained different perspectives from each other based on their respective interactions. Consultation allowed for brainstorming formulation-driven strategies when things were difficult and the opportunity to celebrate successes together. It is often during this phase that staff attitudes toward CT-R change.

Sustainability

Sustainability begins at the start of implementation. To keep CT-R going after the active phase of training requires building it into existing structures (e.g., groups, documentation). In at least two hospitals, rounds sheets were modified to include checkboxes so staff could note engagement in meaningful activities and other CT-R activities. In another, the nursing census board was updated to note which phase in the CT-R process staff were focusing on with each individual. In several units and residences across an entire state system, group therapy and milieu program written descriptions were updated to indicate how the programs align with CT-R targets as well as forensic and/or discharge requirements, making CT-R themes and interventions a core part of the therapeutic curriculum.

Also key to sustainability is identifying primary champions of the approach who can take over the role of guiding CT-R from expert trainers. A measure called the *CT-R Quality Scale* (Beck et al., 2021) can be particularly helpful, as it involves a formalized self-assessment of CT-R strengths and areas for improvement. This measure can be administered at baseline, prior to any training occurring, and then routinely throughout implementation to identify needs and priorities and track progress. Emerging data suggest that full sustainability can often be achieved within one to two years. An interesting theme site should be attentive to is how some of the best, most dedicated teams tend to undersell themselves in self-assessment, while fractured teams may overstate their efforts – perhaps out of concern for castigation. Champions and internal trainers may be best poised to guide more accurate assessments.

Considerations

Though programs build CT-R implementation from their own teams, there are still costs involved with having staff off-line while participating in the workshop and consultations. The hope is that these costs will be offset by reduced costs resulting from fewer incidents, including a reduced need for more intensive levels of staff observation, and increased staff satisfaction (Chang et al., 2014).

Broader systemic challenges that can impact implementation include how participating staff perceive their role and the purpose of their setting. In some systems, for example, inpatient forensic programs fall under the state's department of corrections, whereas other programs fall under the jurisdiction of health and human services departments. This can impact the priorities of the staff. While maintaining safety is paramount in both cases, if the perception of staff is that security, order, and chastisement are the priorities, it can be difficult to get buy-in to implement an approach that frontloads connection and highly interactive interventions. In some systems, the governing authority changes based on evolving streams of funding. Despite high-level changes, often the staff in the facility remain the same and may not readily adjust their philosophy or approach. In these circumstances, administrative buy-in is essential. More than encouraging staff to try the approach, the most successful forensic implementations involve active participation from leadership at every stage, as well as the expectation that CT-R outcomes are captured in internal processes such as treatment planning, documentation, new staff orientation, and supervision sessions. When a recovery-oriented perspective is given precedence, cultural change can occur.

Considering the CT-R approach itself, a common question in implementation is: "Are we setting people up for failure or disappointment when we ask them about their aspirations?" This is especially true when individuals are residing in high-level care or when a return to the community is unlikely. This is where the concentration on meanings underlying aspirations, rather than specific targets, is critical; focusing on how people want to see themselves or be seen by others and values more broadly (e.g., contribution, being skilled) provides the path to finding meaningful, productive action in any setting. Related to this, staff can also feel discouraged when individuals make progress but get demoralized due to restrictions or legal factors outside of everyone's control. CT-R supervision can be an invaluable help here, shifting focus to formulation and together strategizing approaches to meaning-driven positive action. Supervisors remind team members about the fluidity of the CT-R approach and encourage prioritizing connection – a return to accessing and energizing adaptive mode. Guidance on empathizing and the use of collaborative "we" language can offer a reset and reinvigoration when staff need it most. This then extends to the individuals.

CT-R in Action

Consider "Mike," an individual living on a forensic psychiatric unit undergoing a CT-R implementation.[2] Mike's staff is in the consultation stage with CT-R experts. They explain that over the past 20 years, Mike has moved throughout the justice system, bouncing between correctional facilities, hospital units, and community supervision. Currently, he does not engage in conversations about discharge; he expresses hopelessness, saying, for example, "I'll just mess up probation anyway and end up back here or in jail, so none of it matters." The staff report that Mike spends most of his days in his room and feels overwhelmed by voices that tell him others despise him and want to hurt him.

Accessing

The CT-R expert begins with the first strategy: establish connection and trust with Mike. The intervention is for staff to learn about Mike's interests, hobbies, or areas of expertise or skill. They consider speaking with collateral contacts (e.g., family, friends, providers), reviewing records, or asking Mike what he liked to do before he became justice-involved. Because of Mike's guardedness, the consultant advises they make brief but frequent attempts at connection, prioritizing approaches that help Mike experience control, such as seeking recommendations on music, video games, or other areas of popular culture from times that predate the onset of the challenges.

The consultant explains that success will be observable; people will show both affective and behavioral shifts. She tells the team to look for smiling, laughing, or engaging verbally, and to be prepared to help Mike notice these shifts and positive beliefs that may be activated. For example, staff could ask, "It seems like you're smiling more when we talk about sports, do you notice that, too?" or "it seems like you really know a lot about this topic, what do you think?"

On the unit, staff observe Mike occasionally watching sports games, writing rap lyrics in his journal, and helping at mealtimes. Following these observations, they put the CT-R strategy in place to form a connection by talking about recent sports games, watching highlights of games when possible, and asking for his advice on recipes. The team learns that in the community, Mike used to enjoy playing pick-up basketball and spending time with his neighbors having cookouts on the weekends. Mike brightens during interactions when he talks about sports or cooking. The staff observe that in those moments Mike experiences positive beliefs such as being capable and having something valuable to offer, though this quickly turns to hopelessness ("I'll never be able to do those things again").

To help the team generalize, the consultant emphasizes that everyone – whether hospital clinicians or direct care staff, correctional staff, community providers, or court stakeholders (e.g., judges, probation/parole offices) – can engage an individual in a conversation or activity that will bring about their adaptive mode. Individuals in especially restrictive settings can experience the adaptive mode through discussion and visualization of certain topics.

Energizing

Now that they know how to access Mike's adaptive mode, the CT-R expert recommends adjusting the strategy to *energizing* it to help him experience positive emotions and beliefs more often. She explains this can be achieved by expanding who Mike engages in activities with (e.g., other staff, members of the community, peers). It could also involve increasing the frequency of activities (e.g., multiple times per day, on different shifts) and trying to engage in new activities that could generate similar important beliefs (e.g., capability, control).

The team creates more opportunities for Mike to talk to staff about sports. With some, he reflects on recent games, and with one, he teaches the rules of basketball. The team also arranges for Mike to play a predictable role on the unit, setting up the dining room for meals and letting other individuals know it is time to eat. Mike knows that at every meal he'll be able to help, and staff help him observe that he is worthwhile and contributing.

Drawing conclusions at this stage involves noticing the benefits of activity and the momentum gained by doing enjoyable and meaningful activities. Another focus is helping individuals like Mike notice that access to the adaptive mode is not a one-time occurrence, generalizing positive beliefs from "I enjoyed playing cards yesterday" to "people like doing things with me." The consultant suggests staff ask Mike, "if you're able to connect with people here, is it possible you can do it in the community too?" and "you've really been helping a lot lately, what does that say about you?" This ensures he makes meaning from each experience and gradually becomes more comfortable considering possibilities for his future.

Developing

Summarizing the team's progress, the CT-R consultant observes that the team has connected with Mike and learned a lot about him. The next strategy, d*eveloping* the adaptive mode, involves identifying and enriching an individual's aspirations. For justice-involved individuals, aspirations are critical. Not only do they serve as the "why" for navigating challenges (e.g., undesirable forensic requirements, evaluations or court hearings, lengthy sentences), but they also serve as a way for individuals to feel in control of their future and take action toward a desired life regardless of their current forensic status and when/whether they will be in the community again. Enriching an aspiration involves visualizing the details of what an aspiration might look like and understanding the meaning underneath – what are the important parts of it?

When the team asks, Mike shares his aspiration of getting back to his old neighborhood so he can join the weekly barbecues again. A team member asks about the "best part" of this. Mike explains that he values his community, that he could bring people together, and that "people would see I'm still me." Though Mike might not yet be eligible for community discharge, these values can be met wherever he is in the forensic process. Similarly, for those in the community, the meaning of aspirations can guide how a person spends their time as they actively work toward their dreams. This is where aspirations become action and hope turns into purpose.

Actualizing

With Mike's aspirations identified and enriched, the CT-R expert proposes the strategies of (1) collaborating on ways for him to take positive action toward aspirations daily and (2) how to feel empowered when challenges arise. This could include completing short-term steps en route to the aspiration or living the personal meanings realized by aspirations (e.g., helping others, contributing). Individuals who are under judicial oversight may have limited freedoms, such as long-term hospitalization, incarceration, or offender status upon release. She advises prioritizing activities that achieve the meaning of aspirations as a powerful source of forward progress and sustained motivation.

With the team's help, Mike takes actions that express his values of community and bring others together by organizing viewing parties for sports games on the unit and helping to plan the unit's holiday luncheon. Even though he is not in his old neighborhood at a cookout, he is still living out the meaning underneath his aspirations. Momentum builds, and positive action creates a context for talking about discharge, meeting with probation/parole to discuss options, and attending groups focused on managing his voices. Drawing conclusions at this stage involves helping individuals notice the progress they are making in working toward aspirations and underlying values and that it is worth taking difficult or sometimes unappealing steps to get closer to their desired future. The expert proposes that staff help Mike notice accomplishments by asking, "what does it say about you that you planned a successful holiday luncheon?" and "is it worth going to groups and meeting with probation if it gets you closer to being back in your neighborhood to plan cookouts?" Conclusions are also drawn about his successful use of skills for challenges or handling situations differently than he might have in the past.

Strengthening

Throughout consultation, the expert emphasizes the importance of *strengthening* the adaptive mode by asking questions that target key conclusions: positive beliefs and resiliency beliefs. The key question, "what does that say about you?" – can be modified to yes-or-no questions for those who have difficulty with abstraction (e.g., "you're quite helpful, would you agree?"). Any member of a team can pose these questions to catch success and build positive beliefs that help the person sustain positive action. Particularly for justice-involved individuals, strengthening resiliency beliefs acts as a protective factor and cushions against negative beliefs that could lead to setbacks. It also helps to strengthen an individual's identity as a good person or a person who can meaningfully contribute.

By this time, a champion of CT-R is facilitating the internal consultation process. Staff plan to help Mike reflect on how far he has come and what that means about him. As discharge gets closer, staff collaborate with Mike to consider how his strengths and values will help him navigate challenges that come up, such as uncertain timelines and restrictions post-discharge.

Empirical Support

Given the overrepresentation of individuals with serious mental health challenges in the criminal justice system, an important research focus, in recent decades, has been on evidence-based practices that address both criminogenic and mental health needs (Casey & Rottman, 2005; James & Glaze, 2006; Honegger, 2015; Gottfried & Christopher, 2017; DeMatteo, 2019). Cognitive-behavioral therapy (CBT) has emerged as the prominent evidence-based practice in offender rehabilitation (Landenberger & Lipsey, 2005). CT-R can advance this by focusing on an individual's pursuit of both forensic recovery (i.e., reduced risk and recidivism) and mental health conceptualizations of recovery (i.e., meaningful and desired life).

CT-R was validated in a randomized blind clinical trial for individuals given serious mental health condition diagnoses, the majority of whom were black or Hispanic from low-resource communities in a major American city (Grant et al., 2012). Participants who received CT-R demonstrated significantly increased functional outcomes (e.g., educational and vocational involvement, socialization), community participation, and access to motivation, along with improvement of both positive and negative symptoms. These gains were maintained at a six-month follow-up (Grant et al., 2017). CT-R has helped systems move long-institutionalized individuals into less restrictive environments (Grant, 2019) and has led to a notable reduction in the use of instruments of control, such as seclusion and physical and chemical restraints (Chang et al., 2014). Providers trained in CT-R also report lower rates of hospitalization, a reduction in jail days, and increased engagement with community treatment teams for the individuals they serve (Grant, 2019; Beck et al., 2021).

Future Directions

Future program evaluation studies could test the cost-effectiveness of the CT-R approach and its ability to reduce hospitalization and increase days in the community. Specific forensic outcomes, including reduced jail time, an increase in protective factors and a decrease in risk factors, improved competency outcomes, and recidivism reduction, will also be crucial as the reach of CT-R expands throughout the justice system. It is important that forensic programs currently employing CT-R as their primary therapeutic modality engages in ongoing outcomes collection that looks at multiple points of impact, such as changes in participation, participant's beliefs, and progress toward aspirations, in addition to changes in untoward incidents (e.g., aggression, parole violations) and reports of distressing symptoms. It would also be beneficial for these programs to use measures such as the *CT-R Quality Scale* (Beck et al., 2021), which can serve as a mediating variable between the implementation process and individual outcomes.

Finally, the expansion of CT-R applications is a promising future direction and path forward. Given the success of CT-R for individuals in higher levels of care (e.g., secure forensic hospitals) and community residences, the focus of CT-R should mirror the direction of the justice system more broadly and look at applications within diversion programs (e.g., at the point of arrest, problem-solving courts) as a way to keep individuals in the community and living the lives they want and a mechanism for decreasing entrenchment within the justice system.

Notes

1 A note about language: To respect the requests of individuals with lived experience, we try to use person-first, recovery-oriented language that reduces implications of judgement. We use the term 'individual' rather than 'patient,' and phrases such as 'given a diagnosis of…' to acknowledge not all will agree with certain labels. We continually aim to improve our language when communicating to and about people and their experiences.

2 This example involves a hospital setting, but can be extrapolated to correctional or residential settings.

References

Arya, D., Connolly, C., & Yeoman, B. (2021). Black and minority ethnic groups and forensic mental health. *BJPsych Open*, 7(Suppl 1), S123. https://doi.org/10.1192/bjo.2021.357

Baillargeon, J., Hoge, S. K., & Penn, J. V. (2010). Addressing the challenge of community reentry among released inmates with serious mental illness. *American Journal of Community Psychology*, 46, 361–375.

Beck, A. T. (1963). Thinking and depression: I. Idiosyncratic content and cognitive distortions. *Archives of General Psychiatry*, 9(4), 324–333.

Beck, A. T. (1996). Beyond belief: A theory of modes, personality, and psychopathology. In P. M. Salkovskis (Ed.), *Frontiers of cognitive therapy* (pp. 1–25). New York: Guilford Press.

Beck, A. T. (1999). *Prisoners of hate: The cognitive basis of anger, hostility, and violence.* New York, NY: Harpers Collins, Inc.

Beck, A. T. (2019). A 60-year evolution of cognitive theory and therapy. *Perspectives on Psychological Science, 14*(1), 16–20.

Beck, A. T., Finkel, M. R., Beck, J. S. (2021). The theory of modes: Applications to schizophrenia and other psychological conditions. *Cognitive Therapy & Research, 45*, 391–400.

Beck, A. T., Grant, P. M, Inverso, E., Brinen, A. P., & Perivoliotis, D. (2021). *Recovery-oriented cognitive therapy for serious mental health conditions.* New York, NY: Guilford Press.

Beck, A. T., & Haigh, E. A. P. (2014). Advances in cognitive theory and therapy: the generic cognitive model. *Annual Review of Clinical Psychology,* 10, 1–24.

Beck, A. T., Himelstein, R., & Grant, P. M. (2019). In and out of schizophrenia: Activation and deactivation of the negative and positive schemas. *Schizophrenia Research, 203*, 55–61.

Beck Institute Center for Recovery-Oriented Cognitive Therapy (2020). *CT-R Recovery Map available at* https://beckinstitute.org/wp-content/uploads/2021/08/Blank-Recovery-Map-Color.pdf

Campellone, T. R., Sanchez, A. H., & Kring, A. M. (2016). Defeatist performance beliefs, negative symptoms, and functional outcome in schizophrenia: A meta-analytic review. *Schizophrenia Bulletin, 42*(6), 1343–1352.

Casey, P. M., & Rottman, D. B. (2005). Problem-solving courts: Models and trends. *Justice System Journal, 26*(1), 35–56.

Chang, N. A., Grant, P. M., Luther, L., & Beck, A. T. (2014). Effects of a recovery-oriented cognitive therapy training program on inpatient staff attitudes and incidents of seclusion and restraint. *Community Mental Health Journal, 50*, 415–421.

Davidson, L., Harding, C., Spaniol, L., Rowe, M., Tondora, J., O'Connell, M. J., & Lawless, M. S. (2008). *A practical guide to recovery-oriented practice: Tools for transforming mental healthcare.* Oxford: Oxford University Press.

Davidson, L., Rakfeldt, J., & Strauss, J. (2011). *The roots of the recovery movement in psychiatry: Lessons learned.* Hobokin, New Jersey: John Wiley & Sons.

DeMatteo, D., Heilbrun, K., Thornewill, A., & Arnold, S. (2019). *Problem-solving courts and the criminal justice system.* New York, NY: Oxford University Press.

Dorkins, E., & Adshead, G. (2011). Working with offenders: Challenges to the recovery agenda. *Advances in psychiatric treatment, 17*(3), 178–187. https://doi.org/10.1192/apt.bp.109.007179

Gable, P. A., Poole, B. D., & Harmon-Jones, E. (2015). Anger perceptually and conceptually narrows cognitive scope. *Journal of Personality and Social Psychology, 109*(1), 163–174.

Gottfried, E. D., & Christopher, S. C. (2017). Mental disorders among criminal offenders: a review of the literature. *Journal of Correctional Health Care, 23*(3), 336–346. https://doi.org/10.1177/1078345817716180

Grant, P. M. (2019). *Recovery-oriented cognitive therapy: A theory-driven, evidence-based, transformative practice to promote flourishing for individuals with serious mental health conditions that is applicable across mental health systems.* Alexandria, VA: National Association of State Mental Health Program Directors.

Grant, P. M., & Beck, A. T. (2009). Defeatist beliefs as a mediator of cognitive impairment, negative symptoms, and functioning in schizophrenia. *Schizophrenia Bulletin*, *34*(4), 798–806.

Grant, P. M., & Beck, A. T. (2010). Asocial beliefs as predictors of asocial behavior in schizophrenia. *Psychiatry Research*, *177*(1), 65–70.

Grant, P. M., & Beck, A. T. (in preparation). *Keys to their kingdom: The theory of modes -- A theoretical structure supporting holistic treatment of serious mental health conditions*.

Grant, P. M., & Best, M. (2019). It is Always Sunny in Philadelphia: The adaptive mode and positive beliefs as a new paradigm for understanding recovery and empowerment for individuals with serious mental health challenges. *International CBT (Cognitive Behavioral Therapy) for Psychosis Annual Meeting*, Philadelphia, PA

Grant, P. M., Bredemeier, K., & Beck, A. T. (2017). Six-month follow-up of recovery-oriented cognitive therapy for low-functioning individuals with schizophrenia. *Psychiatric Services, 68*(10), 997–1002. https://doi/10.1176/appi.ps.201600413

Grant, P. M., Huh, G. A., Perivoliotis, D., Stolar, N. M., & Beck, A. T. (2012). Randomized trial toevaluate the efficacy of cognitive therapy for low-functioning patients with schizophrenia. *Archives of General Psychiatry*, *69*(2), 121–127. https://doi.org/10.1001/archgenpsychiatry.2011.129

Grant, P. M., & Inverso, E. (2023). Recovery-oriented cognitive therapy: Changing lives with a whole-person approach. *Psychiatric Times*, *40*(1), 29–31.

Hicks, J. A., Fields, S., Davis, W. E., & Gable, P. A. (2015). Heavy drinking, impulsivity and attentional narrowing following alcohol cue exposure. *Psychopharmacology*, *232*(15), 2773–2779.

Honegger, L. N. (2015). Does the evidence support the case for mental health courts? A review of the literature. *Law and Human Behavior*, *39*(5), 478.

James, D. J., Glaze, L. E. & United States Bureau of Justice Statistics. (2006). *Mental Health Problems of Prison and Jail Inmates*. [Washington, DC: U.S. Dept. of Justice, Office of Justice Programs, Bureau of Justice Statistics] [Web]. Retrieved from https://bjs.ojp.gov/content/pub/pdf/mhppji.pdf.

Landenberger, N. A., & Lipsey, M. W. (2005). The positive effects of cognitive–behavioral programs for offenders: A meta-analysis of factors associated with effective treatment. *Journal of Experimental Criminology*, *1*(4), 451–476.

Mann, B., Matias, E., & Allen, J. (2014). Recovery in forensic services: Facing the challenge. *Advances in Psychiatric Treatment*, *20*(2), 125–131. https://doi.org/10.1192/apt.bp.113.011403

Morales Vigil, T., Grant, P. M., & Inverso, E. (2022). *Recovery-oriented cognitive therapy: Group manual*. Bala Cynwd: Beck Institute.

President's New Freedom Commission on Mental Health. (2003). Achieving the promiseTransforming mental health care in America (Final Report: Pub SMA-03-3832). Rockville, MD: U.S. Department of Health and Human Services. Retrieved from www.sprc.org/sites/default/files/migrate/library/freedomcomm.pdf

Raugh, I. M., Chapman, H. C., Bartolomeo, L. A., Gonzalez, C., & Strauss, G. P. (2019). A comprehensive review of psychophysiological applications for ecological momentary assessment in psychiatric populations. *Psychological Assessment, 31*(3), 304–317.

Reddy, L. F., Horan, W. P., Barch, D. M., Buchanan, R. W., Gold, J. M., Marder, S. R., Wynn, J. K., Young, J., & Green, M. F. (2018). Understanding the association between negative symptoms and performance on effort-based decision-making tasks: The importance of defeatist performance beliefs. *Schizophrenia Bulletin, 44*(6), 1217–1226.

Stirman, S. W., Spokas, M., Creed, T. A., Farabaugh, D. T., Bhar, S. S., Brown, G. K., Perivoliotis, D., Grant, P. M., & Beck, A. T. (2010). Training and consultation in evidence-based psychosocial treatments in public mental health settings: The ACCESS model. *Professional Psychology, Research and Practice, 41*(1), 48–56. https://doi.org/10.1037/a0018099

Thomas, E. C., Luther, L., Zullo, L., Beck, A. T., & Grant, P. M. (2017). From neurocognition to community participation in serious mental illness: The intermediary role of dysfunctional attitudes and motivation. *Psychological Medicine, 47*(5), 822–836.

US Census Bureau, American Community Survey 2019 tables BO2001 & BP05. Accessed from https://www.census.gov/programs-surveys/acs/data/data-tables.html

15 People with Paraphilia as Targets of Sexual Offence Prevention Strategies in Czechia

Recent Developments and Future Directions

Marek Páv, Lucie Krejčová, and Kateřina Klapilová

Prevalence of Paraphilia and Sexual Offending in Czechia

Sexual preference determines both our sexual inclinations and who we tend to be emotionally attracted to. This innate sexuality programming cannot be changed. Therefore, the aim of early intervention is to help individuals with paraphilia accept their sexuality and not act on fantasies and urges that are socially unacceptable (i.e., there is a pattern of preference connected with an inappropriate mating object or sexual activity).

There is a long-standing public view of paraphilia as an unusual or rare pattern of sexuality (see the earlier term, "sexual deviance"). However, new representative studies, including a large-scale survey of the Czech population (10.7 million inhabitants) in 2016, shed light on this common myth. Over 10,000 Czech citizens answered questions on all dimensions of sexual experiences within a specific paraphilic pattern: sexual preference, sexual fantasies in the last six months, pornography use in the previous six months, and experience with paraphilic behavior. The data showed that 31.3% of men and 13.6% of women admitted to having at least one paraphilic preference (in the dimension of self-identified paraphilic preference). Less than 1% (0.6%) of men reported pedophilia, 3.1% reported hebephilia, and 6.5% reported a preference for sexual violence (for the complete list of paraphilic preferences, see Table 15.1; Bártová et al., 2021). The results might be surprising, but they are highly comparable with those of other recent nationally representative surveys (Carpentier, 2017).

These unique data on the prevalence of paraphilia should not be mixed with data on the prevalence of sexual offending. In Czechia, recent data suggest that only 20% of convicted sexually motivated crimes (e.g., rape) were committed by people with a diagnosed paraphilic disorder

DOI: 10.4324/9781003360926-19

Table 15.1 The prevalence of paraphilia in the Czech population in total percentage and accounted for the number of Czech inhabitants at the time of the survey (2021)

Paraphilia	*Prevalence of paraphilia*			*Prevalence of paraphilia*		
(N = 5023 men/5021 women)	*(%)*			*(Number of Czech inhabitants)*		
	Total	*Men*	*Women*	*Total*	*Men*	*Women*
Pedophilia	0.3	0.6	0	26,795	26,136	0
Hebephilia	1.6	3.1	0.1	1,42,905	1,35,037	4,576
Zoophilia	0.5	0.8	0.2	44,658	34,848	9,151
Fetishism	6.3	10.1	2.4	5,62,687	4,39,960	1,09,812
Voyeurism	11.5	16.6	6.4	10,27,128	7,23,103	2,92,832
Exhibitionism	2.3	3.0	1.5	2,05,426	1,30,681	68,633
Frotteurism/ Toucherism	8.3	12.7	3.9	7,41,318	5,53,217	1,78,445
Humiliation/ Subordination	2.9	3.5	2.3	2,59,015	1,52,461	105,237
Beating/Torture	1.9	2.1	1.7	1,69,699	91,477	77,784
Biastophilia/Sexual coercion	1.0	1.7	0.4	89,315	74,053	18,302
Immobilization	3.6	5.1	2.2	3,21,536	2,22,158	1,00,661

(Blatníková et al., 2015). However, a paraphilic disorder is a lifelong static factor that increases the risk of problematic sexual behaviors, including offending (Mann et al., 2010).

Sexual Offending and Barriers to Accessing Professional Care

Recent statistics from the Czech police report 3,049 registered sexual offenses, with the highest proportion being rape (773 cases) and abuse of a child for the production of pornography (627 cases) in 2021 (Ministerstvo vnitra ČR, 2022). Online sexual offenses have marked an almost 50% increase in the past five years (479 cases in 2017 vs. 828 cases in 2022). The National Center for Missing and Exploited Children reported nearly 12,000 suspected incidents of sexual exploitation of children online between January and May 2023 in Czechia. When these numbers were compared with the self-reported prevalence of victims in the Czech population, they revealed an alarming number of latent crimes never detected by the system. As suggested by a recent nationally representative study, 9.2% of women and 2% of men were raped, 6.6% of the women were forced into unpleasant sexual practices at least once in their lifetime, and 22.3% of men had encountered sexual violence or sexual harassment (proFEM, 2021). According to the European survey, EU Kids Online 2020 (Smahel et al., 2020), 35% of the boys and 32% of the girls had ever received a message with sexually explicit content (the European countries average is 22%), and 16% of the boys and 31% of the girls were forced to participate in sexual topic communications in Czechia (17% for European countries). The study showed that 25.7% of the respondents aged 15 years had experienced some form of sexual abuse (*N* = 1112) (Smahel et al., 2020).

The above-mentioned Czech survey on the prevalence of paraphilia in the Czech population revealed another alarming result: an extremely low proportion of people with paraphilic preferences seek professional help in Czechia. In total, it was less than 15% across all paraphilic preferences, with the least common experience with professional care observed among men with a preference for minors and the largest (but still low) among men with exhibitionism (Bártová et al., 2021).

These results suggest significant barriers to accessing care in the Czechia. Accordingly, members of the self-supportive pedohebephilic community reported hesitation in seeking help because of concerns that professionals might want to change their preferences (Čepek, 2019; Klapilová et al., 2019). There was also an opinion that healthcare did not offer them a safe space where their problems could be solved. These findings have led to the initiation of the implementation of a network of effective early prevention strategies aimed at supporting at-risk individuals and their loved ones.[1]

This chapter describes multiple aspects of the system that have been developed to implement these strategies, including both judicial and treatment-oriented interventions. These interventions include participation in legally mandated services under certain circumstances (Figure 15.1), as well as voluntary support and treatment opportunities at both local and nationwide levels.

Tertiary and Quaternary Sexual Offending Prevention Strategies in Czechia

Unsurprisingly, presently, most individuals with paraphilic preferences are treated involuntarily through court orders in the Czech system. This is especially true for those who have already committed sexual offenses due to sexual preference disorders or mental illnesses. Two types of legally mandated treatments are available: inpatient and outpatient. It is worth mentioning that specific sex-offender treatment is only given to those who suffer from paraphilia because of the accepted understanding that paraphilia is a medical condition, as indicated within a medical model framework. The healthcare system currently offers various services to individuals

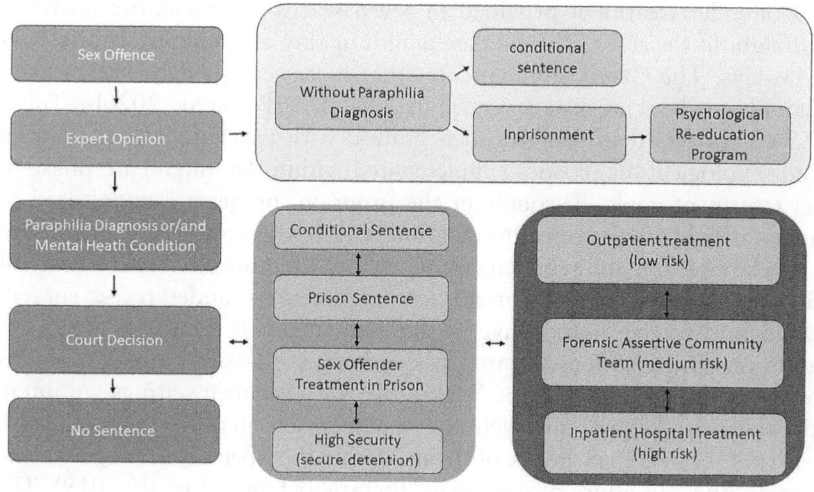

Figure 15.1 Schema of the Czech system of care for sexual offenders with/without paraphilic disorder.

with paraphilic disorders convicted of sexual offenses, such as psychiatric outpatient clinics, sexological outpatient clinics, clinical psychologist outpatient clinics, and institutional inpatient care. From 2010 to 2018, the total number of patients diagnosed with paraphilia and treated in psychiatric departments, outpatient clinics, or sex-offender programs was between 1273 and 1486 per year. Pedophilia was the most common form of paraphilia, with an average of 427 patients annually from 2010 to 2018.

In the following text, we describe the system of interventions in the "pyramid" system, from the most restrictive, selected services providing care to patients who carry the most significant risks to the less restrictive and low-threshold ones. This arrangement reflects the risk-need-responsivity principle, when the most at-risk patients must be given the least significant care (and they also require a significant allocation of resources). However, a preventive approach is no less important with regard to equal access to care and the identification of potentially risky people.

The Inpatient Paraphilia Protective Treatment Program

The Paraphilia Protective Treatment Program (PPTP) was designed for medium-to-high-risk offenders who lack insight into their disorders. As of 2020, there were 839 patients receiving inpatient treatment, with 140 sentenced to sex-offender treatment. The PPTP is a high-intensity inpatient sex-offender treatment provided in seven wards of psychiatric hospitals throughout the state. The average length of stay at Bohnice Hospital was 548 days. The Czech law mandates that forensic sex-offender treatment should only be sentenced to paraphilic offenders (Páv et al., 2020b). Treatment is provided in four regimen grades, with psychological evaluation and sexological diagnostics supplemented within the initial care phase to set treatment goals. Throughout the program, progress is monitored to assess insight, improvements in group psychotherapy, treatment-related task elaboration, and regimen compliance. With more advanced treatment phases, patients receive a broad activity portfolio, undergo less surveillance, and receive home leave in the final stages of treatment. The program targets sex offense-related risk factors, such as paraphilic fantasies or uncontrolled sexual urges. Within the ward regimen settings, an intensive cognitive-behavioral psychotherapeutic program is implemented, with patients receiving six hours of group psychotherapeutic meetings weekly and another six hours of supportive therapy (Klapilová et al., 2019). The PPTP comprises six core modalities that ensure that patients receive comprehensive care, including uncovering psychotherapy, cognitive-behavioral techniques, psychoeducation, biological therapies, social interventions, and community support. Additionally, patients receive social support and participate in prosocial free-time activities supported within the regimen frame during the treatment. Recent data show that the general recidivism rate was 33.1%, which amounts to 42 of 127 offenders who underwent treatment within ten years of follow-up. During this period, the sexual violence re-offence "hands-on" rate was 4.7% (six patients), and the sexual non-violent "hands-off" rate was 11.8% (Páv et al., 2023). The overall rate of sexual recidivism was 16.5% (21 patients). Non-sexual recidivism was also 16.5% (21 patient). When broken down, the non-sexual violence rate was 6.3% (eight patients), whereas the non-sexual criminality (general criminality) rate was 10.2% (13 patients) (Páv et al., 2023). Considering hands-on sexual recidivism, we could argue that the PPTP is a relatively practical approach with a recidivism risk of 4.7%. Concerning general crime, sexual recidivism, or violent recidivism, the PPTP is comparable to other treatment programs (Dennis et al., 2012; Eher et al., 2020).

Protective Treatment In Prison Services

From 1998 to 2018, 413 offenders with protective sex-offender treatment sentences passed through the specialized prison section providing sex-offender treatment programming. It is also worth noting that perpetrators convicted of offenses against children not diagnosed with paraphilia are offered participation in the Guilt Re-education Psychological Program, which is a restorative justice psychological re-education program (Honzek,

2014). The aim of this program is psychoeducational, thereby increasing knowledge and awareness of the specific consequences of criminal activity for victims and the management of guilt. Another pathway of inpatient protective sex-offender treatment is its realization during the execution of a prison sentence, carried out for convicts who, in addition to an unconditional prison sentence, have been imposed with protective treatment and ordered to carry it out. However, the capacity of this service is limited to 37 people, and within 25 years of operation, it has treated approximately 500 patients, who often continue with institutional protective treatment after discharge from prison service.

Outpatient Services

In Czechia, long-term outpatient facilities have been established to provide health services to patients with paraphilia. These services are designed to provide integrated therapeutic and medical interventions involving drug treatment, focusing on calming down patients and reducing the urgency of sexual urges. Meanwhile, psychotherapy aims to reduce the distress associated with paraphilic fantasies and desires, providing information on the possibilities of realizing one's sexuality within the relationship and especially providing insight into one's paraphilia. However, the capacity of these services is currently insufficient to meet the needs of the target population, and there is no space to provide psychotherapeutic treatment at the required frequency. Moreover, some regions lack such services due to insufficient expertise. Sadly, there is a trend toward a decline in the service network, with the number of providers decreasing from 77 in 2010 to 64 in 2020, as reported by the Institute of Health Information and Statistics of the Czech Republic (UZIS) in 2021 (UZIS, 2021).

From Reactive to Early Prevention Approach in Sexual Offending

Early intervention is crucial for preventing inappropriate or criminal behavior, especially for those at an increased risk of sexual offending (Knack et al., 2019). The lack of secondary prevention strategies across Europe is acknowledged by the current European Commission EU strategy for a more effective fight against child sexual abuse (European Commission, 2020), which emphasizes the need to introduce missing interventions aimed at persons at increased risk of problematic sexual behavior (e.g., persons with paraphilia) and specific active preventive strategies (e.g., targeted addressing of people with problematic behavior online through internet providers) across European countries. Even if we put aside the ethical aspects, the early prevention of sexual delinquency has an essential economic basis. Within the framework of secondary and tertiary prevention, society incurs high costs in the care of victims of sexual violence, including the consequences that the victims carry with them throughout their lives. There are also considerable economic costs associated with abuse. Worldwide, the estimated annual costs associated with child sexual abuse are as follows: in the United States, USD 124 billion (Fang et al., 2012), in Australia, AUD 3.9 billion (Taylor et al., 2008), and in the United Kingdom, £ 3.2 billion (Saied-Tessier, 2014). The estimated cost incurred by one adult female victim in the United States in 2015 was $282,734 (Letourneau et al., 2018). The estimated annual cost of gender-based and intimate partner violence against women in the Czech Republic in total is EUR 4,701,951,720 (Walby, et al., 2014); an estimate of expenses for a child victim of sexual abuse online and offline is not available.

Improving access to mental healthcare is crucial for addressing the current state of mental health services and prevention strategies in the Czechia. Increasing awareness in and education on mental health can help reduce stigma and encourage more people to seek care when needed.

Early Prevention Strategies in Czechia: Forensic Assertive Community Treatment Teams

Owing to the shortcomings of outpatient care services' limited ability to support clients with multiple needs through standard outpatient services, the overall care provision trend is to provide it through a multidisciplinary team, especially regarding court-ordered treatment. Forensic Assertive Community Treatment (FACT) is a widely studied evidence-based mental health service delivery model. FACT programs may improve justice outcomes, such as the number of days spent in jail (Goulet et al., 2022). The FACT model was recently implemented in Czechia, where it provides crisis assessment and intervention, pharmacotherapy and behavioral interventions, recovery, social support services, vocational and housing services, and substance use treatments (Cuddeback et al., 2020). This complex service portfolio is designed to fill the gap in caring for people suffering from paraphilia who have multiple needs and are challenging to handle in general outpatient services because of higher risk levels or problematic cooperation and behavior.

Pilot FACT (in our conditions Centrum Duševního Zdraví pro Ochranné Léčení (CDZ-OL) was built adjacent to the inpatient program to satisfy the multiple needs of this target group in Czechia and ensure the interconnectedness of services. The pilot development of the service was ensured by the Ministry of Health of the Czech Republic's project for the development of new services in the mental health field. Currently, two such teams are operating (in Bohnice and Dobrany Hospitals). The Bohnice team presently provides care to 70 patients with paraphilia and 170 patients in total. Patients with newly ordered protective treatment, those who were converted to institutional protective treatment, and those from regular outpatient clinics were taken into the team's care. The Department of Health decree stipulates the standard of care provided (MZČR, 2022). CDZ-OL aims to provide community and multidisciplinary services aimed at preventing hospitalization or shortening it and helping to reintegrate people undergoing forensic treatment into the community. The multidisciplinary team of the CDZ-OL works in case management and provides flexible, individualized services to patients or clients in need. Some CDZ-OL services are provided to patients or clients in their natural environment. As part of the provision of health services, CDZ-OL provides patients or clients with preventive, curative, and rehabilitative healthcare. To ensure medical and medical rehabilitation care, the CDZ-OL cooperates with other members of the health service system and providers of healthcare.

An essential aspect of providing health and social services is the CDZ-OL point-of-contact function for persons who are potential bearers of significant risks (e.g., currently delinquent persons with paraphilic preferences). This methodology contains a wide array of early intervention services provided by the CDZ-OL, including low-threshold counseling, telephone consultations with self-identified clients (including anonymous contacts), and consulting activities for other experts or institutions, such as schools, outpatient clinics, psychiatric inpatient facilities, community assertive teams, school psychotherapeutic facilities, and social facilities (MZČR, 2022). The CDZ-OL is also commissioned to actively search for clients at increased risk of committing sexual offenses. In addition, the CDZ-OL is responsible for the implementation of awareness-raising and educational activities in their natural region to prevent violent behavior, including sexual violence. The team is also tasked with training workers from other professions to assess and manage the risk of violent acts, including sexual violence (MZČR, 2022).

In addition, the utilization of risk assessment for the identification of higher risk individuals and the implementation of more targeted interventions is relatively undeveloped in Czechia. Structured professional judgment tools, such as Sexual Violence Risk-20 Version 2 (SVR-20), Historical Clinical and Risk Management, and Structured Assessment of Protective Factors for violence risk for risk mapping and care planning, are introduced into teamwork (Halouzková et al., 2020; Páv et al., 2020a; Vňuková et al., 2020). Translation, adaptation, and pilot training in working with these tools were provided by the Ministry of Health of the Czech Republic, and further training is currently being provided through the Institute of Postgraduate Education of the Czech Republic. This assessment is paid for through general health insurance within the care model provided by the CDZ-OL, and this service is guaranteed to be sustainable. The collection of pilot data continues, which will enable a comparison of the effectiveness of newly introduced services with existing services, both from the point of view of reducing the occurrence of sexual violence and cost-effectiveness.

Early Prevention Strategies in Czechia: Project Parafilik

The identification of paraphilic preferences with sexual delinquency is a myth that is problematic not only for diagnostic practice (i.e., sexual delinquents are automatically labeled as paraphilic) but also with regard to increasing the stigmatization of individuals with paraphilic preferences in society. In Great Britain, equating paraphilia with child abuse crimes has resulted in high levels of hostility and the stigmatization of people with pedophilic preferences (Harper & Hogue, 2015). Therefore, the increased stigmatization of people with paraphilic preferences is one of the most significant barriers preventing them from seeking professional care (Levenson et al., 2017).

Early intervention strategies are aimed at helping individuals at risk of sexual offending not act on their fantasies and urges. In response to the lack of early intervention strategies and services in the Czech Republic, the pilot prevention project, Parafilik, was developed between 2019 and 2023 at the National Institute of Mental Health (NIMH). It has established a system of early interventions for people at increased risk of sexual offending online and offline, namely, individuals with paraphilia (and their close associates). It currently provides a complex system of four intervention modes available anonymously and free of charge (belonging to the secondary and tertiary prevention stages) and evaluates its effectiveness. The low-threshold services include the website Parafilik.cz with basic psychoeducation and information on destigmatization (68.000+ visits in years 2021–2023), online counseling (text responses with a five-day limit, allowing continuous individualized anonymous responses; more than 380 clients in 2021–2023), and the helpline Parafilik, which serves the purpose of counseling and crisis intervention (more than 200 clients in 2021–2023).

Contact healthcare services offer long-term therapy in a group or individual setting run by trained specialists (duration between 6 and 12 months, with aftercare options). The goal of the treatment is to improve the client's well-being (including mental well-being), social skills, and the management of sexual fantasies, impulses, and behavior by increasing protective factors (e.g., empathy and self control) and reducing risk factors (e.g., cognitive distortions, loneliness, and isolation). The therapeutic frequency and target are based on complex sexological examinations, individual demands, and standardized risk assessment tools (with people in high-priority groups receiving treatment more frequently according to risk-need-responsivity principles). The STATIC-99, STABLE-2007, and

ACCUTE-2007 (Hanson et al., 2015) assessments are introduced within the treatment plans and used for the evaluation of treatment outcomes. In 2021–2023, more than 70 people with paraphilia (and more than 10 close associates) attended the contact intervention. The results on the effectiveness of the interventions (including cost-effectiveness) will be available in 2023, and continuous annual reports are available at https://www.projektparafilik.cz/materialykprojektu.

In addition, the media and destigmatization campaign led to more than 80 press releases (2021–2023), and three original TV spots were created for the project (https://parafilik.cz/). The "deterrence messaging," which involved warning messages with invitations to health care services, targeted people with problematic behavior online and was implemented in 2022 in cooperation with porn websites (e.g., Pornhub), Google ads, and the Czech hotline cz.nic. The Parafilik team has also developed long-term professional training courses and supervision for healthcare specialists to build a network of certified specialists across all Czech regions and increase the number of competent professionals in the field.

Currently, the project is moving toward sustainability. Most of the interventions developed to address these issues are built into the Czech care system. Healthcare interventions are provided by trained specialists within the Czech healthcare system. The helpline and online counseling were transferred to the Czech social care system as part of the newly established national helpline for sexual health provided by the NIMH. However, there is a lack of finances for online low-threshold interventions (deterrence messaging and destigmatization campaigns). Additionally, the development of other low-threshold services (e.g., self-management and self-supportive platforms for people with paraphilia or problematic online behavior) is dependent on EU findings in the field (Martinec Nováková et al., 2023).

People with Paraphilia and Prevention Strategies in Czechia: Conclusion

Early prevention services for paraphilia are becoming more prevalent in various countries. However, their availability and quality vary depending on a country's health, legal, and social systems. Supplementing well-established services with preventive programs, such as those provided by multidisciplinary teams or interventions based on the Parafilik Project, is the logical next step in the development of a comprehensive service environment. The Czechia is on a sound track with this philosophy, promoted by current EU strategies. In addition to a well-functioning system of care for convicted sexual offenders, multidisciplinary teams that offer long-term forensic care and community support with cost-effective potential are being introduced. They also offer various early intervention services within their catchment areas. In addition, Project Parafilik might serve as an example for implementing early intervention strategies in Central and Eastern European countries. Czechia also took initial steps to implement the risk-need-responsivity principle to improve further service integration, identify high-risk patients, and promote standardized risk tools that would enable accurate risk identification and facilitate communication between health professionals, law enforcement agencies, and justice officials. We continue to evaluate the pilot service outcomes to create a basis for cost-effectiveness calculations and facilitate decision-making in disseminating system-wide services. The evolving network of services described in this chapter provides increasing avenues of support and treatment for people presenting risks, as well as those who have already engaged in paraphilic behaviors in Czechia.

Note

1 Throughout the text we refer to the four prevention stages (primary/secondary/tertiary and quaternary) as defined in the current report of the European Commission Joint Research Center on classification criteria for child sexual abuse and exploitation prevention programs (Di Gioia, 2022).

References

Bártová, K., Androvičová, R., Krejčová, L., Weiss, P., & Klapilová, K. (2021). The prevalence of paraphilic interests in the Czech population: Preference, arousal, the use of pornography, fantasy, and behavior. *Journal of Sex Research*, *58*(1), 86–96.

Blatníková, Š., Faridová, P., & Zeman, P. (2015). *Znásilnění v ČR-trestné činy a odsouzení pachatelé*. Institut pro kriminologii a sociální prevenci.

Carpentier, J. (2017). The prevalence of paraphilic interests and behaviors in the general population: A provincial survey. *Journal of Sex Research*, *54*(2), 161–171.

ČEPEK. (2019). *Průzkum v rámci Československé pedofilní komunity*.

Cuddeback, G. S., Simpson, J. M., & Wu, J. C. (2020). A comprehensive literature review of Forensic Assertive Community Treatment (FACT): Directions for practice, policy and research. *International Journal of Mental Health*, *49*(2), 106–127.

Dennis, J. A., Khan, O., Ferriter, M., Huband, N., Powney, M. J., & Duggan, C. (2012). Psychological interventions for adults who have sexually offended or are at risk of offending. *The Cochrane Database of Systematic Reviews*, *12*, CD007507. https://doi.org/10.1002/14651858.CD007507.pub2

Di Gioia, R. Beslay, L., Cassar, A., & Pawula, A., (2022). *Classification criteria for child sexual abuse and exploitation prevention programmes*. Publications Office of the European Union.

Eher, R., Hofer, S., Buchgeher, A., Domany, S., Turner, D., & Olver, M. E. (2020). The predictive properties of psychiatric diagnoses, dynamic risk and dynamic risk change assessed by the VRS-SO in forensically admitted and released sexual offenders. *Frontiers in Psychiatry*, *10*, 922.

European Commission. (2020). *EU Strategy for a more effective fight against child sexual abuse*.

Fang, X., Brown, D. S., Florence, C. S., & Mercy, J. A. (2012). The economic burden of child maltreatment in the United States and implications for prevention. *Child Abuse & Neglect*, *36*(2), 156–165.

Goulet, M. H., Dellazizzo, L., Lessard-Deschênes, C., Lesage, A., Crocker, A. G., & Dumais, A. (2022). Effectiveness of forensic assertive community treatment on forensic and health outcomes: A systematic review and meta-analysis. *Criminal Justice and Behavior*, *49*(6), 838–852.

Halouzková, L., Sejbalová, P., Páv, M., Vňuková, M., & Ptáček, R. (2020). *SVR-20, Česká adaptace: Boer, Douglas P., SVR 20 V2 manual for version 2 of the sexual violence risk-20*. Ministerstvo zdravotnictví ČR.

Hanson, R. K., Helmus, L. M., & Harris, A. J. (2015). Assessing the risk and needs of supervised sexual offenders: A prospective study using STABLE-2007, Static-99R, and Static-2002R. *Criminal Justice and Behavior*, *42*(12), 1205–1224.

Harper, C. A., & Hogue, T. E. (2015). The emotional representation of sexual crime in the national British press. *Journal of Language and Social Psychology*, *34*(1), 3–24.

HONZEK, Lumír. Percepce standardizovaného programu GREPP vybranou skupinou odsouzených ve výkon trestu odnětí svobody, Ostrava, 2014. Bakalářská práce. Ostravská univerzita, Pedagogická fakulta.

Klapilová, K., Demidova, L. Y., Elliott, H., Flinton, C. A., Weiss, P., & Fedoroff, J. P. (2019). Psychological treatment of problematic sexual interests: Cross-country comparison. *International Review of Psychiatry*, *31*(2), 169–180.

Knack, N., Winder, B., Murphy, L., & Fedoroff, J. P. (2019). Primary and secondary prevention of child sexual abuse. *International Review of Psychiatry*, *31*(2), 181–194.

Letourneau, E. J., Brown, D. S., Fang, X., Hassan, A., & Mercy, J. A. (2018). The economic burden of child sexual abuse in the United States. *Child Abuse & Neglect*, *79*, 413–422.

Levenson, J. S., Willis, G. M., & Vicencio, C. P. (2017). Obstacles to help-seeking for sexual offenders: Implications for prevention of sexual abuse. *Journal of Child Sexual Abuse*, *26*(2), 99–120.

Mann, R. E., Hanson, R. K., & Thornton, D. (2010). Assessing risk for sexual recidivism: Some proposals on the nature of psychologically meaningful risk factors. *Sexual Abuse*, *22*(2), 191–217.

Martinec Nováková, L., Krejčová, L., Potyszová, K., & Klapilová, K. (2023). Held back by limited experience, training, and therapeutic confidence: Self-perceptions of Czech mental health professionals about addressing paraphilic-related concerns. *Sexual and Relationship Therapy*, 1–27. DOI: 10.1080/14681994.2023.2232318

Ministerstvo vnitra ČR. (2022). *ZPRÁVA O SITUACI V OBLASTI VNITŘNÍ BEZPEČNOSTI A VEŘEJNÉHO POŘÁDKU NA ÚZEMÍ ČESKÉ REPUBLIKY V ROCE 2021.*

MZČR. (2022). *Věstník Ministerstva Zdravotnictví České Republiky.*

Páv, M., Sebalo, I., Brichcín, S., & Perkins, D. (2023). Outcome evaluation of a treatment program for men with paraphilic disorders convicted of sexual offenses: 10-year community follow-up. *International Journal of Offender Therapy and Comparative Criminology*, 0306624X231165416.

Páv, M., Skřivánková, P., Vňuková, M., & Ptáček, R. V. J. (2020). Hodnocení rizika násilného jednání. *Ceská a Slovenská Psychiatrie*, *116*(2), 66–73.

Páv, M., Skřivánková, P., Wiseman, C., Vňuková, M., Blatníková, Š., & Hollý, M. (2020). Forensic treatment services in the Czech Republic: Current state and future challenges. *International Journal of Forensic Mental Health*, *19*(3), 269–282.

proFEM. (2021). *Zkušenost obyvatel ČR se sexuálním násilím a sexuálním obtěžováním: výzkumná zpráva.* www.profem.cz

Saied-Tessier, A. (2014). *Estimating the costs of child sexual abuse in the UK.* https://calio.dspacedirect.org/handle/11212/1637

Smahel, D., Machackova, H., Mascheroni, G., Dedkova, L., Staksrud, E., Ólafsson, K., Livingstone, S., Hasebrink, U., Smahel, D., Mascheroni, G., Dedkova, L., Staksrud, E., Ólafsson, K., & Livingstone, S. (2020). *EU Kids Online 2020: Survey results from 19 countries.*

Taylor, P., Moore, P., Pezzullo, L., Tucci, J., Goddard, C., & De Bortoli, L. (2008). *The cost of abuse in Australia.* https://calio.dspacedirect.org/handle/11212/873

UZIS. (2021). *Psychiatrická péče 2021.*

Vňuková, M., Ptáček, R., Páv, M., & Vevera, J. (2020). *HCR-20v3 : hodnocení rizika násilí. Česká adaptace: Boer, Douglas P., HCR 20 - assessing for risk violence version 3*. Ministerstvo zdravotnictví České Republiky.

Walby, S., & Olive, P. (2014). Estimating the costs of gender-based violence in the European Union. Publications Office of the European Union.

16 Community Re-entry Needs and Solutions

An Overview of Innovative and Emerging Initiatives in New Jersey

Dione Johnson

New Jersey is a national forerunner in implementing community models of supervision for adjudicated individuals. Since 2016, New Jersey has been enacting legislation and carrying out sweeping grassroots reforms. Bail reform and restorative justice models, for adults and juveniles, respectively, are ever-evolving in New Jersey as ways to re-imagine and re-interpret how to lessen the likelihood of oversentencing individuals in ways that are not commensurate with the infractions. More attention is being given to economic and racial disparities in how individuals are sentenced, contributing to changes in how our current legal system responds to individuals who commit drug-related and nonviolent offenses.

A "one-size-fits-all" approach has been applied within each population as it relates to sentencing practices. However, there is a need to clarify and distinguish between what are the most effective changes to make between and within adult and juvenile populations and to consider whether there are certain times and instances in which bail reform and restorative justice interventions are not appropriate.

Ongoing shifts at both the legislative and grassroots levels are preventing incarcerations and lessening the length of incarceration stays and rates. There are very specific differences in the re-entry needs of juveniles compared to adults, as well as several significant similarities within each group that current reform targets. In particular, the rates of juveniles and adults who are incarcerated due to drug-related offenses and nonviolent offenses are comparable.

In the state of New Jersey, it is estimated that there are 4400 juveniles and adults on parole and probation. Between 2014 and 2016, New Jersey State Police report 20,026 juvenile (ages 16–24) juvenile arrests with 52% afforded the opportunity to participate in diversion to incarceration programs for those arrested for the first time. Similar arrest and early-release

DOI: 10.4324/9781003360926-20

rates for adults have also been implemented. The overall goal for both juveniles and adults who are low risk, nonviolent offenders is to lower recidivism by providing community alternatives for treatment.

There is a need to maintain public safety while identifying appropriate alternatives that are commensurate to someone's infraction(s). This chapter will explore and compare the implications of emerging alternatives to incarceration in New Jersey, assess efficacy rates, and outline additional areas of policy reform and community changes that will continue to be impactful.

There are numerous social, cultural, and political undertones that relate to the current consideration of bail reform, and to the management of the co-occurring mental health and legal needs of those in our society. Over the last five-ten years, particularly during the last four years at the height of the global pandemic, the United States has experienced dramatic and ongoing civil unrest and protest regarding law enforcement encounters with community members, and regarding lessening the likelihood of criminalizing the poor and mentally ill. Also, the impetus of the national health crisis and global pandemic contributes to heightened awareness regarding ways to mitigate the risk of disease due to overcrowding in our jails and prison populations. The following exploration in this chapter is not to argue in favor of, or against, any political position or sociocultural agenda. Rather, such frameworks will be critiqued by outlining some of the most salient perspectives and strategies to integrate policy reform with community mental health best practices.

Current Challenges

Managing public safety in many of our cities is an ongoing concern. Such safety concerns relate to criminal and community supervision requirements pertaining to both juvenile and adult populations. For adults, New Jersey's incarcerated population has dropped by 38% (Atmonavage, 2021), as noted by a 39% reduction in Black inmates and a 45% reduction in Latinx inmate population. However, most individuals who are labeled as felons are at an increased risk of re-arrest via parole and probation violations. According to the Bureau of Justice Statistics study, approximately 30% of individuals released from prison on conditional release were re-arrested within six months of release (Travis, 2002). Nearly 68% were re-arrested for a new offense within three years of conditional release. Travis (2002) further comments that the vast majority of those re-arrested for new charges and/or parole/probation violations are not for violent crimes but rather for property offenses, drug offenses, and offenses against the public order.

It is important to note that most people who are under correctional control are not incarcerated in prisons. Glaze (2010) reports that approximately 20% of said individuals are in prison. The majority of individuals live under various community and conditional supervision arrangements. Moreover, regarding individuals who are under probationary community supervision, "the most common offense for which probations are under supervision is a drug offense" (Glaze, 2010). The highest rates of new commitments in the state prison system are not for violent offenses such as homicide. Most state inmates are convicted of violent offenses due to lengthier sentences and fewer opportunities to be considered for parole or early release. In the federal system, those convicted of violent offenses such as homicide account for less than 10% of the population (West & Sobol, 2009). Throughout the country, many individuals who are arrested, convicted, and conditionally released into the community are arrested for drug offenses. In some states, those convicted of drug offenses constitute the single largest category of people admitted to prison, and more importantly, afforded the opportunity at conditional community release (i.e. parole, probation).

Similar to their adult counterparts, Pelletier and Harvell (2017) noted that most youth in New Jersey are incarcerated for nonviolent offenses such as disorderly persons offenses (e.g. criminal mischief, shoplifting), violations of probation, drug charges, etc. Black youth comprise up to 73% of youth incarcerated, although they are 14% of the youth population in the state. In addition, most justice-involved youth in the state are between the ages of 17 and 19; youth on probation tend to be slightly younger. Most of the justice-involved youth in New Jersey are male, and approximately 42% of committed youth and 41% of youth on probation receive special education services (Juvenile Justice Commission, 2017).

Problems That Are Specific to Adults

In 2022, there were 1.9 million individuals incarcerated in state prisons, county jails, and federal facilities in the United States. Of the approximately 52% of adults incarcerated in state prisons, half of them were incarcerated for nonviolent offenses, and one-quarter of that total were for various nonviolent drug charges (Prison Policy Initiative, 2022). Since 2000, New Jersey's prison population has reflected similar trends compared to national statistics. However, grassroots initiatives have helped to facilitate legislation aimed at addressing the prevalence of systemic factors that contribute to race-based disparities. One study has been radical in its premise that the entire increase in the prison population from 1980 to 2001 can be explained by sentencing policy changes (Mauer, 2013). Conversely, it is plausible to suggest that further revisions to said policy changes have helped to dramatically reduce the prison population. For example, legislation passed in 2021 is noteworthy. New Jersey prosecutors must now waive mandatory minimum prison sentences for nonviolent drug offenses (Catalini, 2021). This legislation is the culmination of efforts spearheaded by a state Criminal Sentencing and Disposition Commission since 2019 to eliminate minimum sentences for nonviolent drug offenses. From a practical perspective, plea bargains no longer include mandatory minimum sentences for current and future nonviolent drug offenders. Individuals who are serving prison sentences under these guidelines could now qualify for a chance at early release.

The consequences of mandatory minimum sentence impositions being repealed continue to impact racial disparities. Black residents account for 14% of New Jersey's nine million state population but comprise 61% of the state's prison population. For those incarcerated on possession charges, the sentencing changes mean that it is no longer an indictable offense to be in possession of 6 oz. or less of marijuana or about three-fifths of an ounce of hashish. It is also not a crime to be under the influence of marijuana or hashish or to be in possession of it while operating a motor vehicle.

In 2020, New Jersey Governor Phil Murphy signed into law legislation to drastically shift the way nonviolent adult offenders convicted of drug offenses qualify for release. The new law, S761, is known as the "Earn Your Way Out Act." The Act creates "administrative parole," allowing certain inmates convicted of nonviolent offenses to forgo a full parole hearing and be released on parole after a review by a hearing officer and certification by a member of the State Parole Board (SPB).

S761 seeks to expedite the parole process via the development of comprehensive plans that are developed shortly after intake into the Department of Corrections (DOCs). The Act requires that both the New Jersey DOC and the SPB coordinate resources that help qualified inmates incarcerated in state prisons earn compliance credits and be deemed as parole-eligible. The bill requires plans to address different domains such as medical, psychological, substance abuse, social rehabilitation, etc. For the purposes of this chapter and in order to maintain parsimony, the most relevant of the four criteria under which an inmate can be administratively released are the following: "the inmate has not been convicted of certain violent crimes, certain other crimes committed with firearms, or certain sex offenses" and

> the inmate has not committed any prohibited acts that resulted in a conviction during the current term of incarceration or any prohibited act that is considered the most serious and results in the most severe sanctions within the previous two years.
>
> (New Jersey State Legislature, 2020)

S761 bill establishes compliance credits allowing parolees to earn time reduction from their parole terms, in addition to earning commutation credits for time served in county jail.

The Earn Your Way Out initiative seeks to accomplish the goals of reducing the prison population and decreasing recidivism rates for nonviolent offenders via the following method employed in many clinical therapy processes: work toward discharge planning at intake or the onset of incarceration. The law requires DOC to analyze each person's criminogenic needs, or those traits or problems that contribute to a person committing a crime and reoffending (O'Dea, 2021). Individuals are immediately placed into necessary rehabilitative programming after the plan development. The S761 bill has immediate and necessary consequences within the DOC and for the community at large. The bill lowers administrative parole costs for the SPB and DOC operating costs via reduced caseloads and expenditures. The bill provides a holistic approach to parole. Individuals can earn parole credits while incarcerated, contingent upon not committing any serious infractions. This can reduce their time on parole by as many as five days for each month they remain in compliance. Individuals are not away from their families, homes, and jobs if they potentially would be without this opportunity to lower their incarceration time. The ability to re-enter society sooner stands to lower homelessness, reduce unemployment rates, and lessen the number of out-of-home placements and placements in settings away from blood relatives for dependents under age 18. The implications of Earn Your Way Out legislation are crucial in identifying more effective alternatives to incarceration, treatment options to address co-occurring substance abuse problems, and ways to mitigate re-offense risk.

Problems That Are Specific to Juveniles

In the United States, high school dropouts commit 75% of crimes (Smiley, 2014). More than any other factor in the last 40 years, the primary contributor to higher percentages of youth arrested and incarcerated are changes in the ways criminal and at-risk behaviors are responded to in schools. Many have traced the exponential increase of incarcerated and justice-involved Black and Brown youth to practices that stem from the "War on Drugs." Called "Zero tolerance policies," legislative policies and practices emerged during the larger shifts during the "War on Drugs" and strict crime laws that significantly increased mass incarceration in the United States during the 1980s and 1990s. The expansion of these policies, intended to address crime among juveniles in school environments, led to what educational and social justice advocates now call the 'school-to-prison' pipeline. Originating in 1994 in public schools, these zero-tolerance policies started with the Gun-Free School Act (GFSA). The GFSA mandated a year-long out-of-school suspension for any student caught bringing a weapon to school. As states began adopting these zero-tolerance policies, the number of suspensions and expulsions increased (Nelson & Lind, 2015). The GFSA led to the expansion of zero-tolerance policies to include other offenses, with a more significant consequence of increased reporting to law enforcement agencies. School districts adopted stricter policies and harsher forms of punishment for less serious offenses in order to preemptively lessen the likelihood of students engaging in more serious crimes.

While juvenile crime and incarceration rates have been decreasing, school discipline policies are moving in the opposite direction. The introduction of School Resource Officers (SROs) – police officers stationed in schools – has contributed to higher rates of court referrals. When SROs arrest students, this immediately introduces them to the juvenile justice system. The presence of SROs makes it much more likely for students to develop arrest records. Out-of-school suspensions have increased by more than 10% since 2000 (Nelson & Lind, 2015). Schools with officers have five times as many arrests for "disorderly person" as schools without them. Students most impacted by the pipeline are those from marginalized groups (American University, 2021).

Arrested students have common risk factors such as poor academic performance, gang membership, substance misuse, and low socioeconomic status. It is important to note that when such risk factors co-occur with reading and writing grade standards between grades nine and ten, in addition to overall ninth grade performance, students are more likely to drop out of the educational system (Education Research & Data Center, 2019). Such students, who are more vulnerable to delinquency, have co-occurring learning and behavior problems in the school setting that can be traced back to academic records at least two years prior to their entry into the justice system.

Growing numbers of districts employ SROs to patrol school hallways, often with little or no training in working with youth (American Civil Liberties Union, 2023). As a result, children are far more likely to be subject to school-based arrests, the majority of which are for nonviolent offenses such as disruptive behavior. When these students present with disciplinary actions that result in court referrals, suspensions, or expulsions, these interactions increase the likelihood of students dropping out of school and entering the juvenile justice system.

There are major consequences relating to school suspensions to consider. For example, students who are suspended are more likely to drop out than students who are not (Nelson & Lind, 2015). A seminal Texas study that examines school discipline policies looked at data from every seventh-grader in the state in 2000, 2001, and 2002, then tracked their academic and disciplinary records for six years. Students who are disciplined by schools are more likely to also end up in the juvenile justice system. The Texas study found that, of students disciplined in middle or high school, 23% of them ended up in contact with a juvenile probation officer. There is often a contrast between-a drift away from the original intention and inception of an idea or innovation versus how it is implemented and evolves over time. "Zero-tolerance" policies criminalize minor infractions of school rules, while police in schools lead to students being criminalized for behavior that should be handled within the school's disciplinary structure. Students of color are especially vulnerable to push-out trends and the discriminatory application of discipline. The literature (American Civil Liberties Union, 2023; Nelson & Lind, 2015; Pelletier & Harvell, 2017) is clear that Black and Brown students remain disproportionately impacted and more likely to be referred to the juvenile court system vis-a-vis zero-tolerance policies in schools.

In New Jersey, most youth incarcerated for nonviolent offenses are high school-age males in grades 10–12 (Juvenile Justice Commission, 2022). The overall mission of the juvenile justice system in New Jersey has followed the principles of the majority of the United States' jurisdictions in the last 25 years (Lento, 2023). Juvenile offenders are handled in a manner that has transitioned away from the "custody and control" approach often seen in the adult justice system. The goal is to provide care and treat juvenile offenders using a rehabilitative model that seeks to encourage youths to lead responsible and productive adult lives in the community. Incarcerating youths in secured correctional facilities is largely viewed as a "last resort" that is employed only when a juvenile offender is determined to be a danger to public safety.

In New Jersey, youth are incarcerated in three secure care facilities operated by the state's Juvenile Justice Commission (JJC). The JJC also operates 11 residential community homes where youth are housed in a less restrictive environment (Juvenile Justice Commission, 2017).

Members of law enforcement may detain a juvenile in custody with probable cause. Whether or not an alleged offender remains in detention during the adjudication process is based on 2A:4A-34 guidelines (criteria for placing juveniles in detention). The juvenile system does not use bail or bonds as a means of increasing the likelihood that the offender will return for their court date. In most cases, the minor is released to their parents or guardian. The court must generally approve whether the youth will remain detained. Those who have previously failed to appear for a hearing or those deemed a threat to public safety are the most likely to be detained. Crimes such as assault, sexual contact, or those involving weapons are among those that create safety concerns. Children may remain in court-designated custody if a parent or guardian is unable to be contacted or refuses to assume custody. Hearings for juvenile offenders may be held in family courts.

Reducing Incarceration and Recidivism, Increasing Social Support, and Treatment

Data abounds that illustrates the current complexities encountered by individuals afforded the opportunity for community supervision. The ability to facilitate interventions and methods that proactively lessen the likelihood of offending and time in detention is equally complex. There are numerous policy components that are emerging that impact the practical application of conditional release. However, such policy components are also built around theoretical models. The most prominent model from which current policy and supervision efforts derive stems from legislation that remains socially, economically, and politically impactful.

In her seminal historical and cultural offering, *The New Jim Crow* (2010), Michelle Alexander carefully outlines the multi-faceted ways that language has been crafted since the inception of chattel slavery in this country to justify the mass incarceration of Black men. Alexander argues that language remains one of the primary ways to promote and gain support for implicit racist policies and practices within our judiciary. Phrases such as "law and order" have morphed over the last two centuries and continue to be used to evoke fear and bias in justifying arrest and incarceration practices that collectively group and disproportionately impact African Americans at significantly higher rates than their white counterparts. For example, initiatives and language to be "tough on crime" during the 1980s and 1990s gained momentum as politicians and legislators were faced with increased pressure and demands from community members to legally intervene with solutions to the increased violence and deaths from drug-related activities.

One of the most consequential and contemporary effects of the "War on Drugs" and getting "tough on crime" policies are mandatory minimum sentencing laws. The Anti-Drug Abuse Act, passed in 1986 by Congress, established very long mandatory minimum prison terms for low-level drug dealing and possession of crack cocaine (Alexander, 2010). The impact of this Act still ripples through adjudication processes and sentencing guidelines throughout the United States at the federal and state levels. For the purposes of this chapter, the focus will be at the state level. State legislatures, including in New Jersey, have supported measures that remain consistent with establishing and maintaining a punitive stance, including harsh drug laws, including the "three strikes" laws that mandate a life sentence for those convicted of any third offense.

Concerns over the effectiveness of the War on Drugs and increased awareness of the racial disparity of the punishments meted out by it led to decreased public support of the most draconian aspects of the drug war during the early 21st century. Consequently, state reforms were enacted during that time, such as the legalization of recreational marijuana. The passage of the Fair Sentencing Act of 2010 reduced the discrepancy between crack-to-powder possession thresholds for minimum sentences from 100 to 1 to 18 to 1. Prison reform legislation enacted in 2018 further reduced the sentences for some crack cocaine-related convictions. While the War on Drugs is still technically being waged, it is done at a much less intense level than it was during its peak in the 1980s.

The "War on Drugs" was positioned to target high-level drug traffickers and suppliers. However, the majority of those incarcerated secondary to this initiative are drug users and small-time drug dealers with few resources. A notable feature of mandatory minimums was the massive gap between the amounts of crack and powder cocaine that resulted in the same minimum sentence: possession of five grams of crack led to an automatic five-year sentence, while possession of 500 grams of powder cocaine triggered that sentence. Since approximately 80% of crack users were African Americans, mandatory minimums led to an unequal increase in incarceration rates for nonviolent Black drug offenders, as well as claims that the War on Drugs was a racist institution. Countless numbers of poor people go to jail every year without ever talking to a lawyer. Or, if given the opportunity to consult with a lawyer for a drug offense, there is not much time allotted to identify or carefully consider options before deciding; "approximately 80% of criminal defendants are indigent and thus unable to hire a lawyer" (Mauer, 2006). Plea-bargaining with drug addicts who often have limited psychological reserve and financial resources, are stressed due to an inability to make bail, and are worn out due to imposed detox from lengthy jail stays, coupled with no and/or cursory consultation with defense attorneys, has contributed to an inordinate number of pleas offered and accepted.

The inception of the Federal Bail Reform Act of 1966 led judicial systems throughout the United States to face the decision of determining whether to release someone from pretrial detention. The Bail Reform Act of 1984 repealed the initial reform and set forth new bail reform. In exchange for release, the courts retained money as a bond. The 1984 Amendment authorizes a judicial officer to consider the safety of any person or the community when making a pretrial release determination. The implementation of the 1984 Act has not been without challenges. Many who were unable to provide cash bail of even modest amounts (e.g., $500) have been retained in prison. The results of cash bail have had an inverse effect on its intended purpose. There has been an increase in overcrowdedness and incarceration of the poor, many of whom are Black and Brown. To address this trend, a 2014 constitutional amendment was approved in NJ and later took effect in 2017. This amendment gives judges the ability to order certain criminal suspects to be detained without bail and, conversely, not hold individuals for minor offenses while awaiting trial (Biryukov, 2017). Replicated studies since 2017 illustrate that the number of pretrial inmates held on bail for $2,500 or less has steadily declined since the new rule went into effect, with only 2.4% of pre-trail individuals under these new parameters eligible for bail under the updated criteria remaining incarcerated. In 2013, the New Jersey Drug Policy Alliance completed a study of New Jersey's jail population. The report found that on a single day in 2012, 12% of New Jersey's jail population, or approximately 1,500 people, were detained because of their inability to meet bail of $2,500 or less. Of this group, 800 people could not meet bail of $500 or less. Moreover, African Americans and Latinos comprised 71% of the population in jail unable to make bail under the previous guidelines. These individuals had been in jail for an average of 314 days awaiting trial (Bernstein, 2020).

It is important to carefully define metrics and outcomes to identify the changes reforms are hoped to produce. At the fore, bail reform serves to reduce pretrial detention rates while also not increasing the risk to the community of those afforded community release. Data indicate that there has been an increase in the rate of violent crime by <1% and a decrease of less than 3% of defendants who fail to appear at their scheduled court hearings. Despite these changes, bail reform is considered successful in reducing the number of people being held pretrial due to an inability to make cash bail. However, the positive shifts in bail reform and other legislation are not without critique. Police unions and bail bond companies, several of the most outspoken opponents of the new model of cash bail, raised concerns that the reform would contribute to an increase in crime and missed court dates.

The overarching ideology of the "War on Drugs" and decades of legislation related to said paradigm are not without concern. Many law enforcement agencies across the country are partnering with community-based crisis-response teams to facilitate a pre-emptive mental health response diverting individuals away from detention as and when needed. The recorded death of George Floyd due to the actions of former police officer Derek Chauvin in 2020 sparked an international discussion and protests on policing. "Defund the police," Clarion calls about police overreach and corruption that arose throughout the country after Floyd's death. The inception of "Blue Lives Matter" as a defense of the value of police in response to "Black Lives Matter" ideology illustrates a major polarization between the police and community policing in many of our communities. Every instance of reform seems to leave room for an adjusted approach.

In New Jersey, for those who are adjudicated, one of the most current and practical adjusted approaches is the Earn Your Way Out bill noted above. Discharge planning begins at intake. The paradigm is one that guides the clinical and therapeutic process for many mental health professionals. A shift in thinking about discharge planning and termination at the outset of treatment helps to remind the clinician and client that services will eventually end, to consistently assess progress toward stated goals, and to place a more pronounced emphasis on the transfer of skills from the provider to the clinician. In a correctional context, the law requires the state DOCs to develop re-entry plans for inmates to ease their transition out of prison. Each plan is to serve as a road map for the services an individual needs and is to be drafted on entry into the system to help guide an inmate into programs available during their confinement as well as when they are released (O'Dea, 2021).

It should also be noted that the global COVID-19 pandemic also provided additional impetus to implementing laws that may reduce the spread of viruses by reducing overcrowding. Concerns that there are not sufficient social services to meet the needs of an increased number of newly released individuals persist. Preliminary data show that approximately one year after the first 2,500 individuals were released in late 2020, 9% of those were reincarcerated (Yi, 2022). The data also show about 230 individuals released in November or December of 2020 were reincarcerated in state or county facilities, with most of them held on parole violations. Dr. Todd Clear, a professor at Rutgers University who specializes in criminal justice, notes that the 9% re-incarceration rate is consistent with additional research that looks at recidivism among early releases (Yi, 2022). Further, Clear reports that reducing someone's time by a few months does not exacerbate recidivism. Currently, New Jersey's three-year recidivism rate is 30%, which is lower than the national average of 50%. New Jersey's growing numbers of re-entry programs work in tandem to help lower re-incarceration.

It is equally important to understand the origins of our country's current sentencing and supervision paradigms for juveniles. Grassroots, community members, and state legislators remain focused on and determined to identify alternative responses to imposing sentences that are excessively punitive and that result in incarceration. Similar to the data on adult incarceration rates, there are trends in youth detention rates that illustrate racial disparities. For example, while youth incarceration rates have continued to decrease since 2011, most of the justice-involved youth in New Jersey are Black (Pelletier & Harvell, 2017).

Cost-efficient methods to improve community reintegration and decrease recidivism among the juvenile population are important. Milieu treatment models are consistent with best practices as a primary intervention strategy. For example, implementing family therapy has been shown to save up to $13 in benefits for every dollar spent and reduce recidivism by up to 23%. New Jersey is notable for its efforts to reduce the pretrial detention of youth through the Juvenile Detention Alternatives Initiative (JDAI; Mendel, 2014). The JDAI focuses on juvenile justice with the aim of decreasing the use of juvenile incarceration nationwide. The COVID-19 pandemic, grassroots and civic organizations such as the New Jersey Institute for Social Justice's (NJISJ) efforts to close youth detention facilities, and legislation that aims to decrease racial disparities in incarceration rates have contributed to the launch of the Restorative and Transformative Justice for Youth and Communities Pilot Program in the JJC. Continued racial disparities and three-year recidivism rates close to 30% are the impetus for the bill. The pilot program is the result of 2019 legislation that allows for the allocation of Department of Education funds to implement the law. The Commission signed the program, NJ S2924, into law in August 2021 as part of ongoing efforts to overhaul and reform juvenile justice. S2924 creates a two-year restorative and transformative justice pilot program focused on reducing initial and repeat youth involvement with the youth justice system.

Restorative justice is a system that brings victims, community members, and youth who have engaged in harm together. Rather than seeing detention and/or community supervision as the final disposition, restorative models aim to build stronger community relationships and improve public safety. Transformative justice addresses conflicts and harms at the individual level, community level, and within broader social structures. Transformative justice offers alternatives to our current systems and aims to transform the conditions that help create acts of violence or make them possible. Restorative justice and transformative justice offer two different perspectives of justice that seek to identify interpersonal and consensual resolutions. Moreover, transformative justice also works to incorporate system-level change. In addition, restorative justice seeks to address the underlying causes of misbehavior, repair damage, and build a sense of community. Nationally, restorative justice and transformative justice programs and practices have been recognized as best practices for keeping young people out of the youth justice system and successfully reintegrating them into their home communities after being released from out-of-home placements.

The purpose of the Restorative and Transformative Justice for Youth and Communities Pilot Program is to develop innovative restorative and transformative justice continuums of care in four target cities that include two components: restorative justice hubs and community-based enhanced re-entry wraparound services. The target cities are Camden, Newark, Paterson, and Trenton. The first component of the pilot program involves establishing restorative justice hubs, one for each pilot program municipality. The second component of the pilot program involves establishing community-based enhanced re-entry wraparound services within each restorative justice hub. These services are to be designed as an emergency response provider for those young people being released from juvenile facilities due to the COVID-19 pandemic. They may also provide long-term programming for young people released from a facility. Community-based enhanced re-entry wraparound services are expected to include, but not be limited to, the following services: mental health, housing assistance, educational supports, preventive monitoring, and substance use disorder treatment and recovery.

Over 3 million students are reportedly suspended, and over 100,000 are expelled every year from school throughout the country. In 2022, 56,000 students were reportedly suspended in New Jersey. In addition to diverting away from the JJC, justice hubs also act to preempt and balance some of the negative consequences in the lives of suspended students, such as increased behavior problems and higher arrest and incarceration rates, in favor of more solution-focused and conflict resolution methods (Stamato & Jaffee, 2023). Mediation, along with accountability for wrongdoing, are seminal aspects of the process. Mediation helps provide a context to keep conflict from becoming destructive. With the hope of helping students and schools rely less on punitive measures and forms of consequences, restorative justice programs aim to implement more constructive strategies to address conflict, de-escalate situations, and improve social cohesion.

Restorative justice hubs are physical spaces in the community where youth and their families can heal, reconnect, and build healthy relationships. The current goals of the hubs are to address the problems of youth justice from an integrated and systems perspective. The hubs help to resolve local conflicts through dialogue instead of punitive measures. Within the larger legislative pilot program, hubs function to establish working relationships with local law enforcement agencies, courts, prosecutors, and defense attorneys to support the diversion of youth away from arrests and prosecution toward participation in restorative justice services provided in the hubs. School districts in New Jersey are also incorporating restorative justice methodology to increase student safety and success and counter high suspension rates, racial and special education disparities in suspension, and high levels of violence. Restorative justice is a viable and necessary alternative to address the negative effects of zero-tolerance policies as an alternative approach to school discipline that has the potential to uncover the underlying causes of misbehavior and improve student outcomes.

Preliminary data on the efficacy rates of restorative justice hubs as a strategy in New Jersey schools to reduce suspension rates is not yet available. However, school mediation programs throughout the country illustrate a 50% reduction in suspension rates for students who go through mediation and later become mediators. Moreover, data show in follow-up interviews that up to 90% of mediation agreements remain intact.

What Still Needs to Be Done

There are many strides that New Jersey is making to facilitate the success of adults and juveniles transitioning from juvenile justice facilities, prisons, and jails to community-based supervision. The global pandemic, concerns with overcrowding in facilities, and socio-political protests because of several very publicized deaths of unarmed Black people in police custody all keep to the fore the importance of assessing the methods by which individuals come into police contact, are sentenced, and are afforded the opportunity for conditional release. All the changes remain fraught with ideological and political concerns. Given the inception of policing and incarceration in this country, it is reasonable to expect that any additional changes in our methods and practices will not occur within the isolation of said systemic and cultural influences. Organizations such as the NJISJ and legislators across the political divide have been able to implement salient policies that impact practical application. Bail reform and the Earn Your Way Out bill remain two of the most important changes in the adult correctional system. Contrary to opposing concerns, recidivism and violence rates have not significantly escalated. Initiatives incorporating restorative and transformative justice models are providing new opportunities for support and treatment for juvenile justice-involved individuals. Preliminary data for the impact of justice hubs in schools to interrupt the school-to-prison pipeline and change the way conflict and violence are responded to is promising.

References

Alexander, M. (2010). *The New Jim Crow: Mass Incarceration in the Age of Colorblindness*. New York: The New Press.

American Civil Liberties Union (2023). School-to-prison pipeline. https://www.aclu.org/issues/juvenile-justice/juvenile-justice-school-prison-pipeline

American University (2021). Who is most affected by the school to prison pipeline? Who is most affected by the school-to-prison pipeline (american.edu).

Atmonavage, J. (2021). NJ continues to have worst racial disparities, nationwide in its prisons. https://www.nj.com/news/2021/10/nj-continues-to-have-worst-racial-disparities-nationwide-in-its-prisons-report-says.html

Bernstein, (2020). How New Jersey made a bail breakthrough- Was the prefect the enemy of the good? https://paw.princeton.edu/article/how-new-jersey-made-bail-breakthrough

Biryukov, N. (2017). Bail reform pays dividends as number of low-risk defendants jailed pre-trial drops again. https://newjerseymonitor.com/2021/10/11/bail-reform-pays-dividends-as-number-of-low-risk-defendants-jailed-pre-trial-drops-again/

Catalini, M. (2021). Its time to act: NJ to waive minimum sentences for nonviolent drug charges. https://www.nbcphiladelphia.com/news/local/new-jersey-waives-minimum-terms-non-violent-drug-cases/2784281/

Education Research & Data Center (2019). Education outcome characteristics of students admitted to juvenile detention. https://erdc.wa.gov/publications/justice-program-outcomes/education-outcome-characteristics-students-admitted-juvenile

Glaze, L. (2010). Correctional Populations in the United States, 2009. Bureau of Justice Statistics, December 2010.

Juvenile Justice Commission (2017). Juvenile Justice Commission. State of New Jersey, Office of the Attorney General. http://www.nj.gov/oag/jjc/index.html.

Juvenile Justice Commission (2022). NJ Office of the Attorney General. Juvenile Justice Commission. Juvenile Demographics and Statistics. https://www.nj.gov/oag/jjc/stats/2022-1230-Juvenile-Demographics-and-Stats.pdf

Lento, J. (2023). Juvenile offenses in New Jersey. https://www.njcriminaldefensellc.com/juvenile-offenses-in-new-jersey

Mauer, M. (2006). *Race to Incarcerate, revised edition*. New York: The New Press.

Mauer, M. (2013). *Race to Incarcerate*. New York: The New Press.

Mendel, R. (2014). *Juvenile Detention Alternatives Initiative progress report 2014*. Baltimore, MD: The Annie E Casey Foundation.

Nelson, L. and Lind, D. (2015). The school-to-prison pipeline, explained. https://www.vox.com/2015/2/24/8101289/school-discipline-race

New Jersey State Legislature (2020). https://trackbill.com/bill/new-jersey-senate-bill-761-earn-your-way-out-act-requires-doc-to-develop-inmate-reentry-plan-and-establish-information-database-establishes-administrative-parole-release-and-provides-compliance-credits/1530656/

O'Dea, C. (2021). New law aims for dramatic shift in how NJ inmates will get ready for life outside prison. https://www.njspotlightnews.org/2021/02/new-law-aims-for-dramatic-shift-in-how-nj-inmates-will-be-helped-to-prepare-for-life-outside-prison/

Pelletier, E. and Harvell, S. (2017). Data snapshot of youth incarceration in New Jersey. https://www.urban.org/sites/default/files/publication/91561/data_snapshot_of_youth_incarceration_in_new_jersey_0.pdf

Prison Policy Initiative (2022). https://www.prisonpolicy.org/profiles/NJ.html#:~:text=New%20Jersey%20has%20an%20incarceration,in%20New%20Jersey%20and%20why.

Smiley, T. (2014). Fact sheet: Is the dropout problem real? http://www.pbs.org/wnet/tavissmiley/tsr/education-under-arrest/fact-sheet-drop-out-rates-of-african-american-boys/.

Stamato, L. and Jaffee, S. (2023). Suspending students isn't the answer. Restorative justice programs in schools are a better solution. https://www.nj.com/opinion/2022/03/suspending-suspensions-restorative-justice-programs-in-schools-are-showing-promise-i-opinion.html

Travis, J. (2002). *But They All Come Back: Facing the Challenges of Prisoner Reentry*. Washington, DC: Urban Institute Press.

West, H. and Sobol, W. Prisoners in 2009. Bureau of Justice Statistics, December 2010.

Yi, K. (2022). A year after NJ released thousands early from prison, only 9% are back in custody. https://gothamist.com/news/year-after-nj-released-thousands-early-prison-only-9-are-back-custody

17 Behavioral Health Transformation under Judicial Oversight

Systemic Change in Washington State's Forensic Mental Health System

Russell S. Horton and Aura MacArthur

Introduction

Critically important, even vital systemic changes, often begin in significant failure as various internal and external forces act and resist from within and without, resulting in the maintenance of system stasis (Katz & Kahn, 1966). Inertia provides that systems, especially larger and bureaucratic systems, prefer to remain at their status quo (Katz & Kahn, 1996). Decades of insufficient public investment in behavioral health, at all levels, following nationwide de-institutionalization led to an increasingly unsustainable situation in Washington State's forensic mental health system heading through the late 2000s and into the early-to-mid-2010s. The state's public system neared a bifurcation point but had until then responded insufficiently to the modest changes and investments made in the early 2010s. Forces for change, through that time, would briefly and incrementally move the system before re-freezing in a new equilibrium (Anderson, 2012; Hatch & Cunliffe, 2006). The catalyst needed for potentially transformational change at a systemic level arrived in 2014, when several appellants filed a lawsuit against the state of Washington, alleging the state was taking too long to provide competency services for pre-trial defendants who awaited those services in jail.

In April 2015, a federal court found in *Trueblood et al. v. Washington State DSHS* ("Trueblood") that the Washington State Department of Social and Health Services (DSHS) was taking too long to provide these competency, evaluation, and restoration services. (Trueblood, Dkts. 1 & 131, 2014 & 2015). As a result of this case, the state was ordered to provide court-ordered in-jail competency evaluations within 14 days and inpatient competency evaluation and restoration services within seven days of receipt of a court order. Trueblood's class members, referred to throughout

DOI: 10.4324/9781003360926-21

this chapter, are those people who are detained in jails awaiting competency evaluation or restoration services. Generally, this detention occurs pre-trial.

Despite the court's order, demand for competency services continued to increase significantly, outstripping new state investments in greater system capacity. In 2016 and 2017, the federal court found the state in contempt of court and imposed significant daily fines. Plaintiffs filed a third motion for contempt of court, which resulted in a substantive negotiation process between the parties leading to the eventual formation of a comprehensive Trueblood Contempt Settlement Agreement.

On December 11, 2018, the court approved the settlement agreement related to the contempt findings in this case, as amended. The settlement agreement's design, generally, has moved the state closer to compliance with the court's injunction and included a plan for phasing in new programs and services. In each phase, the state has focused its efforts on specifically identified geographic regions. The settlement agreement included three initial phases of two years each and can continue through additional phases. Services and regions implemented in each phase are evaluated and continued into future phases of the settlement. Phases run parallel to the legislative biennia and began with the 2019–2021 biennium. Phase 1 is completed as of June 30, 2021. Phase 2 concluded on June 30, 2023. As of fall 2023, Phase 3 is the current active settlement implementation phase. The Thurston/Mason region, consisting of Thurston and Mason Counties, and the Salish region, consisting of Clallam, Jefferson, and Kitsap Counties, comprise the Phase 3 implementation regions.

This chapter provides an overview of Washington State's forensic mental health system, discusses key state laws that regulate the system, and sets the stage for the Trueblood lawsuit by discussing the "2014 current state" of forensic behavioral health in Washington State. The 2014 current state evolves into the Trueblood lawsuit, its escalation, and subsequent findings of civil contempt against the state of Washington. Following discussion of the court's contempt findings, the chapter discusses the parties' negotiated Contempt Settlement Agreement's framework before concluding with an update on the status of the Trueblood case as of fall 2023.

Washington State's Forensic Mental Health System and Key Laws

Washington State's involuntary commitment system for persons suffering from grave mental illness or disability generally operates along two tracks: (1) a pre-trial forensic track for individuals alleged to have committed criminal offenses; and (2) a non-criminal civil track for individuals who are either not involved in the criminal justice system or for individuals whose criminal charges are dismissed with subsequent referral to the civil system. Two main laws regulate these tracks. The Revised Code of Washington (RCW) is the body of law for the state, containing duly enacted legislation through the state's legislative process. RCW 10.77 regulates the pre-trial forensic cases that constitute Trueblood class members, and RCW 71.05 regulates civil commitment (RCW 10.77 Criminally Insane – Procedures & RCW 71.05 Behavioral Health Disorders).

All criminal defendants have a constitutional right to assist in their own defense. If a court believes a mental disability may prevent a defendant from assisting in their own defense, or from understanding the proceedings against them, the court puts the criminal case on hold while an evaluation is completed to determine the defendant's competency. Generally, if the evaluation finds the defendant competent, they are returned to stand trial; but if the court finds the evaluation shows the person is not competent, the court may order the defendant to receive competency restoration services. DSHS is the state agency tasked with providing such competency services in Washington State. Defendants ordered to receive competency restoration services typically join a waiting list for a bed that best matches their needs.

The 2014 "Current State" of Forensic Behavioral Health in Washington State

Prior to legislation enacted in 2012, the state traditionally experienced a 5–8% annual increase in competency evaluation and restoration referrals. In early 2012, in response to the growing situation in Washington State, the Governor signed Senate Bill 6492 with the goal of improving the timeliness of services. The legislation enacted targets for DSHS to offer timely admissions and the requirement of an annual legislative report where DSHS would document any missed targets and action plans to address issues that prevented meeting timeline targets moving forward.

Repeated show cause hearings around the state over the next two years and individual trial court orders brought additional attention to the problems while further straining DSHS' limited resources, but those actions failed to drive meaningful systemwide change.

By summer 2014, DSHS' struggle to keep up with the demands from courts to admit patients waiting in jails for inpatient competency evaluation and restoration was well documented.

Although Washington State did not find itself in an entirely unique situation, surging demand levels for evaluation and restoration services overwhelmed the modest attempts to improve the system, as represented by legislation like Senate Bill 6492. During the ten-year period from July 2012 through June 2022, total annual jail orders doubled in the first six years, from just under 3,050 to more than 6,100. After leveling off for two years during the COVID-19 pandemic, orders skyrocketed by 40% in a single fiscal year to nearly 8,600 per year. Similarly, competency evaluations for clients waiting in jail tripled during the 10-year period from more than 2,050 orders to approximately 6,200 orders per year, and inpatient evaluation orders for clients who waited in jail for those services also tripled from nearly 700 orders in 2012 to more than 2,100 annually in 2022. The substantial year-over-year increases in pre-trial competency cases have frequently increased faster than new staff and infrastructural resources can be added.

In August 2014, with approximately 100 people waiting for competency restoration at Western State Hospital in jails across the state, the original bench trial demand was filed for what would eventually become the Trueblood lawsuit. It was supported by Carney Gillespie Isitt PLLP, Disability Rights Washington, the Public Defender Association, and the ACLU of Washington Foundation. That filing was later amended, and amended again, into class action lawsuit *A.B. By and Through Trueblood et al v. Washington State DSHS, No. 14-1178 MJP*, simply referred to hereafter as "Trueblood" (Trueblood, Dkt. 1).

Once formalized as a class action lawsuit, class members were defined as "[a]ll persons who are now or will be in the future charged with a crime in the State of Washington" (Trueblood, Dkt. 24, September 12, 2014, p. 6) to include persons:

a) [W]ho are ordered by a court to either be evaluated for competency or to receive competency restoration services;
b) [W]ho have waited for court-ordered competency evaluation or restoration services for seven or more days from the date on which the court order was entered (Trueblood, Dkt. 24, p. 6).

The original demands of the lawsuit focused on competency restoration, but the final amended class action suit included both in-jail and inpatient competency evaluations along with inpatient competency restoration. The federal court filed a permanent injunction on April 2, 2015, requiring the defendants to cease violating the constitutional rights of plaintiffs and class members by providing inpatient competency restoration services in the "therapeutic environment of a psychiatric hospital" (Trueblood Dkt. 131 at 22, April 2, 2015).

At that time, Washington State had two main state psychiatric hospitals, one on each side of the state. The Center for Forensic Services at Western State Hospital, the largest of the state's psychiatric hospitals, had 270 beds, 120 of which were designated for pre-trial evaluation and restoration and for civil conversions, with the remaining beds serving those found not guilty by reason of insanity (DSHS, December 1, 2014, p. 3). Washington State's other psychiatric hospital on the east side of the state was much smaller, with 95 beds and only 25 of those dedicated to pre-trial forensics (DSHS, p. 3).

Escalation of the Trueblood Lawsuit

From 2014 through 2017, the state invested "tens of millions of dollars to solve the problems plaguing Washington's failing forensic mental health system" (Trueblood, Dkt. 289, July 7, 2016). In addition to paying millions of dollars in fines to the federal court, the legislature provided funding to make improvements to the portions of the behavioral health system managed by the state. This included funds to hire additional staff like forensic evaluators, add beds at both psychiatric hospitals, open two temporary residential treatment facilities, Yakima and Maple Lane, to provide competency restoration services, increase outreach, further enhance DSHS data systems, and for other efforts. The legislature also provided funds to other areas of the system not managed by the state. One example was funding provided to the Washington Association of Sheriffs and Police Chiefs (WASPC) to administer and issue grants to local communities to stand up mental health field response teams. The plan was that teams comprised of law enforcement and mental health professionals could successfully divert people in a behavioral health crisis away from incarceration.

In addition to providing funds, the legislature also passed bills they expected would lead to an improved behavioral health system in Washington State. One example was Senate Bill 5311 in 2015, which set a goal that 25% of all peace officers assigned to patrol duty in Washington State complete 40 hours of crisis intervention training (CIT).

Executive agencies did not remain idle during this time. In addition to implementing many program improvements, bed additions, and other activities directed by legislative funding, DSHS created the Office of Forensic Mental Health Services (OFMHS) within its Behavioral Health Administration in 2015 to consolidate focus on the forensic services and programs within DSHS and to prioritize goals of accuracy, prompt service to the court, quality assurance, and integration with other services (RCW 10.77.280 – OFMHS).

During that same time, the federal court, presided over by Judge Marsha Pechman, adjudicated numerous Trueblood filings. Subsequent orders resulted, in part, in requirements that the state provide competency evaluations within 14 days, competency restoration admission within seven days, and the production of monthly reports. Additionally, two of the plaintiff's filings generated the court's first two contempt findings against the state, which levied the fines enumerated below:

- Inpatient competency services (2016, *as revised*): $500 per day for each class member in jail between 8 and 13 days; $1,000 per day for each class member waiting in jail beyond the 14-day mark (Trueblood Dkt. 289, July 7, 2016).
- In-jail evaluations contempt order: $750 per day for each class member in jail beyond the 14-day mark; $1,500 per day for 21 days or more of waiting (Trueblood Dkt. 506, October. 17, 2017).

Those fines added up quickly. In 2016, the court ordered that the money paid in fines be spent on programs that could keep class members out of jail. Disability Rights Washington, the Court Monitor, DSHS, and others came together to create a Trueblood Diversion Workgroup. Their purpose was to manage the advertisement and selection of funding proposals and the eventual disbursement of funds to successful providers and programs around the state. The first disbursement supported programs started in July 2017, the second group started in March 2018, the third group started in July 2018, and the most recent group was funded effective in July 2021. As the state continues to pay fines, this work is expected to continue.

Despite the combined efforts of the executive, legislative, and judicial branches, as well as the communities and service providers at the local levels around Washington State, the status at the end of 2017 was bleak. Wait times were worse than when the lawsuit was originally filed, and the efforts to bolster the system and divert people from incarceration had not achieved the timeline goals set by the federal court.

In late 2017, dissatisfied with the services being provided at Yakima and Maple Lane and frustrated by the fact that these two temporary facilities were not only operational past the original 12-to-18-month plan but that the state was planning to invest additional money to expand the Yakima facility, plaintiffs filed a third motion for contempt. In that motion, they asked the court to stop DSHS' planned expansion at the Yakima facility and to increase contempt sanctions for class members at the Yakima facility to $4,000 per class member per day (Trueblood Dkt. 458-1, August 24, 2017).

In an environment of rapid and unpredictably increasing demand for services, the state realized that adding more beds and hiring more staff alone was not a viable solution. In January 2018, the parties met and began discussing an idea to enter into a Contempt Settlement Agreement, one where the focus would be on reducing demand for forensic competency services by developing, implementing, and supporting diversionary programs and other efforts that would reform the forensic mental health system. The parties hoped to craft a plan that would "dramatically reduce the number of individuals with mental illness entering the criminal justice system" (Trueblood, Dkt. 534-1, February 1, 2018).

Together, the parties filed and then amended a motion with the court in February 2018 requesting that the court approve a plan for the parties to negotiate a Contempt Settlement Agreement (Trueblood, Dkt. 535-1, 2018). As part of that plan, DRW withdrew their enhanced contempt fines motion, and the state stopped pursuing expansion of the Yakima Competency Restoration Center (Trueblood, Dkt. 535-1, p. 2). Further, they asked the court to use contempt fines already paid by the state to fund the building of what would become the Fort Steilacoom Competency Restoration Program, a 30-bed residential treatment facility on the grounds of Western State Hospital that would be focused on competency restoration

(Trueblood, Dkt. 535-1, p. 2). They also proposed an ambitious timeline to develop, negotiate, and file a settlement agreement by August 16, 2018.

Contempt Settlement Agreement Overview

Once the motion was approved, the parties launched their efforts by holding a series of stakeholder issue and solution input meetings around the state. Those engagements were used to gather a fuller understanding of the systemic challenges and barriers and to compile a list of potential best practices and/or solutions that could be implemented to reduce systemic pain points and to reduce the demand for forensic competency services.

Armed with their learnings, the parties developed five key substantive elements that needed to be addressed in the resulting Contempt Settlement Agreement. Those included:

a) Competency Evaluations
b) Competency Restoration
c) Crisis Triage and Diversion Support
d) Education and Training
e) Workforce Development (Substantive Elements, May 4, 2018).

From May 2018 until August 16, 2018, the parties met and negotiated the details of the substantive elements, crafting a 54-page proposed Contempt Settlement Agreement that outlined improvements to the existing forensic system, including proposing the creation of new programs and services that had never existed in Washington State. They believed their proposal would support the aim of providing the right care at the right time, in the right place, and at the right cost. Their goal was to reduce the number of people who become or remain class members and to timely serve those who do become class members (Trueblood, Dkt. 599, October 25, 2018).

The court reviewed the proposal; the parties amended the proposal; and the court subsequently re-reviewed and approved the Contempt Settlement Agreement in December 2018.

Following that approval, DSHS worked quickly to seek funding from the legislature during the legislative session that launched in January 2019 and to pursue statutory changes that would allow those new programs to operate. The legislature was very supportive, and both funding and statutory changes (in the form of Senate Bill 5444) were approved.

Moving forward, the parties referred to the programs and services included in the Contempt Settlement Agreement simply as "elements." One way to categorize the elements of the agreement is by utilizing the original five substantive elements, described previously, that parties used at the start of negotiation (Substantive Elements, May 4, 2018). Another way to categorize the elements is through the lens of the U.S. Department of Health and

Human Services Substance Abuse and Mental Health Services Administration's (SAMHSA) Sequential Intercept Model (SIM). The SIM details how individuals with mental and substance use disorders encounter and move through the criminal justice system. SAMHSA's visual model is a process map broken into six different intercept stages as a person moves through the various behavioral health, crisis, law enforcement, court, jail, prison, and community correction systems. The SIM's Intercept model is detailed below:

Intercept 0 – community behavioral health services; voluntary crisis services;
Intercept 1 – law enforcement involvement;
Intercept 2 – initial detentions; first court appearance; includes competency services; diversion;
Intercept 3 – jail; specialty courts; trials; prison services; involuntary commitment;
Intercept 4 – re-entry with supportive services;
Intercept 5 – community corrections; parole; probation with supportive services. (SAMHSA Criminal & Juvenile Justice website).

Prior to the Contempt Settlement Agreement, the state's primary efforts to resolve the lawsuit centered on Intercept 2. The agreement focused on getting upstream, so many programs and efforts of the agreement targeted earlier intercept points.

This included substantial investments in the crisis system. The Washington State Health Care Authority received additional funding so they could negotiate program enhancements at existing crisis facilities in each region that would allow them to accept police drop-offs, funding for construction and operations to stand up additional 16-bed crisis facilities, funding for emergency housing vouchers for use by crisis facilities, and funding to increase the number of mobile crisis response teams (Senate Bill 5444, 2019).

Investments in law enforcement included more funds to WASPC for their mental health field response teams grants, increased funding to the Washington State Criminal Justice Training Commission (CJTC) for CIT for law enforcement officers, and funding to the CJTC for CIT for 911 dispatchers and correctional officers (House Bill 2892, 2018).

New programs put forward as part of the agreement included standing up Outpatient Competency Restoration[1] providers, creating a brand new Forensic Navigator program, which would provide integrated communication and support between state systems, the courts, and the communities, creating forensic models of the existing HCA Projects for Assistance in Transition from Homelessness, Housing and Recovery Through Peer Services, and developing enhanced peer certifications that focused on behavioral health and criminal court systems and then embedding staff with those certifications in many of the Trueblood programs and services (Senate Bill 5444, 2019).

Finally, there were significant additions to the existing forensic system, including hiring additional forensic evaluators, adding beds to both state psychiatric hospitals, a timeline for the closure of the temporary Maple Lane and Yakima facilities, the creation of a best practices guidebook and ongoing training for jails, workforce development support, and several gap analyses on different parts of the behavioral health system (Trueblood, Dkt. 679-1, June 27, 2019).

Because of the breadth and complexity of the intentionally intertwined programs and services outlined in the agreement, the parties developed a phased implementation of the Contempt Settlement Agreement. Phases are tied to the two-year state budget cycle, so the first phase, Phase 1, began July 1, 2019, and ran through June 30, 2021. Phase 1 included three different regions of the state, both rural and urban, while Phase 2 focused on the most populated region of the state and the biggest consumer of competency services, King County. The Contempt Settlement Agreement intentionally left future phases for future decisions as there was a recognition that the complex plan, built of known and unknown elements, might not have the desired impact that everyone at the negotiation table was hoping for. The Contempt Settlement Agreement contained language that required an intentional pause and evaluation at the end of Phase 2 to determine if the state should go back and significantly change what was deployed during the first two phases, keep everything the same and move forward to a third phase, or do a combination of the two (Trueblood, Dkts. 679-1 & 838-1, 2019 & 2021).

The state and DRW met, and after discussion and evaluation, they decided to move forward with two additional regions in Phase 3. Based on feedback and results within the first two phases, the parties adjusted some of the programs and services both in the new Phase 3 implementation regions and retroactively for the Phases 1 and 2 regions. In June 2023, the parties filed their joint Phase 3 implementation plan with the court.

Status of the Contempt Settlement Agreement – Fall 2023

Phase 3 implementation of the Trueblood Contempt Settlement Agreement began per the terms of the court-filed Phase 3 Final Implementation Plan (FIP) on July 1, 2023. Implementation continues through June 30, 2025. The two-year implementation period runs concurrent with two state fiscal years, consistent with Washington State's multi-year budgeting process. The Phase 3 FIP's implementation period is also consistent with the agreed-on time periods for Phases 1 and 2 of the Contempt Settlement Agreement (Trueblood, Dkt. 1002-1, May 31, 2023).

Phase 3 implementation covers two of the 10 Behavioral Health Administrative Service Organization regions (BHASO), the Thurston/Mason region and the Salish region, and includes five of Washington State's 39 counties (BHASO Services Fact Sheet), Thurston, Mason, Kitsap, Clallam, and Jefferson Counties. This brings enhanced Trueblood programming to six of the 10 BHASO regions and 16 of the 39 counties in Washington State (BHASO Map with Counties). As discussed in the previous section, Phase 3 provided an opportunity to evaluate the Phases 1 and 2 implementation and consider new programming options for Phase 3 as well as new programming to add to the existing suite of enhanced Trueblood services implemented in the Phases 1 and 2 regions.

Many of the problems with untimely competency services can be prevented if fewer people experiencing mental illness enter the criminal justice system and instead receive community-based treatment. People who get the treatment they need when they need it are less likely to become involved with the criminal justice system. A major goal of many of the innovative programs being developed and implemented in the phased Trueblood Contempt Settlement Agreement is to provide variable levels of care to prevent overuse of the highest and most intensive level of care and to provide outpatient care in the community whenever possible and appropriate. Expansion, acceptance, and greater utilization of these alternatives to inpatient care at the state hospitals would open more beds to the most acutely ill and potentially increase inpatient bed throughput. To that end, Phase 3 programming offers entirely new diversion-focused programming to try and mitigate demand for competency services. Additionally, new statute changes during the 2023 legislative session place additional limits on eligibility for the types of alleged crimes eligible for restoration services as well as the number of allowable periods of restoration, and DSHS received permission to launch a pilot program in partnership with a regional jail offering class members medically supervised stabilization services while patients await inpatient restoration (Senate Bill 5440, 2023). Many of the programs created through the Trueblood Contempt Settlement Agreement also target people who have previously received competency evaluation and restoration services, who are released, and who are at risk for re-arrest or re-institutionalization.

Statewide demand for competency services continues to rise year-over-year at very high rates. Even with enhanced services provided by Trueblood, demand increases have often blunted the potential impact of new programs, improved staffing, and other historic investments in the state's behavioral health systems. DSHS' research unit, Research and Data Analysis (RDA) provides ongoing evaluation and data monitoring services associated with Trueblood implementation. Sufficient time has elapsed to study the longer-term impact of Trueblood programs in Phases 1 and 2 regions compared against the balance of the state. As of September 2023, results included three periods of analysis. The results, especially for the Phase 2 region, are preliminary and may change over time. Analyses included impact on the number of competency referrals and assessment of behavioral health access and social outcomes metrics (Trueblood SAR, September 29, 2023). Overall, results are mixed. Findings include statistically significant decreases in competency evaluation orders in the Phase 1 regions, while the Phase 2 region showed a highly significant but preliminary decrease in restoration orders. Likewise, Phase 1 regions showed "a significant increase in the rate of mental health treatment among people with at least one competency evaluation order in Phase 1 regions compared to the balance of the state" (Trueblood SAR, September 29, 2023, p. 23). As implementation continues, further time elapses, and program resources allow, RDA plans to continue studying and releasing updated program impact analyses.

Parallel to collaboratively developing and finalizing the Phase 3 implementation plan, plaintiffs also filed a motion with the court seeking to find the state in material breach of the Contempt Settlement Agreement for an alleged ongoing lack of compliance with the Contempt Settlement Agreement's terms. Among other items, the plaintiff's motion requested:

- Fine amounts imposed but suspended under the current Contempt Settlement Agreement could potentially be foreclosed upon; and
- Significant additional conditions and sanctions will be applied to the department (Trueblood Dkt. 938, December 22, 2022).

The department filed its response to the plaintiff's motion on January 11, 2023, and the plaintiff's filed their counter-response on January 16 (Trueblood Dkts. 943 and 954, January 2023). During the court's regularly scheduled Trueblood Quarterly Status Hearing in January, the court scheduled a series of hearings from March 28–31, 2023, to understand the alleged issues more fully and come to a decision on the plaintiff's motion. The March 28–31 hearings were canceled, and after a series of delays, the hearings were rescheduled for June 12–15. The judge issued her initial ruling on July 7 (Trueblood Dkt. 1009, July 2023). The court's initial order maintained the settlement agreement; however, it found the state in material breach of the settlement agreement for approximately nine months in 2022–2023 and further found the breach had already been cured. As part of the court's July 7 order, the parties met and conferred on various aspects of the order and jointly proposed modified language, which was one of the 17 new conditions ordered by the court. A hearing on the modification language was held on August 7, and the court issued a second order on August 14. The August 14 order clarified the original July 7 order in certain respects. Notably, the August 14 order specifically excludes defendants charged with non-violent criminal acts from being admitted into either state hospital on a civil conversion order (Trueblood Dkt. 1033, August 2023). The state filed a notice of appeal with the federal Ninth Circuit Court of Appeals, and that appeal is pending as of late 2023 (Trueblood Dkt. 1029, August 7, 2023).

Conclusion

Despite the adversarial process and contested court room proceedings, the Trueblood parties have often enjoyed a good working relationship and significantly collaborated on shared interests and goals. Removing the third contempt motion to a negotiated comprehensive Contempt Settlement Agreement, which resulted in a groundbreaking agreement and subsequent court-approved multi-phase implementation process with never-before-tried in Washington State programs, changed the tenor of this lawsuit and allowed the parties to focus on shared interests while keeping sight of the true end goal: utilizing the historic investments, new programs, and legal changes to truly attempt to usher in transformational systemic change.

Trueblood represents a generational opportunity to make a difference and impact the quality of life of those experiencing mental illness at the intersection of behavioral health and the law. Many important changes have occurred in Washington State's forensic behavioral health system, along with historic levels of financial investment, and yet 23 of 39 Washington State counties remain without the full suite of Trueblood program enhancements due to the ongoing phased implementation process. Likewise, change is hard; even incremental change is hard. Obstacles and setbacks along the way emerge frequently. Not the least of which, the COVID-19 pandemic itself was a transformational three-year-long experience that has left indelible impacts on the state's behavioral health system. Post-pandemic, COVID-19 remains endemic in Washington State with periodic flare-ups to manage at DSHS facilities similar to other seasonal illnesses.

The behavioral health system in Washington State has moved from a change-resistant, incrementally moving system at best to an open system undergoing continuous change (Katz & Kahn, 1966). Having emerged from the pandemic in spring 2023 and exited the winter/spring 2023 legislative session with substantial new legal and financial authorizations, the opportunity to further enact and lock in transformative change is substantial over the course of the two-year Phase 3 implementation period. However, the spotlight, the financial resources, the political will, the legal pressure, and other less tangible factors may eventually shift, threatening to leave the system overly intact and threatening to waste a rare opportunity to truly impact people and systems for good.

Note

1 Now that state contracted outpatient competency restoration (OCR) services began July 2020, OCR services must likewise be provided to class members within seven days of receipt of a court order. Class members waiting in jail for OCR services longer than seven days accrue fines to DSHS for each additional day waiting in jail.

References

Anderson, D. L. (2012). *Organizational Development: The Process of Leading Organizational Change.* (2nd Ed.), SAGE Publications, Inc., Thousand Oaks, California.

Cassie Cordell Trueblood, et al., v. Washington State Department of Social and Health Services, et al. Case No. C14-1178 MJP 2014. Washington State Department of Social and Health Services, Washington State Health Care Authority, & Washington State Criminal Justice Training Commission, Semi-Annual Report, 4(2). September 29, 2023. Retrieved from: https://www.dshs.wa.gov/sites/default/files/BHSIA/FMHS/Trueblood%20Semi-Annual%20Report%20Fall%20 2023.pdf

Disability Rights Washington: A.B. By and Through Trueblood v. DSHS: Reforming Washington's Forensic Mental Health System: https://www.disabilityrightswa.org/cases/trueblood/#below

Document 1. In Cassie Cordell Trueblood, et al., v. Washington State Department of Social and Health Services, et al. Case No. C14-1178 MJP, 2014, Complaint, August 4, 2014.

Document 24. In Cassie Cordell Trueblood, et al., v. Washington State Department of Social and Health Services, et al. Case No. C14-1178 MJP, 2014, Second Amended Complaint for Injunctive and Declaratory Relief – Class Action, September 12, 2014, Filed, September 12, 2014.

Document 131. In Cassie Cordell Trueblood, et al., v. Washington State Department of Social and Health Services, et al. Case No. C14-1178 MJP, Findings of Fact and Conclusions of Law, April 2, 2015.

Document 289. In Cassie Cordell Trueblood, et al., v. Washington State Department of Social and Health Services, et al. Case No. C14-1178 MJP, 2014, Order of Civil Contempt July 7, 2016.

Document 458-1. In Cassie Cordell Trueblood, et al., v. Washington State Department of Social and Health Services, et al. Case No. C14-1178 MJP, 2014, (Proposed) Order Granting Motion for Contempt Regarding YCRC Filed, August 24, 2017.

Document 506. In Cassie Cordell Trueblood, et al., v. Washington State Department of Social and Health Services, et al. Case No. C14-1178 MJP, 2014, Filed, October 17, 2017.

Document 534-1. In Cassie Cordell Trueblood, et al., v. Washington State Department of Social and Health Services, et al. Case No. C14-1178 MJP, Revised Agreement Resolving Plaintiffs' Pending Motions and Establishing a Settlement. As submitted with Dkt. 534 Revised Joint Submission of the Proposed Agreement of the Parties – Declaration of Amber L. Leaders, February 1, 2018, Filed February 1, 2018.

Document 535-1. In Cassie Cordell Trueblood, et al., v. Washington State Department of Social and Health Services, et al. Case No. C14-1178 MJP, 2014, Second Revised Agreement Resolving Plaintiffs' Pending Motions and Establishing a Settlement Negotiation Process. As submitted with Dkt. 535 Joint Submission of the Second Revised Proposed Agreement of the Parties – Declaration of Amber L. Leaders, February 5, 2018, Filed February 5, 2018.

Document 599. In Cassie Cordell Trueblood, et al., v. Washington State Department of Social and Health Services, et al. Case No. C14-1178 MJP, 2014, Amended Joint Motion for Preliminary Approval of Amended Settlement Agreement, October 25, 2018.

Document 679-1. In Cassie Cordell Trueblood, et al., v. Washington State Department of Social and Health Services, et al. Case No. C14-1178 MJP, Declaration of Nicholas Williamson, Attachment A. As submitted with Dkt. 679, Trueblood Implementation Plan – Final, June 27, 2019, Filed June 27, 2019. Retrieved from: https://www.dshs.wa.gov/sites/default/files/BHSIA/FMHS/Trueblood/2019Trueblood/679_1_ExhibitA_FinalPlan.pdf

Document 838-1. In Cassie Cordell Trueblood, et al., v. Washington State Department of Social and Health Services, et al. Case No. C14-1178 MJP, Trueblood Phase 2 Implementation Plan – Final. As submitted with Dkt. 838, June 24, 2021, Filed June 24, 2021. Retrieved from: https://www.dshs.wa.gov/sites/default/files/BHSIA/FMHS/Trueblood/2021Trueblood/838_1_Phase2FinalImplementationPlan.pdf

Document 938. In Cassie Cordell Trueblood, et al., v. Washington State Department of Social and Health Services, et al. Case No. C14-1178 MJP, Plaintiff's Motion for Material Breach of Contempt Settlement Agreement and Motion for Civil Contempt, December 22, 2022.

Document 943. In Cassie Cordell Trueblood, et al., v. Washington State Department of Social and Health Services, et al. Case No. C14-1178 MJP, The Department's Response to Plaintiff's Motion for Material Breach of Contempt Settlement Agreement and Motion for Civil Contempt, January 11, 2023.

Document 954. In Cassie Cordell Trueblood, et al., v. Washington State Department of Social and Health Services, et al. Case No. C14-1178 MJP, Plaintiff's Reply on Motion for Material Breach of Contempt Settlement Agreement and Motion for Civil Contempt, January 16, 2023.

Document 1002-1. In Cassie Cordell Trueblood, et al., v. Washington State Department of Social and Health Services, et al. Case No. C14-1178 MJP, Trueblood Phase 3 Implementation Plan. As submitted with Dkt. 1002, May 31, 2023, Filed June 23, 2023. Retrieved from: https://www.dshs.wa.gov/sites/default/files/BHSIA/FMHS/Trueblood/1002_1_Phase3FinalImplementationPlan.pdf

Document 1009. In Cassie Cordell Trueblood, et al., v. Washington State Department of Social and Health Services, et al. Case No. C14-1178 MJP, Findings of Fact and Conclusions of Law on Plaintiffs' Motion for Material Breach of Contempt Settlement Agreement, July 7, 2023.

Document 1029. In Cassie Cordell Trueblood, et al., v. Washington State Department of Social and Health Services, et al. Case No. C14-1178 MJP, Notice of Appeal, August 7, 2023.

Document 1033. In Cassie Cordell Trueblood, et al., v. Washington State Department of Social and Health Services, et al. Case No. C14-1178 MJP, Order

Modifying Order on Motion for Material Breach of Contempt Settlement Agreement, August 14, 2023.

Engrossed Second Substitute Senate Bill 5440, Chapter 453, Laws of 2023: https://lawfilesext.leg.wa.gov/biennium/2023-24/Pdf/Bills/Session%20Laws/Senate/5440-S2.SL.pdf?q=20231011073537

Engrossed Second Substitute Senate Bill 5444, Chapter 326, Laws of 2019: https://lawfilesext.leg.wa.gov/biennium/2019-20/Pdf/Bills/Session%20Laws/Senate/5444-S2.SL.pdf?q=20231004160026

Hatch, M. J., & Cunliffe, A. L., (2006). *Theory in Practice: Modern, Symbolic, and Postmodern Perspectives*. (2nd Ed.), Oxford University Press, Oxford, United Kingdom.

House Bill 2892, Chapter 142, Laws of 2018: https://lawfilesext.leg.wa.gov/biennium/2017-18/Pdf/Bills/Session%20Laws/House/2892.SL.pdf?q=20231003094749

Katz, D., & Kahn, R. L., (1966). *The Social Psychology of Organizations*. New York: John Wiley & Sons.

Second Substitute Senate Bill 5311, Chapter 87, Laws of 2015: https://lawfilesext.leg.wa.gov/biennium/2015-16/Pdf/Bills/Session%20Laws/Senate/5311-S2.SL.pdf?q=20231003093550

Substitute Senate Bill 6492, Chapter 256, Laws of 2012: https://lawfilesext.leg.wa.gov/biennium/2011-12/Pdf/Bills/Session%20Laws/Senate/6492-S.SL.pdf?q=20230826080713

Trueblood v. DSHS Negotiation Agreement, Substantive Elements, May 4, 2018.

U.S. Department of Health and Human Services Substance Abuse and Mental Health Services Administration, Sequential Intercept Model: https://www.samhsa.gov/criminal-juvenile-justice/sim-overview

Washington State Department of Social and Health Services, Behavioral Health and Service Integration Administration, Division of State Hospitals. Report to the Legislature: Timeliness of Services Related to Competency to Proceed or Stand Trial – 2014 Annual Report, December 1, 2014.

Washington State Health Care Authority, Behavioral Health Administrative Service Organization (BH-ASO) Fact Sheet: https://www.hca.wa.gov/assets/program/bhaso-fact-sheet.pdf

Washington State Health Care Authority, Behavioral Health: Administrative Services Organizations (BH-ASO) Map with Counties: https://www.hca.wa.gov/assets/free-or-low-cost/19-0040-bh-aso-map.pdf

Washington State Legislature, Revised Code of Washington, RCW 10.77 Criminally Insane – Procedures: https://app.leg.wa.gov/RCW/default.aspx?cite=10.77

Washington State Legislature, Revised Code of Washington, RCW 71.05 Behavioral Health Disorders: https://app.leg.wa.gov/RCW/default.aspx?cite=71.05

Washington State Legislature, Revised Code of Washington, RCW 10.77.280 Office of Forensic Mental Health Services: https://app.leg.wa.gov/RCW/default.aspx?cite=10.77.280

Index

Note: **Bold** page numbers refer to tables; *italic* page numbers refer to figures and page numbers followed by "n" denote endnotes.